Oncocytic (Hürthle Cell) Thyroid Lesions

Mahmoud Sakr

Oncocytic (Hürthle Cell) Thyroid Lesions

From Diagnosis to Treatment

Springer

Mahmoud Sakr
Department of Surgery, Head, Neck
and Endocrine Surgery Unit
Alexandria University
Alexandria, Egypt

ISBN 978-3-032-03114-3 ISBN 978-3-032-03115-0 (eBook)
https://doi.org/10.1007/978-3-032-03115-0

This Springer imprint is published by the registered company Springer Nature Switzerland AG
The registered company address is: Gewerbestrasse 11, 6330 Cham, Switzerland

To my dear students and colleagues

Preface

Since its description in the nineteenth century to date, Hürthle cell lesions (called "oncocytic" by the WHO in 2022) have been a subject of continuing and evolving controversies and conflicts in nearly all of their aspects, starting from nomenclature to management due to their morphological heterogeneity and uncertain biological behavior. Many recent studies have highlighted important facts relevant to these lesions and have proposed several clinical and nonclinical tools that may help in diagnosis and management. Recent molecular studies have shed light on the distinct oncogenic features of Hürthle cell carcinomas (oncocytic carcinomas of the thyroid), suggesting that they represent a separate pathological entity from both Hürthle cell adenomas (oncocytic adenomas) and follicular cell carcinomas. However, only few facts are established while controversies, challenges, and debates still encompass most of the spectrum of oncocytic (Hürthle cell) lesions. Further research is definitely required to enable surgeons and patients to make an informed decision about the extent of surgical resection for oncocytic/Hürthle cell lesions. In this book, we aim at emphasizing established concepts, displaying the ongoing arguments with a view of clarifying some uncertainties, and making suggestions, which may contribute to further resolving others and helping clinicians to reach the accurate diagnosis and chose the best therapeutic options.

This authored book, in 16 chapters with 73 images, 20 Tables, and 1,186 references, will provide a valuable source of knowledge and reference for all specialists and trainees entrusted with the care of patients suffering from oncocytic (Hürthle cell) lesions of the thyroid gland, whether non-neoplastic or neoplastic, and whether benign or malignant. It addresses a wide range of topics including controversies of nomenclature, origin, and cytology/histology of oncocytic (Hürthle) cells, as well as controversies of oncocytic/Hürthle cell lesion pathogenesis, biological and clinical behavior, diagnosis and management. Regarding oncocytic (Hürthle cell) neoplasms, this book discusses controversies of pathological classification, clinical presentation, diagnostic work-up and therapeutic strategies of oncocytic (Hürthle cell) adenoma and carcinoma. A special chapter is provided addressing the updates in genetic and molecular diagnostics of oncocytic (Hürthle cell) carcinoma. Finally, this book includes also a chapter summarizing the various international guidelines and recommendations published recently related to oncocytic lesions, particularly carcinoma; thus, aiding in decision-making and appropriate management.

It is my collective hope that head and neck surgeons, maxillofacial surgeons, endocrinologists, oncologists, otolaryngolists, and clinicians of other specialties will find this book to be a useful and indispensable resource as they face the most challenging of thyroid gland disorders to help provide individual patients with the best possible outcome.

Alexandria, Egypt Mahmoud Sakr

Acknowledgments I would like to thank all those who helped and encouraged me during the writing, editing, and revision of this book. I would like to express my appreciation and gratitude to my wife and children for their continuous support and unconditioned love.

Contents

1 Oncocytic (Hürthle Cell) Lesions: Overview ... 1
1.1 Oncocytic (Hürthle Cell) Lesions: Definitions ... 1
1.2 Oncocytic (Hürthle Cell) Lesions: Controversies ... 1
References ... 2

2 Oncocytic (Hürthle) Cells in Thyroid Disorders ... 5
2.1 Introduction ... 5
2.2 Chronic Lymphocytic (Hashimoto's) Thyroiditis ... 6
2.3 Graves' Disease ... 6
2.4 Nodular Hyperplasia of the Thyroid Gland ... 6
2.5 Oncocytic Thyroid Neoplasms ... 7
2.5.1 Oncocytic Variant of Papillary Thyroid Carcinoma (PTC) ... 8
2.5.2 Warthin-like Variant of Papillary Thyroid Carcinoma (PTC) ... 11
2.5.3 Tall-Cell Variant of Papillary Thyroid Carcinoma (PTC) ... 12
2.5.4 Oncocytic Follicular Variant of Papillary Thyroid Carcinoma (FVPTC) ... 13
2.5.5 Oncocytic Poorly Differentiated Thyroid Carcinoma (PDTC) ... 15
2.5.6 Oncocytic Variant of Medullary Thyroid Carcinoma (MTC) ... 16
2.5.7 Oncocytic Tumors of Non-thyroid Origin ... 18
References ... 19

3 Oncocytic (Hürthle Cell) Lesions: Controversy of Nomenclature, Origin, and Histology ... 25
3.1 Controversy of Nomenclature ... 25
3.2 Oncocytic (Hürthle) Cells: Controversy of Origin ... 27
3.2.1 Follicular Cell Origin ... 27
3.2.2 Parafollicular Cell Origin ... 27
3.2.3 Conclusion ... 27
3.3 Oncocytic (Hürthle) Cells: Controversy of Histology ... 28
3.3.1 Histological Features ... 28
3.3.2 Impact of Trauma on Histological Appearance ... 28

3.4 Electron Microscopy 29
References 29

4 Oncocytic (Hürthle Cell) Lesions: Controversy of Pathogenesis, Biology, and Clinical Behavior 31
4.1 Controversy of Pathogenesis 31
4.2 Controversy of Biological Behavior 32
4.3 Controversy of Clinical Significance 34
References 34

5 Oncocytic (Hürthle Cell) Lesions: Controversy of Oncocytic (Hürthle) Cells in Cytology 37
5.1 Bethesda System for Reporting Thyroid Cytopathology 37
5.1.1 Introduction 37
5.1.2 Risk of Malignancy (ROM) in Adults 37
5.1.3 Risk of Malignancy (ROM) in Children 38
5.1.4 Format of the Report 39
5.1.5 Nondiagnostic Category (Bethesda I) 39
5.1.6 Benign Category (Bethesda II) 40
5.1.7 Atypia of Undetermined Significance (AUS) Category (Bethesda III) 40
5.1.8 Follicular Neoplasm Category (Bethesda IV) 41
5.1.9 Suspicious for Malignancy (SFM) Category (Bethesda V) 42
5.1.10 Malignant Category (Bethesda VI) 42
5.2 Oncocytic (Hürthle) Cell Cytology Categories: Overview 42
5.3 Cytological Features of Benign Disorders (B-II) 43
5.3.1 Oncocytic (Hürthle) Cell Change in Benign Thyroid Nodules 43
5.3.2 Hürthle Cells in Chronic Lymphocytic (Hashimoto's) Thyroiditis 43
5.4 Cytological Features of Atypia with Unknown Significance (B-III) 45
5.5 Cytological Features in Follicular Neoplasm (B-IV) 46
5.6 Hürthle Cells in Other Pathologies 48
5.6.1 Neoplasms of the Parathyroid Gland 48
5.6.2 Medullary Thyroid Carcinoma (MTC) 49
5.6.3 Non-Hürthle Follicular Cell–Derived Tumors 50
5.6.4 Papillary Thyroid Carcinoma (PTC) 51
5.7 Cytology Limitations of Oncocytic (Hürthle Cell) Lesions 52
5.7.1 Risk of Malignancy in Indeterminate Oncocytic/Hürthle Cell Nodules 52
5.7.2 Role of Morphological Features in Suggesting Neoplasia or Malignancy 53
References 53

6 Oncocytic (Hürthle Cell) Lesions: Controversy of Diagnosis: Neoplastic or Nonneoplastic . . . 57
6.1 The Challenge of Neoplastic or Nonneoplastic . . . 57
6.2 Oncocytic (Hürthle Cell) Lesion: Is It Nonneoplastic? . . . 58
6.2.1 Definition of Nonneoplastic Oncocytic (Hürthle Cell) Lesions . . . 58
6.2.2 Cytological Features of Nonneoplastic Oncocytic (Hürthle Cell) Lesions . . . 59
6.3 Oncocytic (Hürthle Cell) Lesion: Is It Neoplastic? . . . 61
6.3.1 Introduction . . . 61
6.3.2 Gross Appearance . . . 62
6.3.3 Cytological Features of Neoplastic Oncocytic (Hürthle Cell) Lesions . . . 62
6.4 Oncocytic (Hürthle Cell) Lesion: Molecular Biology . . . 65
6.4.1 The Role of Molecular Biology in the Diagnosis of Hürthle Cell Neoplasms. . . . 65
6.4.2 Application of Molecular Testing in Cytologically Indeterminant Oncocytic (Hürthle Cell) Lesions. . . . 66
References. . . . 68

7 Oncocytic (Hürthle Cell) Lesions: Controversy of Management . . . 73
7.1 General Considerations . . . 73
7.2 To Operate or Not to Operate. . . . 74
7.2.1 Whether or Not to Operate. . . . 74
7.2.2 Observation and Surveillance . . . 75
7.3 How Much to Resect . . . 75
7.3.1 Whether Hemithyroidectomy or Total Thyroidectomy . . . 75
7.3.2 Hemithyroidectomy as the Initial Procedure . . . 75
7.3.3 Total Thyroidectomy as the Initial Procedure . . . 76
7.4 To Use or Not to Use Radiotherapy . . . 77
7.4.1 Whether or Not to Use Radioactive Iodine (RAI) . . . 77
7.4.2 Whether or Not to Use External-Beam Radiation Therapy (EBRT). . . . 78
7.5 Conclusion . . . 78
References. . . . 79

8 Oncocytic (Hürthle Cell) Neoplasm: Controversy of Pathological Classification . . . 83
8.1 Thyroid Tumors: Classification . . . 83
8.1.1 Introduction . . . 83
8.1.2 The 2017 World Health Organization (WHO) Classification . . . 83
8.1.3 THE 2022 World Health Organization (WHO) Classification . . . 83
8.1.4 Primary Tumors . . . 86

8.1.5 Changes in Thyroid C-Cell-Derived Tumors and Mixed Tumors . . . 92
8.1.6 Unusual Thyroid Neoplasms . . . 92
8.1.7 Other Primary Tumors . . . 94
8.1.8 Metastatic Tumors . . . 95
8.1.9 Pathological Classification by Grade (Differentiation) . . . 96
8.2 Oncocytic (Hürthle Cell) Neoplasms: Traditional Classifications . . . 96
8.2.1 Hürthle Cell Adenoma (HCA)/Hürthle Cell Carcinoma (HCC) . . . 96
8.2.2 Hürthle Cell Papillary Carcinoma (HCPC) . . . 97
8.2.3 Encapsulated Papillary Oncocytic Neoplasm (EPON) . . . 97
8.2.4 Other Aggressive Oncocytic (Hürthle Cell) Tumors . . . 97
8.3 Oncocytic (Hürthle Cell) Neoplasms: Recent Classifications . . . 98
References . . . 99

9 Oncocytic (Hürthle Cell) Neoplasm: Controversy of Nature: Benign or Malignant? . . . 107
9.1 The Challenge of Benign or Malignant . . . 107
9.1.1 Introduction . . . 107
9.1.2 Incidence . . . 107
9.1.3 Cytology and Histopathology . . . 108
9.1.4 Body Mass Index (BMI) and Fine-Needle Aspiration (FNA) . . . 113
9.1.5 Demographic Data . . . 114
9.1.6 Clinical Features . . . 114
9.1.7 Laboratory Data . . . 115
9.1.8 Ultrasonographic Findings . . . 116
9.1.9 Other Imaging Modalities . . . 117
9.1.10 Studies Evaluating Oncocytic (Hürthle Cell) Neoplasm Criteria . . . 117
9.2 Molecular Tests and Immunohistochemistry (IHC) . . . 119
9.2.1 Molecular Markers/Immunohistochemistry (IHC) . . . 119
9.2.2 Genetic Alterations in Oncocytic/Hürthle Cell Neoplasms . . . 121
9.2.3 Low Frequency of Canonical FDTC Driver Mutations . . . 122
9.2.4 Identification of Mitochondrial Genome (mtDNA) Alterations in Oncocytic/HCC . . . 123
9.2.5 Chromosome Gains and Losses in Oncocytic/HCC . . . 125
9.3 Stratification of Hürthle Cell Carcinoma Risk . . . 126
References . . . 127

10 Oncocytic (Hürthle Cell) Neoplasm: Controversy of Clinical Behavior . . . 135
10.1 Demographic Data . . . 135
10.2 Clinical Presentation . . . 135
10.3 Clinical Behavior Compared to Follicular Carcinoma . . . 137
10.4 Clinical Behavior Compared to Papillary Carcinoma . . . 138
References . . . 138

11 Oncocytic (Hürthle Cell) Adenoma: Controversy of Diagnosis and Treatment . . . 141
11.1 Definition . . . 141
11.2 Risk Factors and Clinical Significance . . . 141
11.3 Workup . . . 142
11.4 Imaging Studies . . . 142
11.4.1 Ultrasonography (US) . . . 142
11.4.2 Computed Tomography (CT) Scan . . . 143
11.4.3 Positron Emission Tomography–Computed Tomography (PET–CT) . . . 144
11.5 Cytology/Histopathology . . . 144
11.5.1 Cytology . . . 144
11.5.2 Histopathology . . . 145
11.6 Differential Diagnosis . . . 145
11.7 Treatment . . . 146
11.8 Hürthle Cell Adenoma in Hashimoto's Thyroiditis . . . 146
References . . . 148

12 Oncocytic (Hürthle Cell) Carcinoma: Controversy of Pathophysiology, Diagnosis, and Treatment . . . 151
12.1 Background . . . 151
12.2 Epidemiology . . . 152
12.2.1 General Incidence . . . 152
12.3 Pathophysiology . . . 153
12.4 Etiology/Risk Factors . . . 155
12.4.1 Etiological Factors . . . 155
12.4.2 Clinical Indicators of Malignancy . . . 156
12.5 Clinical Presentation . . . 156
12.5.1 History-Taking . . . 156
12.5.2 Physical Examination . . . 156
12.6 Differential Diagnosis . . . 157
12.7 Investigations (Workup) . . . 158
12.7.1 Laboratory Studies . . . 158
12.7.2 Imaging Studies . . . 159
12.7.3 Fine-Needle Aspiration (FNA) . . . 167
12.7.4 Macroscopic Features . . . 171
12.7.5 Histological Features/Differential Diagnosis . . . 172
12.7.6 Electron Microscopy . . . 176
12.7.7 Molecular Changes in Hürthle Cell Carcinoma (HCC) . . . 177
12.8 Staging of Hürthle Cell Carcinoma . . . 177
12.9 Treatment of Oncocytic (Hürthle Cell) Carcinoma . . . 178
12.9.1 Surgical Treatment . . . 178
12.9.2 Adjuvant Therapy . . . 181
12.9.3 Systemic Therapy (Chemotherapy) . . . 186
12.9.4 Management of Locoregional Recurrence/Relapse . . . 187

12.9.5 Follow-Up 190
12.9.6 Further Outpatient Care 190
12.9.7 Complications 193
12.9.8 Patient Education 194
References 194

13 Oncocytic (Hürthle Cell) Carcinoma: Updates in Genetic and Molecular Diagnostics 205
13.1 Introduction 205
13.2 Genetic Change in Genes Involved in *RAS/RAF/MAPK* and *PIK3/AKT/MTOR* Pathways 206
13.3 Genetic Rearrangements 207
13.4 Tumor Protein 53 (TP53) Gene Mutation 208
13.5 Telomerase Reverse Transcriptase (*TERT*) Promoter Mutations 208
13.6 Tumor Mutational Burden (*TMB*) and Global Copy Number Diversity 209
13.7 Mutations in Mitochondrial DNA (*mtDNA*) and Related Genes 209
13.8 Other Molecular Changes 210
References 212

14 Oncocytic (Hürthle Cell) Carcinoma: Guidelines and Decision-Making 217
14.1 Introduction 217
14.2 Diagnostic Guidelines 218
14.2.1 Initial Evaluation 218
14.2.2 Ultrasonography (US) 218
14.2.3 Non-ultrasound Imaging Modalities 219
14.2.4 Thyroid Biopsy 221
14.3 Therapeutic Guidelines 225
14.3.1 Clinical Surveillance 225
14.3.2 Surgery 225
14.3.3 Minimally Invasive Techniques 228
14.3.4 Radioactive Iodine (RAI) Therapy 228
14.3.5 Levothyroxine Therapy 231
14.3.6 Follow-Up Strategies 232
14.3.7 Treatment of Recurrent/Metastatic Disease 232
14.3.8 Treatment of Thyroid Nodules and Cancer During Pregnancy 234
14.4 Concluding Remarks and Future Perspectives 235
References 235

15 Oncocytic (Hürthle Cell) Carcinoma: Controversy of Prognosis 241
15.1 Survival 241
15.2 Distant Metastases 242
15.3 Locoregional Recurrence 242
15.4 Age, Metastases, Extra-thyroid Extension, Stage [AMES] 244
15.4.1 Old Age [A] 244

15.4.2 Metastases [M] 245
15.4.3 Extra-thyroid Extension [E] 245
15.4.4 Stage [S] 246
15.5 Effect of Gender/Stage 246
15.6 Microscopic Morphology 247
15.7 Impact of Management 248
15.8 Prognostic Nomogram 248
References 249

16 Oncocytic (Hürthle Cell) Lesions: Conclusions 253
16.1 Nomenclature 253
16.2 Cell of Origin 253
16.3 Pathogenesis and Biological Behavior 254
16.4 Cytology 254
16.5 Histopathology 255
16.6 Diagnosis 255
16.7 Management 256
16.8 Prognosis 256
16.9 Future Perspectives 257
References 258

Oncocytic (Hürthle Cell) Lesions: Overview

1

1.1 Oncocytic (Hürthle Cell) Lesions: Definitions

"Oncocytic" cells or "Hürthle" cells are large thyroglobulin-producing epithelial cells that are present in both nonneoplastic and neoplastic thyroid lesions, which encompass pathological entities ranging from hyperplastic nodules with oncocytic/Hürthle cell metaplasia to oncocytic/Hürthle cell carcinomas (HCCs).

Oncocytic/Hürthle cell lesions are rather uncommon, accounting for only 4.5–10% of all thyroid neoplasms and up to 6% of all differentiated thyroid cancer (DTC) [1, 2]. Oncocytic/Hürthle cell lesion is defined as a "hyper-cellular lesion with a predominance of oncocytic/Hürthle cells (more than 75%) and a paucity of colloid on cytological examination" [3].

1.2 Oncocytic (Hürthle Cell) Lesions: Controversies

Since its description in the nineteenth century to date, oncocytic/Hürthle cell lesions have been a subject of continuing and evolving controversies and conflicts in nearly all of their aspects, starting from nomenclature to management. Many recent studies have highlighted important facts relevant to these lesions and have proposed several clinical and nonclinical tools that may help in diagnosis and management. However, only few facts are established while controversies, challenges, and debates still encompass most of the spectrum of oncocytic/Hürthle cell lesions. Further research is definitely required to enable surgeons and patients to make an informed decision about the extent of surgical resection of these lesions.

Thyroid nodules are exceedingly common, occurring in 5–8% of the population on physical examination, increasing to 15–67% when high-frequency ultrasound (US) is employed [4, 5]. Many pathological conditions of the thyroid gland can manifest by nodules. These range from hyperplastic or adenomatous (nonneoplastic) nodules, including nodular goiter and chronic lymphocytic thyroiditis

M. Sakr, *Oncocytic (Hürthle Cell) Thyroid Lesions*,
https://doi.org/10.1007/978-3-032-03115-0_1

(Hashimoto's thyroiditis), to encapsulated neoplasms such as benign follicular adenomas, to malignant neoplastic disease, including well-differentiated thyroid cancers (WDTC), medullary thyroid cancer (MTC), and metastases from various sources. Nodules may be discovered on routine physical examination when they begin to cause symptoms of compression, or as incidental findings on imaging studies performed for other reasons.

Fine-needle aspiration biopsy (FNAB) has become an invaluable tool and the gold standard in the evaluation of thyroid nodules; however, there is a tremendous variability reported in the results from different institutions [6]. Among the descriptions employed by cytopathologists in the interpretation of FNAB are those of Hürthle cell neoplasm (HCN), Hürthle cell change, and variations thereof. The dilemma facing the clinician is how to proceed from there. What findings are significant and warrant surgical evaluation/intervention? Which may be observed?

Oncocytic or Hürthle cells (HCs) and HC change, as well as the frequently employed synonyms "oncocytes/oncocytic change" or "oxyphils/oxyphilic change," are not infrequently described on fine-needle aspiration biopsy (FNAB) reports of thyroid lesions. Not all oxyphilic cells are true HCs and not every aspirate containing HCs is or should be considered equivalent to a Hürthle cell neoplasm (HCN) or as currently termed oncocytic neoplasm [7].

There are many benign thyroid lesions associated with HCs or HC change. A skilled and experienced cytopathologist is invaluable in discriminating the subtle features that distinguish these lesions from those warranting a more aggressive approach. The diagnosis of oncocytic/Hürthle cell carcinoma (HCC) relies on histopathological scrutiny and evidence of capsular and/or vascular invasion or metastasis to lymph nodes (LNs) or distant organs. Many investigators have sought clinical, radiographic, cytological, genetic, and other factors to attempt to discriminate preoperatively between benign and malignant HCNs. To date, none has been definitively proven to be reliable [8].

References

1. McLeod MK, Thompson NW. Hürthle cell neoplasms of the thyroid. Otolaryngol Clin N Am. 1990;23:441–52.
2. Cooper DS, Schneyer CR. Follicular and Hürthle cell carcinoma of the thyroid. Endocrinol Metab Clin N Am. 1990;19:577–91.
3. LiVolsi VA. Surgical pathology of the thyroid. Philadelphia: WB Saunders; 1990.
4. Yeung MJ, Serpell JW. Management of the solitary thyroid nodule. Oncologist. 2008;13:105–12.
5. American Thyroid Association (ATA) Guidelines Taskforce on Thyroid Nodules and Differentiated Thyroid Cancer, Cooper DS, Doherty GM, Haugen BR, Kloos RT, Lee SL, Mandel SJ, et al. Revised American Thyroid Association management guidelines for patients with thyroid nodules and differentiated thyroid cancer. Thyroid. 2009;11:1167–214.

6. Mijovic T, Rochon L, Gologon O, Hier MP, Black MJ, Young J, et al. Fine-needle aspiration biopsies in the management of indeterminate follicular and Hürthle cell thyroid lesions. Otolaryngol Head Neck Surg. 2009;140:715–9.
7. Baloch ZW, Asa SL, Barletta JA, Ghossein RA, Juhlin CC, Jung CK, et al. Overview of the 2022 WHO classification of thyroid neoplasms. Endocr Pathol. 2022;33(1):27–63.
8. Cannon J. The significance of Hurthle cells in thyroid disease. Oncologist. 2011;16:1380–7.

Oncocytic (Hürthle) Cells in Thyroid Disorders

2

2.1 Introduction

When confronted with thyroid fine-needle aspiration (FNA) samples containing oncocytic cells (Hürthle cells) it is important to keep in mind that oncocytic changes may be encountered also in other thyroid lesions than oncocytic/Hürthle cell neoplasms. Hürthle cells can be observed in a wide variety of benign and malignant conditions of the thyroid gland; they are not specific to any particular pathology. The mechanism behind mitochondrial abundance in these conditions is not completely understood; however, it is likely a reflection of excessive mitochondrial proliferation and/or mitophagy [1].

Oncocytic/Hürthle cells are commonly found in older individuals, and in thyroids of patients that have been treated with head and neck irradiation and systemic chemotherapy, and in patients with long-standing nodular goiters, Graves' disease, and chronic lymphocytic thyroiditis (Hashimoto's disease or thyroiditis) [2–8]. The classical definition of Hashimoto's disease calls for the triad of lymphocytes, plasma cells, and Hürthle cells [9, 10]. In some instances, one can often find an entire nodule composed of oncocytes and the distinction of hyperplasia from neoplasia can be problematic.

Most of the conditions associated with oncocytic/Hürthle cell change are "chronic," suggesting the possibility that alteration in the follicular epithelium to take on Hürthle cell or oncocytic histology requires chronic stimulation [2, 5]. Because they are more commonly seen in older individuals, it was believed that the oncocytic/Hürthle cell is a result of senescent change. These show limited thyroglobulin production and contain high levels of oxidative enzymes [11–14].

M. Sakr, *Oncocytic (Hürthle Cell) Thyroid Lesions*,
https://doi.org/10.1007/978-3-032-03115-0_2

2.2 Chronic Lymphocytic (Hashimoto's) Thyroiditis

Hashimoto's thyroiditis (chronic lymphocytic thyroiditis) is, in most cases, a diffuse process, but in some instances discrete nodules may be dominant. Follicular cell metaplasia, ranging from pale pink cells with abundant cytoplasm to true oncocytic/Hürthle cells (HCs) with the characteristic granular, deeply eosinophilic cytoplasm, is commonly seen [15]. Reflecting the apparent need for cells to accumulate significant numbers of mitochondria over a prolonged period of time, oncocytic/HC metaplasia is rarely seen in the "juvenile" form of Hashimoto's disease [16].

2.3 Graves' Disease

Although the disease entity in which Askanazy first described HCs, diffuse toxic goiter (Graves' disease), typically does *not* contain an abundance of HCs, they may be seen in cases of long-standing Graves' disease, in older individuals with the disease, or in patients with a history of Graves' disease who have undergone radioactive iodine (RAI) ablation and subsequently develop nodular thyroid disease [9]. The basis for this change is considered to be a response to cellular stress induced by the inflammation, or probably exhaustion in the hyper-stimulated follicular cells of Graves' disease. These oncocytic follicular cells retain their normal intercellular adhesion and polarity, but they are enlarged and have abundant eosinophilic granular cytoplasm. Their nuclei tend to be large but round, and they have prominent cherry-red macro-nucleoli.

Graves' disease is the most common cause of hyperthyroidism accounting for 60%–80% of hyperthyroid cases. It has been reported to be associated with aggressive thyroid carcinomas, 88% being papillary thyroid cancers (PTCs). Some studies noted an increased mortality in patients with differentiated thyroid cancer (DTC) associated with Graves' disease when compared to euthyroid controls. Oncocytic/Hürthle cell carcinoma (HCC) is a rare thyroid malignancy and is uncommonly seen in conjunction with Graves' disease [17]. Clinical follow-up ranging from 7 to 22 years (median = 16 years) of 39 such patients showed no evidence of recurrence, metastasis, or malignant transformation [18].

2.4 Nodular Hyperplasia of the Thyroid Gland

Nodular hyperplasia of the thyroid, also known as "sporadic, non-endemic nodular goiter," is one of the most common thyroid pathologies encountered in surgical practice. It is thought to be caused by a combination of environmental factors (such as lack of iodine) and genetic factors (such as autosomal dominant inheritance). The follicles in conventional nodular hyperplasia can be of micro-follicular, macro-follicular, or normo-follicular type, but the follicular cells lining the nodules are generally similar to those seen in the surrounding uninvolved normal thyroid [19].

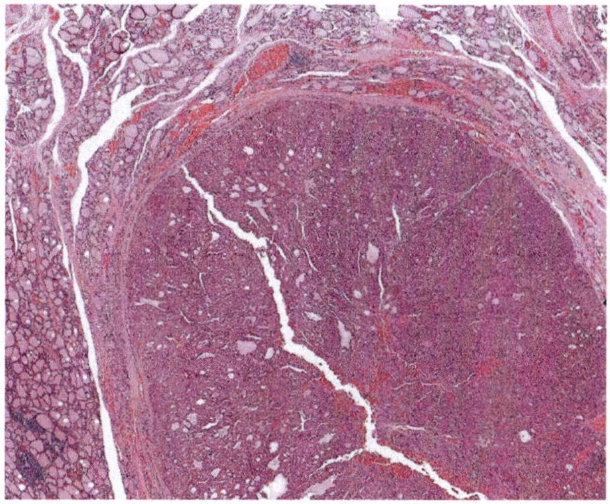

Fig. 2.1 Microscopy showing multifocal benign proliferations of thyroid follicular epithelium demonstrating extensive oncocytic cytology, but retaining the uniform, round, and homogeneous nuclear morphology of benign thyroid follicular epithelium. H&E stain

Oncocytic change is seen in follicular nodular disease (Fig. 2.1). It can be diffuse or focal [20, 21]. The presence of oncocytic change results in nuclear features that are *not* "normal"; however, the presence of only enlarged nuclei with prominent cherry red macronucleoli should *not* be of concern. Other nuclear atypia, such as irregular nuclear contours, peripheral margination of chromatin, nuclear pseudo-inclusions, and crowding with overlap and molding should indicate malignancy as in other follicular thyroid neoplasms [15, 22]. The presence of invasive behavior, into or beyond tumor capsule, lymphatics, and/or blood vessels, is also universally accepted as a criterion of malignancy.

Recently, Suster et al. [18] studied a series of 45 patients (39 women and 6 men, aged 25–69 years with a mean of 50.3 years) with clinically multinodular goiters (MNGs) in which the thyroid gland was abnormally enlarged due to a proliferation of multiple well-circumscribed and mostly non-capsulated nodules composed of a monomorphous population of oncocytic (Hürthle) cells against a background of chronic lymphocytic thyroiditis (CLT) [18]. The nodules varied from microscopic to 5 cm and appeared to compress the surrounding thyroid parenchyma. Most of the lesions lacked a well-defined capsule. In 26 lesions, the nodules displayed a predominantly follicular pattern of growth; in 8 cases, there were admixtures of follicular and trabecular patterns with focal solid areas devoid of follicles.

2.5 Oncocytic Thyroid Neoplasms

Hürthle cells are also seen in neoplastic diseases of the thyroid, both benign and malignant, including oncocytic adenoma (Hürthle cell adenoma–HCA), oncocytic carcinoma (Hürthle cell carcinoma–HCC), variants of papillary thyroid carcinoma (PTC), and the oncocytic variant of medullary thyroid carcinoma (MTC), and oncocytic variant of poorly differentiated thyroid carcinoma (PDTC), among others. Oncocytic/oxyphilic change (HC change), focal or diffuse, may be described. Oxyphilic cells may be seen in metastatic renal cell carcinoma (RCC) to the thyroid; however, these are not "true" oncocytic/HCs because they are *not* derived from thyroid follicular epithelium [23].

Oncocytic thyroid carcinomas are thought to represent a category of thyroid tumors with genetic and clinical characteristics that differ from non-oncocytic thyroid cancers [9, 24, 25]. Oncocytic changes are commonly seen, at least focally, in conventional papillary thyroid carcinoma (PTC); they are even more widespread in the oncocytic, Warthin-like, and tall-cell variants. Medullary thyroid carcinoma (MTC) and parathyroid lesions can also exhibit oncocytic changes. Immunocytochemistry may be useful for resolving at least some of these differential diagnoses. For example, cells derived from MTC are positive for calcitonin, but negative for thyroglobulin (Tg), whereas cells from an oncocytic/Hürthle cell carcinoma (HCC) are negative for calcitonin, but positive for Tg [26].

It has been suggested that only 10–38% of oncocytic thyroid carcinomas take up radioactive iodine (RAI); thus, the use of RAI in this population has been inconsistent in the literature [26, 27]. Recent evidence suggests that RAI may improve overall survival in patients with differentiated oncocytic follicular cell thyroid carcinomas [28–30], whereas others argue that there is no evidence to support its use [31, 32]. Review of data on "Hürthle cell" carcinomas in the National Cancer Data Base from 1998 to 2006 identified that the use of RAI improved survival at 10 years from 65.0% to 74.4% ($p < 0.001$) [29]. A recent retrospective study by Amouri et al. (2019) showed uptake by metastatic disease in greater than 70% of patients with distant metastasis at presentation supporting the use of RAI in this patient population [33]. These data suggest that there may be an indication for the use of RAI in the management of patients with oncocytic thyroid cancers, although there remains ongoing uncertainty.

2.5.1 Oncocytic Variant of Papillary Thyroid Carcinoma (PTC)

The Hürthle cell (oncocytic) variant of papillary thyroid carcinoma (PTC) (also known as oncocytic PTC and PTC with complex papillary architecture) is a part of the differentiated thyroid carcinoma (DTC) spectrum and there remains significant controversy about its biological behavior and optimal management [34]. It is a rare subtype accounting for 1–11% of all PTCs [34–37]. The histological and cytological criteria for its diagnosis have not been clearly determined. These tumors should be distinguished from other oncocytic thyroid neoplasms because of its different biological behavior and prognostic implications [35].

This tumor is characterized histologically by the presence of oncocytic cells with the classical nuclear features of PTC usually arising in a background of chronic lymphocytic thyroiditis (Hashimoto's thyroiditis) with oxyphilia [35, 38–42]. Most lesions are well-circumscribed and encapsulated, and often show at least a focal

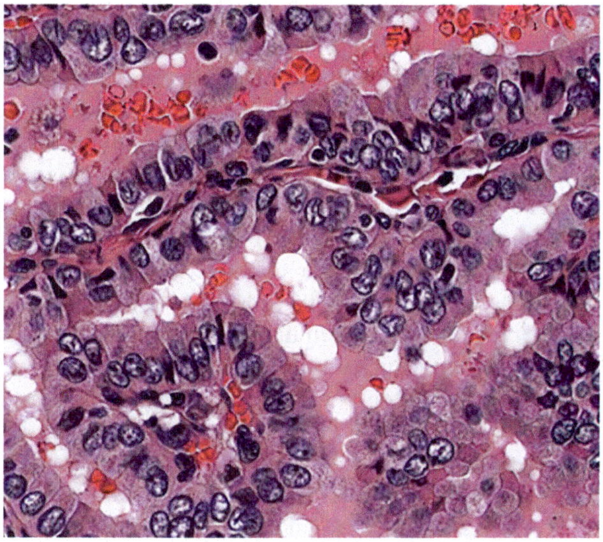

Fig. 2.2 Microscopy showing oncocytic classical variant papillary thyroid carcinoma (PTC) exhibiting the classical (papillary) architecture along with nuclear features of PTCs in the absence of tumor necrosis or increased mitotic activity. H&E stain

papillary growth pattern. There may be areas of follicular growth and in some cases the follicular pattern may be the predominant growth pattern.

Cytologically, the tumor cells of the oncocytic variant of PTC show abundant eosinophilic cytoplasm and the classical PTC nuclear features, namely, fine powdery chromatin, grooves, and pseudo-inclusions [43, 44] (Fig. 2.2). These oncocytic cells are arranged in irregular clusters or papillary aggregates. Oncocytic papillary carcinomas are characterized by a distinct mahogany brown appearance and may have a papillary or follicular architecture. Occasional tumors of oncocytic type may appear gray-white. Papillary tumors are characterized by complex branching papillae in which oncocytic cells cover thin fibro-vascular stromal cores [35, 39, 42, 45].

By molecular analysis, the oncocytic variant of PTC shows *RET/PTC* gene rearrangements [46, 47]. Trovisco et al. (2004) [46] identified *BRAF* mutations in oncocytic variants with papillary or papillary/follicular growth, whereas tumors with just follicular growth did not show *BRAF* mutations suggesting that the follicular oncocytic variants are genetically different from the papillary oncocytic variants. Abrosimov et al. (2007) [48] observed MUC1 and cyclin D1 expression (a target of the Wnt pathway) in 100% of tall-cell, columnar-cell, and oncocytic variants of PTC and almost 80% of Warthin's variants, but only in 27% of follicular variants. These data again show that the follicular variants appear to be distinct genetically from the oncocytic variants.

The biological behavior of the oncocytic variant of PTC seems quite variable, based on different series reported in the literature. It is believed that these discrepancies might reflect the lack of more precise histological criteria to define these neoplasms, leading to inclusion of a broad range of oncocytic tumors within such studies [44]. Berho et al. (1997) found that oncocytic PTC does not appear to behave more aggressively than conventional PTC [35]. Similar findings were reported more recently by Carr et al. (2018) [49] and Han et al. (2015) [50]. They reported that the oncocytic variant of PTC tends to be infiltrative; they metastasize to lymph nodes (LNs) and they harbor *BRAFV600E* mutations or *RET/PTC* gene rearrangements.

The differential diagnosis of oncocytic variant of PTC includes other oncocytic/Hürthle cell neoplasms (HCNs), other variants of PTC, and the oncocytic variant of medullary thyroid carcinoma (MTC). Both benign and malignant HCNs, have a tendency to show pseudo-papillary change, which is believed to be an artifact from fixation and tissue processing. The oncocytic/Hürthle cell variant of PTC shows true papillae with fibrovascular cores in addition to the classical nuclear changes of PTC. The eosinophilic cells in Hürthle cell variant are *not* twice as tall as they are wide, a feature that aids in distinguishing this histological variant of PTC from the tall-cell variant, which usually behaves in a much more aggressive fashion. Although the lesions are often confined to the thyroid, extra-thyroid extension (ETE), and lymph node (LN) metastases have been reported [51]. The distinction between oncocytic variant of PTC and oncocytic poorly differentiated thyroid carcinoma (PDTC) is based on lack of necrosis and mitoses that are characteristic of high-grade malignancies. The oncocytic variant of MTC is characterized by a solid or follicular growth pattern with prominent oncocytic cell changes, absence of the characteristic nuclear features of PTC, and the presence of more conventional areas of medullary carcinoma within the tumor [52, 53].

Importantly, the differential diagnosis of oncocytic solid variant PTC should also include oncocytic parathyroid neoplasms and thyroid paragangliomas with oncocytic change. It should be noted that solid growth in PTCs occurs in both RAS-like and BRAF-like tumors, as well as carcinomas with oncogene fusions that fall into these molecular subgroups.

The use of radioactive iodine (RAI) in the setting of oncocytic PTC is variable due to the suggestion that there is reduced capacity to uptake RAI and hence limited benefit due to less response to RAI therapy [35, 39, 41, 42]. Lucovic et al. (2021) reported that approximately 50% of their patients with oncocytic PTC received RAI. In that study, the clinical factors predictive of RAI use were similar to non-oncocytic PTCs and included large lesions (>4 cm), widely invasive disease, and angioinvasion. There was no difference in overall survival or disease-free survival in the group of patients with differentiated oncocytic PTC based on receipt of RAI [34]. This is similar to the observed behavior of non-oncocytic PTC, with published data suggesting no benefit of RAI in patients with low-risk disease [54–56].

Mai et al. (2005) [57] examined 19 cases of encapsulated Hürthle cell neoplasms with papillary architecture that lacked nuclear features of PTC. In their study, they identified proliferative activity in the neoplastic cells associated with the papillary architecture and felt the papillary changes were part of the lesion and not a degenerative process as described in some oncocytic tumors. All 19 patients were free of disease with follow-up (1–19 years after diagnosis). This group believes the term papillary variant of oncocytic (Hürthle cell) adenoma should be used to describe these overall benign-acting oncocytic lesions [57].

A wide range of outcomes has been reported for patients with oncocytic PTC, likely secondary to the lack of distinction between various types of oncocytic PTC and heterogenous grouping into "Hürthle cell" thyroid carcinomas. Some authors report that patients with oncocytic PTCs generally have an excellent prognosis with reported 5- and 10-year disease-free survival of 93% and 81%, respectively, and < 10% of patients developing local or distant recurrence [30, 58]. Similar results were reported by Lucovic et al. (2021) with a cumulative incidence of any recurrence (local, regional, or distant) at 10 years of 8.0% [34]. Stage for stage, the prognosis of patients with the oncocytic variant of PTC is similar to that of patients with conventional PTC [30, 49]. In one clinical series, oncocytic PTCs were not significantly different from oncocytic/Hürthle cell thyroid carcinomas with respect to their overall clinico-pathological variables and favorable RAI response [33].

Conversely, a retrospective study from the Mayo Clinic described 5- and 10-year rates of locoregional or distant recurrence of 11 and 28%, respectively [39]. The poorer outcomes seen in the Mayo Clinic study are likely due to changes in treatment guidelines during the 32-year study period as well as inconsistencies and changes to the histological criteria for the diagnosis of various forms of thyroid carcinomas with oncocytic change.

2.5.2 Warthin-like Variant of Papillary Thyroid Carcinoma (PTC)

The Warthin-like PTC (also known as papillary Hürthle cell carcinoma with lymphocytic stroma) is a variant that is characterized by a papillary growth of oncocytic cells with classical nuclear features of PTC and an associated brisk lympho-plasmacytic infiltrate in the cores of papillary stalks [59, 60]. The variant is so named because of its close resemblance to parotid gland Warthin's tumor (papillary cystadenoma lymphomatosum) (Fig. 2.3). These tumors often have an associated chronic lymphocytic thyroiditis (Hashimoto's thyroiditis) with oxyphilia in the background thyroid.

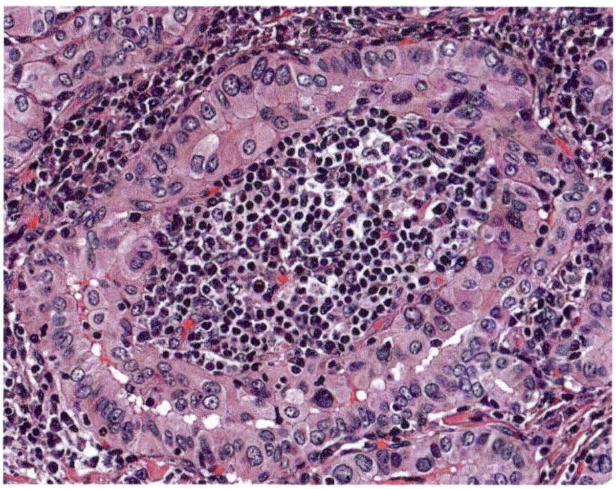

Fig. 2.3 Microscopy showing Warthin-like papillary thyroid carcinoma with a striking lympho-plasmacytic infiltrate in the stroma that yields a resemblance to Warthin's tumor of salivary glands. H&E stain

The FNA specimen and the histological sections from Warthin-like PTC can pose difficulties in distinguishing these lesions from florid chronic lymphocytic thyroiditis itself, oncocytic/Hürthle cell nodules in chronic lymphocytic thyroiditis, Hürthle cell tumors, tall-cell variant of PTC (oncocytic cells in Warthin-like PTC are *not* twice as tall as they are wide), and oncocytic variant of medullary thyroid carcinoma (MTC) [60, 61].

Trovisco et al. (2004) [46] identified *BRAF* mutations in 75% of Warthin-like PTCs versus 46% of usual-type PTCs. In contrast though, Sargent et al. (2006) [62] observed *BRAF* mutations only rarely in a variety of papillary carcinomas arising in a background of chronic lymphocytic thyroiditis and not in Warthin variant.

The biological behavior of these Warthin-like variants of PTC is similar to usual (classical or typical or conventional) PTC when compared for tumor size and stage, and hence the prognosis of this lesion is similar to that reported with typical PTC [9].

2.5.3 Tall-Cell Variant of Papillary Thyroid Carcinoma (PTC)

In 1976, Hawk and Hazard [63] described a variant of PTC that was characterized by carcinoma cells with classical PTC nuclei, but with abundant cytoplasm in which the cells were three times as tall as they were wide (Fig. 2.4). The distinction between this tall-cell variant and the usual variant of PTC proved to be important because the tall-cell variant showed a more aggressive biological behavior and because tumors were large in size, more often showed extra-thyroid extension (ETE), and showed a propensity for vascular invasion [63, 64]. The cells in this tumor are described as tall, with the most recent definition indicating their height is at least three times their width and most of them have an eosinophilic cytoplasm. However, the tumor cells are less granular than oncocytic/Hürthle cells.

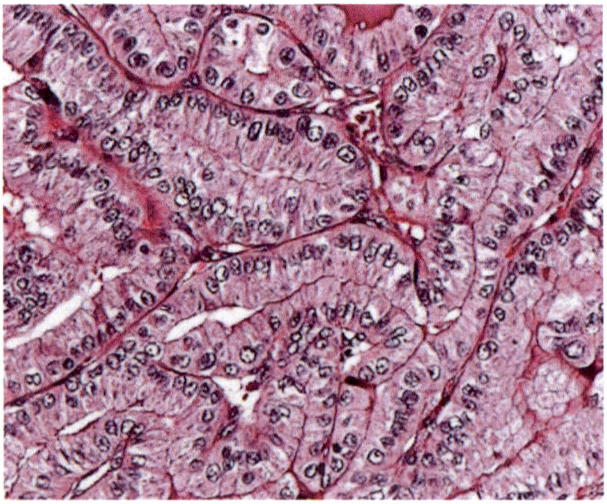

Fig. 2.4 Histology of tall-cell variant of papillary thyroid carcinoma. The carcinoma cells show a height greater than three times its width. H&E stain × 200

Cytology specimens of this tumor usually show elongated cells with sharp cytoplasmic borders, granular eosinophilic cytoplasm, and variably sized nuclei with nuclear features of papillary carcinoma. The nuclear features of PTC are usually abundant in aspirates of tall-cell variant as compared with that of classical PTC. Thus, nuclear grooves and inclusions are readily identifiable. Some authors reported the presence of intraepithelial neutrophils in aspirates from cases of tall-cell variant of PTC. This tumor can be confused with oncocytic/Hürthle cell tumor on cytology due to cytoplasmic eosinophilia; however, the nuclear features should help in differentiating between these two tumors [65].

There has been debate about the amount of tall cells needed to make a diagnosis of tall-cell variant of PTC. Montone et al. (2008) [9] prefer a diagnosis of tall-cell variant when tumors show more than 70% tall cells in the lesion; however, it is wise to mention any tall-cell differentiation if seen in a PTC. In addition, when these lesions show anaplastic transformation, they give rise to spindle-cell squamous carcinomas [66]. Squamous change of the tall cells may be seen in "recurrent" tall-cell PTCs and precede by months or years the development of anaplastic spindle-cell squamous carcinoma.

Ghossein et al. (2007) [67] compared the behavior of tall-cell variant of PTC (defined as >50% tall cells in their study) without ETE with classical-type PTC. They reported that tall-cell variants even without the adverse feature of ETE were more likely to develop LN and distant metastases and they concluded tall-cell variant of PTC without ETE is a more aggressive variant of PTC independent of age, gender, and tumor size. Adeniran et al. (2006) [68] identified *BRAF* mutations more commonly than *RET/PTC* and *RAS* mutations in tall-cell variants of PTC.

2.5.4 Oncocytic Follicular Variant of Papillary Thyroid Carcinoma (FVPTC)

Follicular variant papillary thyroid carcinoma (FVPTC) and follicular thyroid carcinoma (FTC) constitute what is known as "follicular-patterned differentiated thyroid carcinoma." They are distinguished from each other based on the degree of nuclear atypia, which is considered to be mild in FTC, and is more evident in FVPTC [69, 70]. Tumors that used to be classified as FVPTC has been recognized to include two distinct tumors; the invasive variant that frequently harbors *BRAFV600E* mutations and is more akin to classical PTC, and the encapsulated type, which is an expansile lesion that resembles FTC grossly and histologically at low magnification.

Tumors with follicular architecture may be macro- or micro-follicular with variable colloid storage [71]. The tumor may be well-delineated or even encapsulated, but careful evaluation usually identifies at least some degree of infiltration of the surrounding capsule; some lesions are frankly and widely invasive. The diagnosis of the oncocytic variant is based on the nuclear features of these lesions, which are identical to those seen in papillary carcinomas of the conventional type. These include nuclear enlargement, oval shape, elongation, and overlap, with clearing, resulting in a ground glass appearance, and irregular nuclear contours with nuclear pseudo-inclusions and grooves. The oncocytic cells are usually polygonal but may be columnar; they have abundant granular eosinophilic cytoplasm [72].

Molecular analyses showed that FTC and encapsulated FVPTC are both RAS-like lesions [73, 74] that are now classified as (1) minimally invasive with tumor capsular invasion only, (2) angioinvasive, but with no widely invasive growth, and (3) widely invasive and often angioinvasive with more aggressive behavior [75]. Indeed, the distinction between FTC and the encapsulated FVPTC is in question since the management approach to both entities overlaps [76, 77]. Noninvasive tumors without nuclear atypia are classified as "adenomas," whereas those with nuclear atypia are "noninvasive follicular tumors with papillary-like nuclei" (NIFTP) [78].

Follicular-patterned neoplasms including FTC and FVPTC, can exhibit oncocytic cytology (Fig. 2.5). When classified using rigid criteria and in the setting of exclusive follicular growth and absence of dedifferentiation, the oncocytic counterparts of FTC and encapsulated FVPTC represent thyroid neoplasms classified as one type of "oncocytic (Hürthle) cell carcinoma" [75].

As in non-oncocytic tumors, these neoplasms are classified as (1) minimally invasive oncocytic carcinoma (tumor capsular invasion only), (2) angioinvasive encapsulated oncocytic carcinoma (angioinvasion with no widely invasive growth), and (3) widely invasive oncocytic carcinoma (often angioinvasive) [75]. Oncocytic lesions that have nuclear atypia, but lack invasion, fall into the category of NIFTP [79]. However, this remains controversial since it has been reported in the literature by several authors that oncocytic tumors with follicular architecture and nuclear atypia that lack overt invasion in sections examined can metastasize [80–82].

Several molecular analyses of oncocytic tumors have classified these lesions only based on their oncocytic cytology and failed to consider other relevant criteria of more aggressive thyroid carcinomas such as predominant solid growth, necrosis, and high mitotic activity (>3/2mm^2), creating potential challenges that may explain

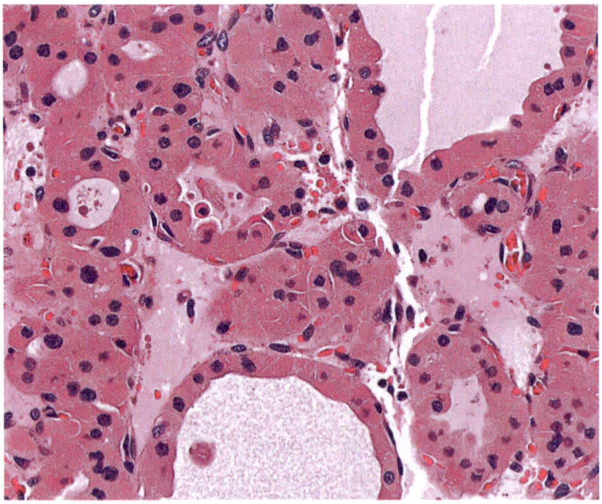

Fig. 2.5 Microscopy showing oncocytic FVPTC exhibiting exclusive follicular architecture along with nuclear features of PTCs in the absence of classical architecture, solid growth, tumor necrosis, or increased mitotic activity. Nuclear alterations of PTC are characterized by nuclear membrane irregularities in enlarged nuclei. H&E stain. *FVPTC* follicular variant papillary thyroid carcinoma

relatively lower rates of RAS-like molecular profiles and higher rates of high-risk molecular alterations in these studies [83–85]. These findings emphasize the importance of the accurate distinction of a poorly differentiated oncocytic thyroid carcinoma from a well-differentiated oncocytic carcinoma based on growth pattern and proliferation. Nevertheless, a consistent finding is that oncocytic FTCs have mitochondrial DNA (mtDNA) mutations [86–88] as well as chromosomal gains and losses, and occasional *EIF1AX, RAS, PTEN,* and *PIK3CA* mutations [83, 85, 89].

2.5.5 Oncocytic Poorly Differentiated Thyroid Carcinoma (PDTC)

Compared with patients with oncocytic PTCs, those with oncocytic poorly differentiated thyroid carcinoma PDTC in the recent Lucovic et al. study (2021) (34) were older, more likely to be male, and had worse outcomes in terms of any recurrence; the 5-year and 10-year cumulative incidence of any recurrence was 24.4% and 53.7%, respectively. Two additional retrospective studies confirmed these results and reported that oncocytic PDTCs follow a more aggressive course [90, 91]. Bai et al. (2015) reported that oncocytic PDTC patients had higher tumor-specific mortality and exhibited more extensive vascular invasion than other differentiated oncocytic cell thyroid carcinoma patients. At final follow-up (4–120 months) 17% of patients had a recurrence and 83% had distant metastases [90]. Papotti et al. (1996) reported previously similar findings—oncocytic PDTCs were more aggressive than stage-matched well-differentiated oncocytic FTCs [91]. In their study, 37% of patients had local recurrences or distant metastases at final follow-up. Skeletal muscle infiltration and extensive vascular invasion were markers of poor prognosis in that series [91]. Lucovic et al. found metastases to be more common in patients with oncocytic PDTCs [34].

A subset of classical “Hürthle cell carcinoma—HCC” actually represents a poorly differentiated thyroid carcinoma (PDTC) (also known as “insular thyroid carcinoma” because of the solid nesting growth pattern) [92] with predominant solid growth and widely invasive behavior, often with a well-delineated nidus [20, 21, 87]. These tumors tend to exhibit focal necrosis and have prominent mitoses (Fig. 2.6).

Immunohistochemical biomarkers supportive of dedifferentiation can help to distinguish PDTC, including focal areas of dedifferentiation indicative of tumor progression [93]. The oncocytic variants of this entity tend to be very aggressive and, like their non-oncocytic counterparts, rarely respond to radioactive iodine (RAI) therapy. In addition to the mitochondrial DNA (mtDNA) mutations, chromosomal gains and losses, and occasional mutations characteristic of DTCs, they harbor *TERT* promoter mutations and occasional mutations of *ATRX* and/or *DAXX* [83, 85]. *TERT* promoter mutation indicates a more aggressive clinical course with distant metastatic spread and reduced iodine uptake. The clinical relevance of recognizing this tumor classification has been highlighted by a recent study by Metovic et al. (2020) showing a distinctive immune-related gene expression profile of oncocytic PDTCs, not only confirming that this is a more aggressive cancer subtype but also pointing to a potential therapeutic role of immunotherapy [94].

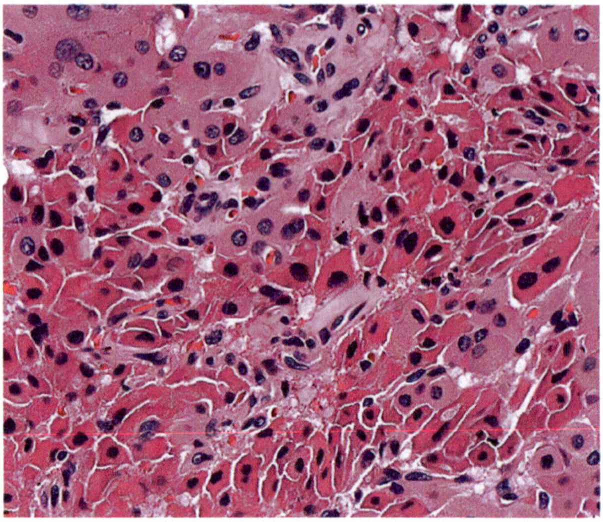

Fig. 2.6 Microscopy of an oncocytic poorly differentiated thyroid carcinoma showing solid/trabecular/insular growth in association with tumor necrosis and/or increased mitotic activity. H&E stain

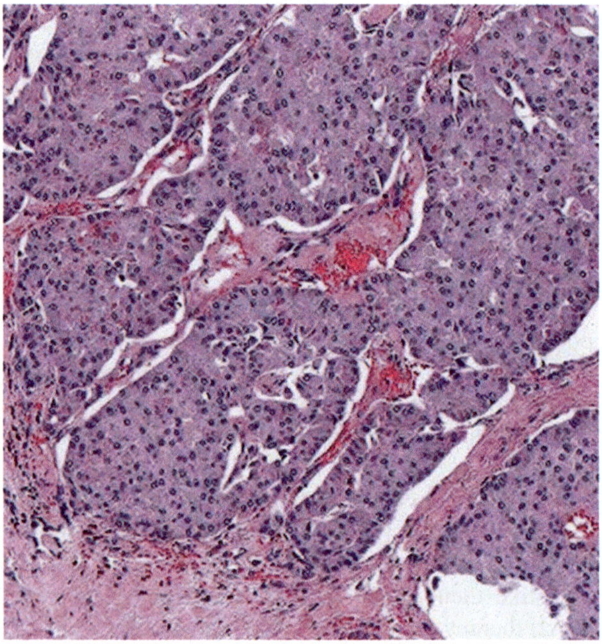

Fig. 2.7 Microscopy of an oncocytic medullary thyroid carcinoma (MTC) showing characteristic oncocytic (Hurthle cell) cytology (easily misdiagnosed as Hurthle cell neoplasm). H&E stain

2.5.6 Oncocytic Variant of Medullary Thyroid Carcinoma (MTC)

The existence of oncocytic medullary thyroid carcinoma (MTC) is well documented in the literature [15, 22, 95]. Some MTCs are composed of large cells with finely granular cytoplasm (Fig. 2.7) and the lesion is often misdiagnosed as HCC [96].

However, the nuclear characteristics are different because most MTCs have uniform, small nuclei unlike the pleomorphic nuclei in the Hürthle cell tumors. The cytoplasmic granularity is less pronounced in medullary lesions, and the latter rarely demonstrate intense eosinophilia. Moreover, lack of cellular cohesiveness and the presence of basophilic to amphophilic cytoplasmic granularity are features that should suggest the possibility of an oncocytic MTC.

In any questionable case, confirmation of this diagnosis should be based on the identification of diffuse positivity for monoclonal CEA (rather than thyroglobulin) as well as reactivity for calcitonin (Fig. 2.8) and/or calcitonin gene-related peptide (CGRP). It is noteworthy that some MTCs lack calcitonin expression, but can express CGRP, whereas others, usually more aggressive tumors that show dedifferentiation, can be negative for both calcitonin and CGRP, while they preserve diffuse staining with monoclonal antibodies to CEA [15]. The importance of CEA as a biomarker is also emphasized by the fact that calcitonin and CGRP can be expressed in various other neuroendocrine neoplasms, including those originating in lung, pancreas, head and neck, as well as rare examples of paragangliomas and parathyroid carcinomas [97]. Little is known in the literature about the molecular

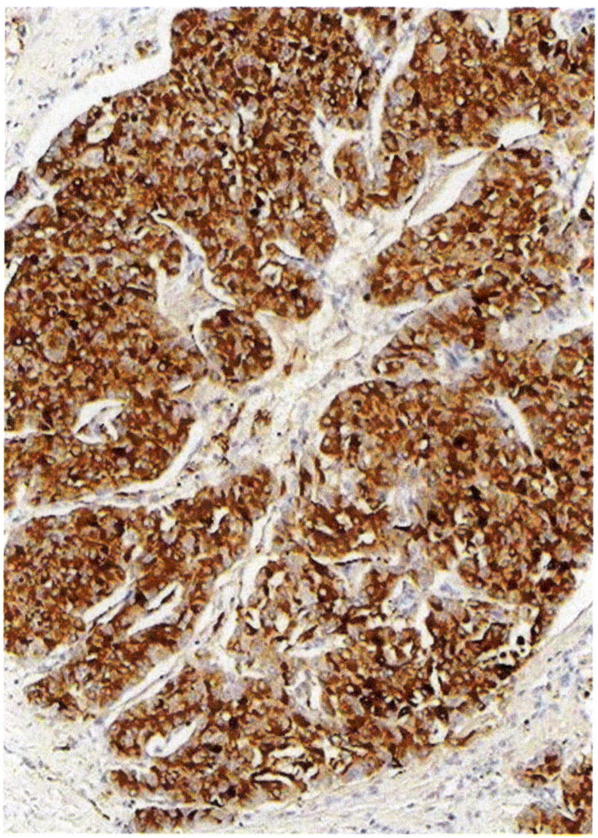

Fig. 2.8 Microscopy of an oncocytic variant of medullary thyroid carcinoma with immunohistochemistry (IHC) confirming the expression of calcitonin

alterations that underlie the whole molecular alterations that underlie the oncocytic variant in addition to the frequent *RET* mutations and less common *RAS* mutations that occur in non-oncocytic MTCs.

2.5.7 Oncocytic Tumors of Non-thyroid Origin

2.5.7.1 Granular Cell Tumor

Granular cell tumor (historically known as "granular cell myoblastoma" and "Abrikossoff tumor") is a rare tumor most likely of "Schwann cell" origin. Approximately 50% of the cases have been reported in the head and neck region. They can occur in other organs, including respiratory tract, gastrointestinal tract, genitourinary tract, vulva, and breast. Rarely, these tumors can occur in the thyroid gland or adjacent to the thyroid and clinically present as thyroid masses [98]. Most reported tumors in the thyroid occur in women, behave in a benign fashion, and can be treated with lobectomy.

In 2022, Srivastava et al. confirmed that thyroid granular cell tumors also harbor V-ATPase component inactivating mutations that characterize these tumors, and that additional PI3K pathway alterations may not necessarily predict aggressive behavior [99].

2.5.7.2 Metastatic and Invasive Oncocytic Tumor

The presence of oncocytic change is not unique to the thyroid gland. Thus, the identification of an oncocytic tumor in the thyroid must also include consideration of a possible metastatic oncocytic neoplasm, including renal and other primary sites, as well as an infiltrating oncocytic tumor, such as a parathyroid, salivary gland, or thymic tumor arising in the region of the thyroid. Renal cell carcinoma metastases tend to be vascular, often with extravasated blood lakes, and nuclear atypia is more prominent than that of granular cell tumor [100].

2.5.7.3 Oncocytic Parathyroid Adenoma

It is difficult to distinguish oncocytic/Hürthle cell thyroid and parathyroid tumors on cytology due to overlapping cytomorphological features [101]. Both tumors comprise epithelial cells with a micro-follicular pattern on a colloid or colloid-like background, and the presence of oxyphil cells and single cells, resembling oncocytic (Hürthle) cells and lymphocytes, respectively [102, 103]. In oncocytic parathyroid adenomas, the cells are very large in size and adherent to each other, nuclei are small and darker, nucleoli are barely visible, with numerous single cells and no colloid, but a similar substance. The monotonous cell population presents indistinct cytoplasmic borders forming large cohesive sheets with pseudo-papillary patterns (Fig. 2.9).

In oncocytic/Hürthle cell thyroid tumors, the cells are less adherent, nuclei are larger, and nucleoli are prominent; single cells are rare, and colloid is present. Correlation with clinical findings and imaging is needed to aid in reaching proper diagnosis. In addition, immunohistochemistry (IHC) for parathyroid hormone

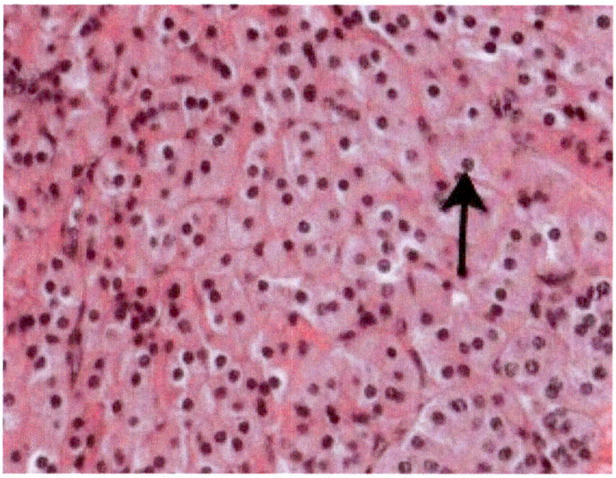

Fig. 2.9 Microscopy showing the presence of cells presenting oncocytic metaplasia (arrow) and normal parathyroid cells. H&E × 200

(PTH), thyroglobulin (Tg) (colloid labeling), and thyroid transcription factor-1 (TTF-1) (nuclear labeling) and GATA-3 can also be performed to confirm clinical suspicion and reach the final diagnosis [102].

References

1. Baloch ZW, LiVolsi VA, Asa SL, Rosai J, Merino MJ, Randolph G, et al. Diagnostic terminology and morphologic criteria for cytologic diagnosis of thyroid lesions: a synopsis of the National Cancer Institute Thyroid fine-needle aspiration state of the science conference. Diagn Cytopathol. 2008;36:425–37.
2. Friedman N. Cellular involution in thyroid gland: significance of Hürthle cells in myxedema, exhaustion atrophy, Hashimoto's disease and reaction in irradiation, thiouracil therapy and subtotal resection. J Clin Endocrinol. 1949;9:874–82.
3. Granter SR, Cibas ES. Cytologic findings in thyroid nodules after 131I treatment of hyperthyroidism. Am J Clin Pathol. 1997;107:20–5.
4. Katz SM, Vickery AL Jr. The fibrous variant of Hashimoto's thyroiditis. Hum Pathol. 1974;5:161–70.
5. Kendal CH, McCluskey E, Meagles JN. Oxyphil cells in thyroid disease: a uniform change? J Clin Pathol. 1986;39:908–12.
6. Kennedy JS, Thomson JA. The changes in the thyroid gland after irradiation with ^{131}I or partial thyroidectomy for thyrotoxicosis. J Pathol. 1974;112:65–81.
7. LiVolsi VA. Surgical pathology of the Thyroid. Philadelphia: WB Saunders; 1990.
8. Rosai J, Cacangiu ML, DeLellis RA. Tumors of the Thyroid gland, 3rd series, fascicle 5. Washington, DC: Armed Forces Institute of Pathology;. Atlas of Tumor Pathology; 1992.
9. Montone KT, Baloch ZW, LiVolsi VA. The thyroid Hürthle (oncocytic) cell and its associated pathologic conditions: a surgical pathology and cytopathology review. Arch Pathol Lab Med. 2008;132:1241–50.
10. Sidhu S. Hürthle cell neoplasm of the thyroid gland. ANZ J Surg. 2008;78:115.
11. Harcourt-Webster JN, Stott NC. Histochemical study of oxidative and hydrolytic enzymes in the human thyroid. J Pathol Bacteriol. 1966;92:291–302.
12. Tremblay G. Histochemical study of cytochrome oxidase and adenosine triphosphatase in Askanazy cells (Hurthle cells) of the human thyroid. Lab Investig. 1962;11:514–7.

13. Tremblay G, Pearse AG. Histochemistry of oxidative enzyme systems in the human thyroid, with special reference to Askanazy cells. J Pathol Bacteriol. 1960;80:353–8.
14. Muller-Hocker J, Jacob U, Seibel P. Hashimoto thyroiditis is associated with defects of cytochrome-c oxidase in oxyphil Askanazy cells and with the common deletion (4,977) of mitochondrial DNA. Ultrastruct Pathol. 1998;22:91–100.
15. Mete O, Asa SL. Oncocytes, Oxyphils, Hurthle, and Askanazy cells: morphological and molecular features of Oncocytic Thyroid nodules. Endocr Pathol. 2010;21(1):16–24.
16. LiVolsi VA. The pathology of autoimmune thyroid disease: a review. Thyroid. 1994;4:333–9.
17. Bhatt PJ, Madhavan P. PSAT296 graves' disease and Hurthle cell carcinoma: a rare presentation. J Endoc Soc. 2022;6(1):A817–8.
18. Suster D, Ronen N, Giorgadze T. Oncocytic nodular hyperplasia of the thyroid. Ann Diagn Pathol. 2022;61:152049.
19. Paschke R. Molecular pathogenesis of nodular goiter. Langenbeck's Arch Surg. 2011;396(8):1127–36.
20. Tallini G. Oncocytic Tumours. Virchows Arch. 1998;433(1):5–12.
21. Tallini G, Carcangiu ML, Rosai J. Oncocytic neoplasms of the Thyroid gland. Acta Pathol Jpn. 1992;42:305–15.
22. Asa SL. My approach to Oncocytic Tumours of the Thyroid. J Clin Pathol. 2004;57(3):225–32.
23. Cannon J. The significance of Hurthle cells in thyroid disease. Oncologist. 2011;16:1380–7.
24. Gross M, Eliashar R, Ben-Yaakov A, Weinberger JM, Maly B. Clinicopathologic features and outcome of the Oncocytic variant of papillary Thyroid Carcinoma. Ann Otol Rhinol Laryngol. 2009;118(5):374–81.
25. Lopez-Penabad L, Chiu AC, Hoff AO, Schultz P, Gaztambide S, Ordonez NG, et al. Prognostic factors in patients with Hurthle cell neoplasms of the Thyroid. Cancer. 2003;97(5):1186–94.
26. Auger M. Hurthle cells in fine-needle aspirates of the Thyroid: a review of their diagnostic criteria and significance. Cancer Cytopathol. 2014;122:241–9.
27. Wenter V, Albert NL, Unterrainer M, Ahmaddy F, Ilhan H, Jellinek A, et al. Clinical impact of follicular Oncocytic (Hurthle cell) Carcinoma in comparison with corresponding classical follicular Thyroid Carcinoma. Eur J Nucl Med Mol Imaging. 2021;48(2):449–60.
28. Yang Q, Zhao Z, Zhong G, Jin A, Yu K. Effect of adjuvant radioactive iodine therapy on survival in rare Oxyphilic subtype of Thyroid cancer (Hurthle cell Carcinoma). Peer J. 2019;7:e7458.
29. Jillard CL, Youngwirth L, Scheri RP, Roman S, Sosa JA. Radioactive iodine treatment is associated with improved survival for patients with Hurthle cell Carcinoma. Thyroid Off J Am Thyroid Assoc. 2016;26(7):959–64.
30. Wenter V, Jellinek A, Unterrainer M, Ahmaddy F, Lehner S, Albert NL, et al. Long-term outcome of rare Oncocytic papillary (Hurthle cell) Thyroid Carcinoma following (adjuvant) initial radioiodine therapy. Eur J Nucl Med Mol Imaging. 2019;46(12):2526–35.
31. Goffredo P, Roman SA, Sosa JA. Hurthle cell Carcinoma: a population-level analysis of 3311 patients. Cancer. 2013;119(3):504–11.
32. Zhou X, Zheng Z, Chen C, Zhao B, Cao H, Li T, et al. Clinical characteristics and prognostic factors of Hurthle cell Carcinoma: a population based study. BMC Cancer. 2020;20(1):407.
33. Amouri W, Charfeddine S, Charfi S, Jardak I, Boudawara T, Guermazi F. Clinicopathological features and outcomes after radioactive iodine treatment of Oncocytic well-Differentiated Thyroid carcinomas. Nucl Med Commun. 2019;40(9):888–93.
34. Lucovic J, Petrovic I, Liu Z, Armstrong SM, Brierly JD, Tsang R, et al. Oncocytic papillary Thyroid Carcinoma and Oncocytic poorly Differentiated Thyroid Carcinoma: clinical features, uptake, and response to radioactive iodine therapy, and outcome. Front Endocrinol. 2021;2:2021.
35. Berho M, Suster S. The oncocytic variant of papillary carcinoma of the thyroid: a clinicopathologic study of 15 cases. Hum Pathol. 1997;28(1):47–53.
36. Selzer G, Kahn LB, Alberttyn L. Primary malignant tumors of the thyroid: a clinicopathologic study of 254 cases. Cancer. 1977;40:1501–11.

37. Woolner LB, Beahrs OH, Black BM, McConahey WM, Keating FR Jr. Classification and prognosis of thyroid carcinoma: a study of 885 cases observed in a 30-year period. Am J Surg. 1961;102:354–87.
38. Herrera MF, Hay ID, Wu PS, Goellner JR, Ryan JJ, Ebersold JR, et al. Hürthle cell (oxyphilic) papillary thyroid carcinoma: a variant with more aggressive biologic behavior. World J Surg. 1992;16(4):669–74.
39. Meissner WA, Adler A. Papillary carcinoma of the thyroid; a study of the pathology of two hundred twenty-six cases. AMA Arch Pathol. 1958;66(4):518–25.
40. Tscholl-Ducommun J, Hedinger CE. Papillary thyroid carcinomas. Morphology and prognosis. Virchows Arch A Pathol Anat Histol. 1982;396(1):19–39.
41. Beckner ME, Heffess CS, Oertel JE. Oxyphilic papillary thyroid carcinomas. Am J Clin Pathol. 1995;103(3):280–7.
42. Hill JH, Werkhaven JA, DeMay RM. Hurthle cell variant of papillary carcinoma of the thyroid gland. Otolaryngol Head Neck Surg. 1988;98(4):338–41.
43. Moreira AL, Waisman J, Cangiarella JF. Aspiration cytology of the oncocytic variant of papillary adenocarcinoma of the thyroid gland. Acta Cytol. 2004;48:137–41.
44. Koseoglu RD, Onuk FN. The Oncocytic variant of papillary thyroid carcinoma. Turk J Med Sci. 2006;36(6):387–92.
45. Ludikova M, Ryska A, Korabecna M, Rydlova M, Michal M. Oncocytic papillary carcinoma with lymphoid stroma–Warthin like tumor of the thyroid. A distinct entity with favourable prognosis. Histopathology. 2001;39:17–24.
46. Trovisco V, Vieira de Castro I, Soares P, Máximo V, Silva P, et al. BRAF mutations are associated with some histological types of papillary thyroid carcinoma. J Pathol. 2004;202(2):247–51.
47. Soares P, Trovisco V, Rocha AS, Lima J, Castro P, Preto A, et al. BRAF mutations and RET/PTC rearrangements are alternative events in the etiopathogenesis of PTC. Oncogene. 2003;22(29):4578–80.
48. Abrosimov A, Saenko V, Meirmanov S, Nakashima M, Rogounovitch T, Shkurko O, et al. The cytoplasmic expression of MUC1 in papillary thyroid carcinoma of different histological variants and its correlation with cyclin D1 overexpression. Endocr Pathol. 2007;18(2):68–75.
49. Carr AA, Yen TWF, Ortiz DI, Hunt BC, Fareau G, Massey BL, et al. Patients with Oncocytic variant papillary Thyroid Carcinoma have a similar prognosis to matched classical papillary Thyroid Carcinoma controls. Thyroid. 2018;28(11):1462–7.
50. Han F, Zhang L, Zhang S, Zhou H, Yi X. Occult Oncocytic papillary Thyroid Carcinoma with lymphoid stroma (Warthin-like tumor): report of a case with concomitant mutations of BRAF V600E and V600K. Int J Clin Exp Pathol. 2015;8(5):5896–901.
51. Johnson TL, Lloyd R, Thompson NW, Beierwaltes WH, Sisson JC. Prognostic implications of the tall cell variant of papillary thyroid carcinoma. Am J Surg Pathol. 1988;12:22–7.
52. Dominquez-Malagon H, Delgado-Chavez R, Torres-Najera M, Gould E, Albores-Saavedra J. Oxyphilic and squamous variants of medullary carcinoma of the thyroid. Cancer. 1989;63:1183–8.
53. Harach HR, Bergholm U. Medullary (C cell) carcinoma of the thyroid with features of follicular oxyphilic cell tumors. Histopathology. 1988;13:645–56.
54. Hundahl SA, Fleming ID, Fremgen AM, Mench HR. A national cancer data base report on 53,856 cases of thyroid carcinoma treated in the US, 1985–1995. Cancer. 1998;83:2638–48.
55. Jonklaas J, Sarlis NJ, Litofsky D, Ain KB, Bigos ST, Brierley JD, et al. Outcomes of patients with Differentiated Thyroid Carcinoma Followign initial therapy. Thyroid. 2006;16(12):1229–42.
56. Vaisman F, Shaha A, Fish S, Michael TR. Initial therapy with either Thyroid lobectomy or Total thyroidectomy without radioactive iodine remnant ablation is associated with very low rates of structural disease recurrence in properly selected patients with Differentiated Thyroid cancer. Clin Endocrinol. 2011;75:112–9.

57. Mai KT, Elmontaser G, Perkins DG, Thomas J, Stinson WA. Benign Hürthle cell adenoma with papillary architecture: a benign lesion mimicking oncocytic papillary carcinoma. Int J Surg Pathol. 2005;13(1):37–41.
58. Besic N, Hocevar M, Zgajnar J, Petric R, Pilko G. Aggressiveness of therapy and prognosis of patients with Hurthle cell papillary Thyroid Carcinoma. Thyroid Off J Am Thyroid Assoc. 2006;16(1):67–72.
59. Apel RL, Asa SL, LiVolsi VA. Papillary Hürthle cell carcinoma with lymphocytic stroma. "Warthin-like tumor" of the thyroid. Am J Surg Pathol. 1995;19(7):810–4.
60. Baloch ZW, LiVolsi VA. Warthin-like papillary carcinoma of the thyroid. Arch Pathol Lab Med. 2000;124(8):1192–5.
61. Solomon A, Gupta PK, LiVolsi VA, Baloch ZW. Distinguishing tall cell variant of papillary thyroid carcinoma from usual variant of papillary thyroid carcinoma in cytologic specimens. Diagn Cytopathol. 2002;27(3):143–8.
62. Sargent R, LiVolsi V, Murphy J, Mantha G, Hunt JL. BRAF mutation is unusual in chronic lymphocytic thyroiditis-associated papillary thyroid carcinomas and absent in non-neoplastic nuclear atypia of thyroiditis. Endocr Pathol. 2006;17(3):235–41.
63. Hawk WA, Hazard JB. The many appearances of papillary carcinoma of the thyroid. Cleve Clin Q. 1976;43(4):207–15.
64. Johnson TL, Lloyd RV, Thompson NW, Beierwaltes WH, Sisson JC. Prognostic implications of the tall cell variant of papillary thyroid carcinoma. Am J Surg Pathol. 1988;12(1):22–7.
65. Das DK, Mallik MK, Sharma P, Sheikh ZA, Mathew PA, Sheikh M, et al. Papillary thyroid carcinoma and its variants in fine needle aspiration smears. A cytomorphologic study with special reference to tall cell variant. Acta Cytol. 2004;48(3):325–36.
66. Bronner MP, LiVolsi VA. Spindle cell squamous carcinoma of the thyroid: an unusual anaplastic tumor associated with tall cell papillary cancer. Mod Pathol. 1991;4(5):637–43.
67. Ghossein RA, Leboeuf R, Patel KN, Rivera M, Katabi N, Carlson DL, et al. Tall cell variant of papillary thyroid carcinoma without extrathyroid extension: biologic behavior and clinical implications. Thyroid. 2007;17(7):655–61.
68. Adeniran AJ, Zhu Z, Gandhi M, Steward DL, Fidler JP, Giordano TJ, et al. Correlation between genetic alterations and microscopic features, clinical manifestations, and prognostic characteristics of thyroid papillary carcinomas. Am J Surg Pathol. 2006;30(2):216–22.
69. Asa SL, de Jesus AC, Kerr D, Mete O, Nose V, Papotti M, et al. Thyroid. In: Mete O, Asa SL, editors. Endocrine pathology. Cambridge University Press; 2016. p. 398–572.
70. Asa SL. The current histologic classification of Thyroid cancer. Endocrinol Metab Clin N Am. 2019;48(1):1–22.
71. Cheung CC, Ezzat S, Freeman JL, Rosen IB, Asa SL. Immunohistochemical diagnosis of papillary thyroid carcinoma. Mod Pathol. 2001;14:338–42.
72. De Lellis RA, Lloyd RV, Heitz PU, Eng C, editors. World Health Organization classification of tumors. Pathology and genetics of tumors of endocrine organs. Lyon: IARC Press; 2004. p. 61.
73. The Cancer Genome Atlas Research Network. Integrated genomic characterization of papillary Thyroid Carcinoma. Cell. 2014;159(3):676–90.
74. Nikiforova MN, Lynch RA, Biddinger PW, Alexander EK, Dorn GW, Tallini G, et al. RAS point mutations and PAX8-PPAR gamma rearrangement in Thyroid tumors: evidence for distinct molecular pathways in Thyroid follicular Carcinoma. J Clin Endocrinol Metab. 2003;88(5):2318–26.
75. Lloyd RV, Osamura RY, Kloppel G, Rosai J. Who classification of Tumours of endocrine organs. 4th ed. Lyon: IARC; 2017.
76. Asa SL. The evolution of Differentiated Thyroid cancer. For Pathol. 2017;49(3):229–37.
77. Asa SL, Giordano TJ, LiVolsi VA. Implications of the TCGA genomic characterization of papillary Thyroid Carcinoma for Thyroid pathology: does follicular variant papillary Thyroid Carcinoma exist? Thyroid. 2015;25(1):1–2.

78. Nikiforov YE, Seethala RR, Tallini G, Baloch ZW, Basolo F, Thompson LDR, et al. Nomenclature revision for encapsulated follicular variant of papillary Thyroid Carcinoma: a paradigm shift to reduce overtreatment of indolent tumors. JAMA Oncol. 2016;2(8):1023–9.
79. Xu B, Reznik E, Tuttle RM, Knauf J, Fagin JA, Katabi N, et al. Outcome and molecular characteristics of non-invasive encapsulated follicular variant of papillary Thyroid Carcinoma with Oncocytic features. Endocrine. 2019;64(1):97–108.
80. Grant CS, Barr D, Goellner JR, Hay ID. Benign Hürthle cell tumors of the Thyroid: a diagnosis to be trusted? World J Surg. 1988;12:488–95.
81. Belchetz G, Cheung CC, Freeman J, Rosen IB, Witterick IJ, Asa SL. Hurthle cell tumors: using molecular techniques to define a novel classification system. Arch Otolaryngol Head Neck Surg. 2002;128(3):237–40.
82. Cheung CC, Ezzat S, Ramyar L, Freeman JL, Asa SL. Molecular basis of Hurthle cell papillary Thyroid Carcinoma. J Clin Endocrinol Metab. 2000;85(2):878–82.
83. Ganly I, Ricarte FJ, Eng S, Ghossein R, Morris LGT, Liang Y, et al. Genomic dissection of Hurthle cell Carcinoma reveals a unique class of Thyroid malignancy. J Clin Endocrinol Metab. 2013;98(5):E962–72.
84. Chindris AM, Casler JD, Bernet VJ, Rivera M, Thomas C, Kachergus JM, et al. Clinical and molecular features of Hurthle cell Carcinoma of the Thyroid. J Clin Endocrinol Metab. 2015;100(1):55–62.
85. Ganly I, Makarov V, Deraje S, Dong YY, Reznik E, Seshan V, et al. Integrated genomic analysis of Hurthle cell cancer reveals oncogenic drivers, recurrent mitochondrial mutations, and unique chromosomal landscapes. Cancer Cell. 2018;34(2):256–70.
86. Maximo V, Soares P, Lima J, Cameselle-Teijeiro J, Sobrinho-Simoes M. Mitochondrial DNA somatic mutations (point mutations and large deletions) and mitochondrial DNA variants in human Thyroid pathology: a study with emphasis on Hurthle cell tumors. Am J Pathol. 2002;160(5):1857–65.
87. Maximo V, Sobrinho-Simoes M. Hurthle cell Tumours of the Thyroid. A review with emphasis on mitochondrial abnormalities with clinical relevance. Virchows Arch. 2000;437(2):107–15.
88. Tallini G, Hsueh A, Liu S, Garcia-Rostan G, Speicher MR, Ward DC. Frequent chromosomal DNA unbalance in Thyroid Oncocytic (Hurthle cell) neoplasms detected by comparative genomic hybridization. Lab Investig. 1999;79(5):547–55.
89. Schark C, Fulton N, Jacoby RF, Westbrook CA, Straus FHII, Kaplan EL. N-Ras 61 oncogene mutations in Hürthle cell tumors. Surgery. 1990;108:994–1000.
90. Bai S, Baloch ZW, Samulski TD, Montone KT, LiVolsi VA. Poorly Differentiated Oncocytic (Hurthle cell) follicular Carcinoma: an institutional experience. Endocr Pathol. 2015;26(2):164–9.
91. Papotti M, Torchio B, Grassi L, Favero A, Bussolati G. Poorly Differentiated Oxyphilic (Hurthle cell) carcinomas of the Thyroid. Am J Surg Pathol. 1996;20(6):686–94.
92. Carcangiu ML, Zampi G, Rosai J. Poorly Differentiated ("Insular") Thyroid Carcinoma. A reinterpretation of Langhans' "Wuchernde Struma". Am J Surg Pathol. 1984;8:655–68.
93. Baloch Z, Mete O, Asa SL. Immunohistochemical biomarkers in Thyroid pathology. Endocr Pathol. 2018;29(2):91–112.
94. Metovic J, Vignale C, Annaratone L, Osella-Abate S, Maletta F, Rapa I, et al. The Oncocytic variant of poorly Differentiated Thyroid Carcinoma shows a specific immune-related gene expression profile. J Clin Endocrinol Metab. 2020;105(12):dgaa655.
95. Asa SL. Survival guide to endocrine pathology. Virginia: Innovative Pathology Press; 2020.
96. Chetty R. Hürthle cell medullary carcinomas of the thyroid gland. S Afr J Surg. 1990;28(3):95–7.
97. Hodgson A, Pakbaz S, Tayyari F, Young JEM, Mete O. Diagnostic pitfall: parathyroid Carcinoma expands the Spectrum of calcitonin and calcitonin gene-related peptide expressing neuroendocrine neoplasms. Endocr Pathol. 2019;30(2):168–72.
98. Baloch ZW, Martin S, Livolsi VA. Granular cell tumor of the thyroid: a case report. Int J Surg Pathol. 2005;13(3):291–4.

99. Srivastava P, Da Cruz PA, Weigelt B, Pareja F, Reis-Filho JS, Yip L, et al. Granular cell tumor of thyroid: a case series with molecular characterization highlighting unique pitfalls. Endocrine. 2022;76(2):395–406.
100. McHugh JB, Hoschar AP, Dvorakova M, Parwani AV, Barnes EL, Seethala RR. p63 immunohistochemistry differentiates salivary gland oncocytoma and oncocytic carcinoma from metastatic renal cell carcinoma. Head Neck Pathol. 2007;1(2):123–31.
101. Paul A, Villepelet A, Lefevre M, Perei S. Oncocytic parathyroid adenoma. Europ Ann Otorhinolaryngol Head Neack Dis. 2015;132(5):301–3.
102. Cibas ES, Ali SZ. The Bethesda system for reporting thyroid cytopathology. Thyroid. 2009;19:1159–65.
103. Paker TI, Yilmazer D, Yandakci K, et al. Intrathyroidal oncocytic parathyroid adenoma: a diagnostic pitfall on fine-needle aspiration. Diagn Cytopathol. 2010;38:833–6.

Oncocytic (Hürthle Cell) Lesions: Controversy of Nomenclature, Origin, and Histology

3

3.1 Controversy of Nomenclature

An "oncocyte" is an epithelial cell defined by the presence of numerous mitochondria imparting a deeply eosinophilic finely granular appearance to the cytoplasm [1].

Mitochondrial proteins, being of basic nature, have avidity to bind acidic dyes like eosin. Because of this staining feature, oncocytes have also been termed "oxyphils." Oncocytes have been found to arise in various tissues, including endocrine glands (thyroid, parathyroid, and pituitary glands), exocrine glands (salivary, lacrimal glands, pancreas, and liver), and secretory epithelia (nasal cavities, buccal mucosa, and larynx) [2, 3]. In the thyroid gland, these cells have also been termed "Hürthle cells" (HCs) or "Ashkanazy cells" [1, 4] after the names of these two scientists, respectively.

James Ewing described a thyroid carcinoma with cells containing finely granular, eosinophilic cytoplasm and suggested that they might be "hypertrophic Hürthle cells." In his study of thyroid tumors, Theodor Langhans had previously (in 1907) published a series of five cases of thyroid tumors that is now considered the first description of Hürthle cell tumors [5]. The name Hürthle cell is widely used because the illustrious and influential James Ewing used the term in the first edition of his textbook *Neoplastic Diseases* [6–8]. The tumors described by Langhans were composed of a distinctly different cell than that described by Hürthle. Nonetheless, since at least 1928, the term "Hürthle cell" has been appended to the cells originally described by the famous pathologist Max Ashkanazy [9–11].

The term "oncocyte" is derived from the Greek word "onkos," meaning "swelling" [4] and was first used in 1932 by Jaffe in the salivary gland, and later adopted in 1936 by Hamperl, describing granular eosinophilic cells and the corresponding neoplasm in a variety of epithelial and glandular tissues, including the thyroid gland [1, 12, 13]. Similar cells were also described in the parathyroid gland by Welsh, who referred to them as "oxyphilic cells." The characteristic red staining of the cytoplasm of these cells on hematoxylin and eosin (H&E)–stained slides is explained by

M. Sakr, *Oncocytic (Hürthle Cell) Thyroid Lesions*,
https://doi.org/10.1007/978-3-032-03115-0_3

the strong affinity of the innumerable cationic (basic) mitochondria in their cytoplasm for eosin, an acidic (anionic) stain [14].

Of note, "oncocyte-like" cells can also exhibit abundant eosinophilic cytoplasm; however, in contrast to "true" oncocytes, which owe their cytoplasmic eosinophilia to mitochondria, the eosinophilia of oncocyte-like cells is a result of the accumulation of other organelles (such as lysosomes, cytofilaments, neuro-secretory granules, smooth endoplasmic reticulum, or a combination of these) [15]. Oncocytes and oncocyte-like lesions can be found throughout the body, mostly in endocrine organs such as the thyroid gland, parathyroid gland, adrenal gland, and pituitary gland, but also in non-endocrine organs such as salivary glands and kidneys [1, 16]. Some authors strongly believe that a distinction should be made between proliferations of true HCs, containing cells with the classical cytological appearance, and smears containing this second similar, but separate, type of cell [17].

Cells with less or incomplete eosinophilic, granular appearance can observed, at least focally, in any thyroid lesions, such as autoimmune thyroiditis, nodular goiter, aging, and irradiated thyroids. These oncocytic, non-Hürthle cells are called "oncocytic metaplasia." Although immunohistochemistry (IHC) using anti-mitochondrial markers can detect focal oncocytic metaplasia [6], there are no quantitative measurements to precisely distinguish between oncocytic metaplasia and non-oncocytic cells. True Hürthle cells have a cytoplasm filled with mitochondria with complete loss of cell polarity, while metaplastic cells do not have a complete loss of cell polarity and have fewer mitochondria at the ultrastructural level.

Although the terms oncocyte, oxyphilic cell, and Hürthle cell are now used interchangeably to indicate cells displaying similar, specific features, independent of their anatomical location, Hürthle cell is used *only* to indicate cells of thyroid follicular origin [18, 19].

The Hürthle cell (HC) is named after the German physiologist and histologist *Karl Hürthle (*March 16, 1860–March 23, 1945), who investigated thyroid secretory function, in canines. However, this is a "misnomer" since what he really described were the "para-follicular" C-cells in the thyroid gland of dogs in 1894 [20]. The oncocytic cells derived from thyroid follicular epithelium (true Hürthle cells) were, in fact, first described in 1898 by the Swiss-German pathologist *Max Ashkanazy* (born on February 24, 1865) in patients with Graves' disease [21]. Despite this historical fact, and despite this being corrected frequently in the literature over the last century, as having been described by Ashkanazy, including a move toward designating these lesions as "oncocytic," more descriptive than ascribed for discovery, the misnomer has taken hold and the term "Hürthle cell" has continued to be used in the literature to refer to thyroid follicular cells with oncocytic features, except in Germany where the term "Ashkanazy cells" is in use.

Recently, in the "2022 WHO classification of Endocrine and Neuro-endocrine Tumors," the term "oncocytic cell" has replaced "Hürthle cell." Accordingly, oncocytic adenoma and oncocytic carcinoma of the thyroid gland are the new names for Hürthle cell adenoma (HCA) and Hürthle cell carcinoma (HCC), respectively [22].

3.2 Oncocytic (Hürthle) Cells: Controversy of Origin

Despite the recent developments in science, the exact origin of oncocytic (Hürthle) cells in the thyroid gland is unclear, in terms of their physiological function and from which progenitor they arise.

3.2.1 Follicular Cell Origin

Detection of thyroglobulin (Tg) immuno-reactivity and thyroid-stimulating hormone (TSH) receptor adenylate cyclase system, unique to the follicular epithelial cell of the thyroid in many oncocytic/Hürthle cell tumors, suggests that these oncocytic/Hürthle cells evolve from the follicular cell (thyrocyte) at some point in their development. However, this appears to take place prior to neoplastic transformation as mixed oncocytic (Hürthle) cell/follicular lesions are *not* typically observed. Oncocytic (Hürthle cell neoplasms—HCNs) have been considered by some investigators as "an orphan disease group in the thyroid" [23].

3.2.2 Parafollicular Cell Origin

A "para-follicular" cell origin of oncocytic (Hürthle) cells was reported in the literature [24] based on the more frequent lymphatic metastasis [25], lower radioactive iodine (RAI) avidity [26], and different oncogene expression when compared to follicular thyroid cancer (FTC) [27].

3.2.3 Conclusion

Given that the hallmark of oncocytic change is mitochondrial proliferation as an adaptive process to a primary nuclear abnormality [4, 28], it can occur in follicular as well as in parafollicular cells. Thus, Hürthle cell neoplasms of the thyroid are generally considered to fall into one of two tumor types, follicular-derived thyroid tumors (FDTT, tumors of thyrocytes) or parafollicular tumors of C-cell/neural crest origin [29]..

In conclusion, Hürthle cell/oncocytic change in the thyroid gland occurs mainly in follicular epithelial cells [30, 31], but also can occur in C-cells and their lesions, and in solid cell nests, the embryological remnants of the ultimobranchial bodies [32].

3.3 Oncocytic (Hürthle) Cells: Controversy of Histology

3.3.1 Histological Features

Oncocytic (Hürthle) cells tend to be polygonal cells with distinct cell borders, larger in size than follicular cells reaching 10-15 μ. The principal features of these oncocytic cells include an eosinophilic granular cytoplasm and a large hyperchromatic round-to-oval nucleus with a prominent nucleolus [18, 33].

Although the actual amount of cytoplasm in oncocytic or Hürthle cells may vary, it is generally sufficient to produce a low nuclear–cytoplasm ratio [1, 9, 17]. The cytoplasm of the oncocytes in oncocytic adenomas (Hürthle cell adenomas) and oncocytic carcinoma of the thyroid gland (Hürthle cell carcinomas) is characterized by an eosinophilic granular nature, which is commonly due to the oncocytes' high content of mitochondria [17]. On Romanowsky stain, the cytoplasm is blue or gray, while on Papanicolaou stain, the cytoplasm can have varying hues, including blue, green, or orange [30, 31, 34].

In 2008, Montone et al. [19] stated that not all oncocytic cells in the thyroid are "true" Hürthle cells and that there is overinterpretation of oncocytic thyroid follicular cells as Hürthle cells in both cytological and histological specimens. Because historically some authors have indicated that all Hürthle cell nodules were potentially malignant, diagnosing or even mentioning these cells in a fine-needle aspiration biopsy (FNAB) report can lead to overreaction by clinicians and excess referrals for surgical excision; the oncocytic follicular cell contains eosinophilic (usually nongranular) cytoplasm and is slightly larger than a normal follicular epithelial cell. These cells commonly occur in nodular goiters and dominant adenomatous or hyperplastic nodules. The authors added that the presence of these cells should *not* engender a diagnosis of an oncocytic/Hürthle cell lesion [19].

3.3.2 Impact of Trauma on Histological Appearance

Trauma as that induced by fine-needle aspiration biopsy (FNAB), especially with associated hemorrhage, can lead to rapid degenerative changes in oncocytic/Hürthle cell lesions, including cystification with papillary architecture, diffuse necrosis, hyalinization, and ossification. These processes that may be triggered following needle biopsy or even palpation can lead to challenges in diagnosis and suggest an extreme sensitivity to tumor hypoxia or other consequences of vasculature interruption. Nuclei may lose their typical appearance and adopt nuclear membrane irregularities, including some clearing and loss of the prominent nucleolus for smaller chromocenters. Oncocytic (Hürthle) cells are known to have occasional intranuclear pseudo-inclusions. Papillary cystic degenerative changes, plus or minus any of the other above changes, could certainly lead to a misdiagnosis of papillary thyroid carcinoma (PTC) [23].

Lack of fibrovascular cores or association of other features of traumatic/degenerative change, including necrosis, hemosiderin deposition, or hyalinization should trigger ancillary testing, including a *BRAF* immunohistochemical stain or molecular testing in particularly challenging/borderline cases. Additional hypoxia-related reactive changes can lead to nearly complete hyalinization or ossification of nodules, in some cases with osseous metaplasia with extramedullary hematopoiesis. Small foci of residual oncocytic (Hürthle) cells may be present, but they may have associated atypia that raise the possibility of oncocytic variant PTC, and again, may trigger immunohistochemical/molecular workup depending upon the size and context of the lesion [23].

Posttraumatic peripheral architectural abnormalities may also be noted especially in tumors with thicker capsules and include intracapsular "coarse" or "eggshell" calcifications, which can push growth of the tumor into the capsule or cause intra-tumoral fibrosis giving the false impression of invasion (pseudo-invasion) [23].

Care should be taken to not overinterpret lesions with fibrosis without overt invasion through the capsule into adjacent parenchyma, trans-capsular invasion. Even in cases with trans-capsular invasion, if linear, consideration to fine needle aspiration site-related changes needs to be considered, especially if linear hemosiderin deposition is noted [23].

3.4 Electron Microscopy

Ultrastructurally, some of oncocytic (Hürthle) cells can be seen containing up to 5000 mitochondria of varying size and shape, whereas a typical eosinophil may contain approximately only 30. Such a huge number of mitochondria fills the cytoplasm to the point of nearly excluding other organelles [30, 31, 34–36]. The mitochondria often show filamentous inclusions, as well as dense core granules under electron microscopy [30, 31, 34–36].

References

1. Wakely PE Jr. Oncocytic and oncocyte-like lesions of the head and neck. Ann Diagn Pathol. 2008;12(3):222–30.
2. Kontaxis A, Zanarotti U, Kainz J, Beham A. Die diffuse Onkozytose der Glandula Parotidea. Laryngo-Rhino-Otologie. 2004;83(03):185–8.
3. Prabakaran SS, Chen F, Aguirre A. Oncocytoma of the parotid gland and its mimickers: a comprehensive review. N Am J Med Sci. 2010;3:171–80.
4. Mete O, Asa SL. Oncocytes, oxyphils, Hurthle, and Ashkanazy cells: morphological and molecular features of oncocytic thyroid nodules. Endocr Pathol. 2010;21(1):16–24.
5. Langhans T. Uber die Epithelialen formen der malignen Struma. Virchows Arch (Pathol Anat). 1907;189:69–152.
6. Ewing J. Neoplastic diseases: a textbook on tumors. Philadelphia: WB Saunders Company; 1919.
7. DeMay RM. Chapter 12: thyroid gland. In: DeMay RM, editor. The art and science of cytopathology, vol. 2. 2nd ed. Hong Kong: ASCP Press; 2012. p. 863–915.
8. Tallini G, Carcangiu ML, Rosai J. Oncocytic neoplasms of the thyroid gland. Acta Pathol Jpn. 1992;42:305–15.
9. McLeod MK, Thompson NW. Hürthle cell neoplasms of the thyroid. Otolaryngol Clin N Am. 1990;23:441–52.
10. Caturegli P, Ruggere C. Karl Hürthle? Now, who was he? Thyroid. 2005;15:121–3.
11. Kauffman PR, Dejax C, de Latour M, Dauplat J. The meaning and predictivity of Hürthle cells in fine needle aspiration cytology for thyroid nodular disease. Eur J Surg Oncol. 2004;30:786–9.

12. Jaffe RH. Adenolymphoma (oncocytoma) of parotid gland. Am J Cancer. 1932;16:1415–23.
13. Hamperl H. Uber das Vorkommen von Onkocyten in verschienden Organen und ihren Geschwulsten. Virchows Arch (Pathol Anat). 1936;298:327–75.
14. Chang A, Harawi SJ. Oncocytes, oncocytosis, and oncocytic tumors. Pathol Annu. 1992;27:263–304.
15. Jaffe RH. Adenolymphoma (onkocytoma) of parotid gland. Am J Cancer. 1932;16:1415–23.
16. Nappi O, Ferrera G, Wick MR. Neoplasms composed of eosinophilic polygonal cells: an overview with consideration of different cytomorphologic patterns. Semin Diagn Pathol. 1999;16:82–90.
17. Schwab M. Encyclopedia of cancer. Berlin/Heidelberg (Germany)/New York: Springer-Verlag; 2011.
18. Asa SL. My approach to oncocytic tumours of the thyroid. J Clin Pathol. 2004;57:225–32.
19. Montone KT, Baloch ZW, LiVolsi VA. The thyroid Hurthle (oncocytic) cell and its associated pathologic conditions: a surgical pathology and cytopathology review. Arch Pathol Lab Med. 2008;132(8):1241–50.
20. Hurthle K. BeitrÃgezurKenntniss des Secretionsvorgangs in der. SchilddrÃse Pflugers Arch Physiol. 1894;56:10–44.
21. Ashkanazy M. Pathologisch-anatomischeBeitr ÃgezurKenntniss des. MorbusBasedowii, insbesondere Ãmber die dabeiauftretende Muskelerkrankung. Dtsch Arch Klin Med. 1898;61:118–86.
22. Baloch ZW, Asa SL, Barletta JA, Ghossein RA, Juhlin CC, Jung CK, et al. Overview of the 2022 WHO classification of thyroid neoplasms. Endocr Pathol. 2022;33(1):27–63.
23. McFadden DG, Sadow PM. Genetics, diagnosis, and Management of Hürthle Cell Thyroid Neoplasms. Front Endocrinol (Lausanne). 2021;12:69638.
24. Johnson TL, Lloyd RV, Burney RE, Thompson NW. Hurthle cell thyroid tumors. An Immunohistochemical study. Cancer. 1987;59(1):107–12.
25. Chen H, Udelsman R. Chapter 14: Hürthle cell adenoma and carcinoma. In: Kebebew OHC-YD, editor. Textbook of endocrine surgery. 2nd ed. Philadelphia: WB Saunders; 2005. p. 123–8.
26. Evans HL, Vassilopoulou-Sellin R. Follicular and Hurthle cell carcinomas of the thyroid: a comparative study. Am J Surg Pathol. 1998;22(12):1512–20.
27. Sanders LE, Silverman M. Follicular and Hürthle cell carcinoma: predicting outcome and directing therapy. Surgery. 1998;124(6):967–74.
28. Masood S, Auguste L-J, Westerband A, Elluco C, Valderama E, Attie J. Differential oncogenic expression in thyroid follicular and Hürthle cell carcinomas. Am J Surg. 1993;166(4):366–8.
29. Stankov K, Romeo G. Oxyphilic carcinoma of the thyroid gland. Arch Oncol. 2003;11(2):81–9.
30. Nesland JM, Sobrinho-Simões MA, Holm R, Sambade MC, Johannessen JV. Hürthle-cell lesions of the thyroid: a combined study using transmission electron microscopy, scanning electron microscopy, and immunocytochemistry. Ultrastruct Pathol. 1985;8:269–90.
31. Sobrinho-Simões MA, Nesland JM, Holm R, Sambade MC, Johannessen JV. Hürthle cell and mitochondrion-rich papillary carcinomas of the thyroid gland: an ultrastructural and immunocytochemical study. Ultrastruct Pathol. 1985;8:131–42.
32. Cameselle-Teijeiro J, Ferreira R, Carames N, Abdulkader I, Máximo V, Soares P, et al. Absence of the BRAF and the GRIM-19 mutations in Oncocytic (Hurthle cell) solid cell nests of the thyroid. Am J Clin Pathol. 2012;137(4):612–8.
33. Cannon J. The significance of Hurthle cells in thyroid disease. Oncologist. 2011;16(10):1380–7.
34. Satoh M, Yagawa K. Electron microscopic study on mitochondria in Hürthle cell adenoma of thyroid. Pathol Int. 1981;31:1079–87.
35. Matias C, Nunes JF, Sobrinho LG, Soares J. Giant mitochondria and intramitochondrial inclusions in benign thyroid lesions. Ultrastruct Pathol. 1991;15(3):221–9.
36. Máximo V, Sobrinho-Simões M. Hürthle cell tumours of the thyroid. A review with emphasis on mitochondrial abnormalities with clinical relevance. Virchows Arch. 2000;437(2):107–15.

4 Oncocytic (Hürthle Cell) Lesions: Controversy of Pathogenesis, Biology, and Clinical Behavior

4.1 Controversy of Pathogenesis

The mechanism behind mitochondrial abundance in oncocytic (Hürthle cell) lesions is *not* completely understood; however, it is likely a reflection of excessive mitochondrial proliferation and/or decreased mitochondrial degradation (mitophagy) [1]. Such changes are reported to be a result of mutations in the mitochondrial DNA (mtDNA) encoding for mitochondrial enzymes, leading to proliferation through stimulation of transcription factors encoded by the nucleus [1–3]. Mitochondrial DNA (mtDNA) alterations were reported by several investigators to include point mutations and large deletions, which were initially detected in early molecular studies of oncocytic/Hürthle cell neoplasms [4–7]. Some authors have identified these mutations as deletions in the mtDNA of oncocytic (Hürthle) cells found in thyroid neoplasms [1]. Interestingly, defects in cytochrome C oxidase (complex IV, the terminal enzyme of the respiratory electron transport chain) and mtDNA deletions have also been associated with oncocytic/Hürthle cell change in chronic lymphocytic thyroiditis (Hashimoto's thyroiditis) [8] and in nonneoplastic thyroid parenchyma with variable oncocytic/Hürthle cell change [4]. These mitochondrial alterations are thought to result in impaired oxidative phosphorylation and ATP synthesis, which may induce a compensatory proliferation of mitochondria [4, 7, 9].

Although specific alterations in nuclear DNA also occur in Hürthle cell neoplasms, they are less frequent than in other follicular cell–derived neoplasms. *RAS* mutations, which are present in 40–50% of follicular thyroid carcinomas (FTCs) [10–12], are found in only 10–15% of oncocytic carcinomas of the thyroid (Hürthle cell carcinomas—HCCs) [13–15]. In addition, *PAX8-PPARγ* rearrangements, which are identified in nearly 33% of FTCs and are frequent in other follicular-patterned tumors [12, 16], appear to be absent in HCCs [14]. *BRAF* V600E mutation, the most common alteration in classic papillary thyroid carcinoma (PTC) [17], is similarly absent in Hürthle cell neoplasms [14, 15]. Widespread loss of heterozygosity by haploidy has instead been demonstrated as a common feature of HCC in two recent

M. Sakr, *Oncocytic (Hürthle Cell) Thyroid Lesions*,
https://doi.org/10.1007/978-3-032-03115-0_4

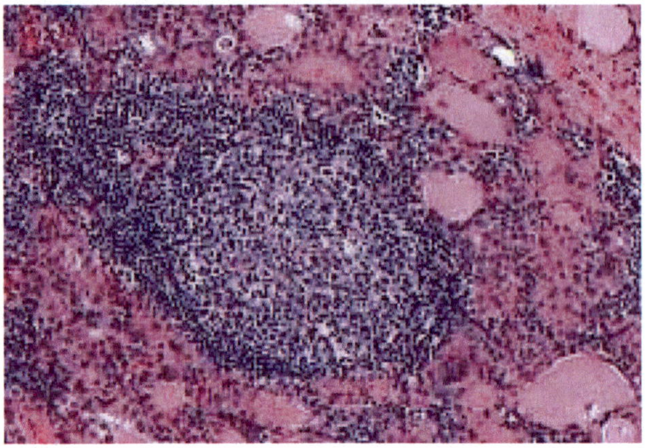

Fig. 4.1 Prominent oncocytic change in chronic lymphocytic thyroiditis. Abundant lymphocytes with germinal center formation are present. H&E × 10

studies by Ganly et al. (2018) [15] and Agrawal et al. (2014) [17]. Ganly et al. [2018) [15] also observed that the near-haploid genome of a subset of tumors, especially those that were widely invasive or clinically aggressive, underwent whole genome duplication, resulting in polysomy or a complex genotype as evidenced by the presence of uniparental disomy. These wide-scale chromosomal changes were absent in *RAS*-mutant tumors, which only occurred with a diploid phenotype.

The recent studies by Ganly et al. (2018) [15] and Gopal et al. (2018) [18] also demonstrated a high rate of mtDNA mutations affecting complex-I subunits of the electron transport chain, consistent with the findings of a previous study by Gasparre et al. (2007) [6]. Although not detected in all HCC, mtDNA mutations were more frequently seen in HCC compared to other cancers [19]. When present, they were found in the majority of tumor mitochondria and were maintained in metastatic sites, suggesting that mtDNA mutations are oncogenic drivers in HCC [19]. Given this association of mtDNA mutations and the widespread chromosomal loss in many HCCs, these tumors appear to be biologically distinct from PTC and FTC.

In the thyroid gland, oncocytic changes are associated with such benign conditions as cell-mediated autoimmune thyroiditis (Hashimoto's disease) (Fig. 4.1), humoral-mediated hyperthyroidism (Graves' disease), and hyperplastic nodules seen in multinodular goiters (MNG). Focal oncocytic trans-differentiation results in neoplasia consisting predominantly of oncocytic (Hürthle) cells that can represent benign oncocytic adenomas (Hürthle cell adenomas) or oncocytic carcinoma of the thyroid (Hürthle cell carcinoma).

4.2 Controversy of Biological Behavior

It was originally believed that the oncocytic (Hürthle) cell is a result of senescent change within the thyroid follicular epithelial cell especially because Hürthle cells are more commonly seen in older individuals; however, that original concept cannot be any further from the truth. Biologically, oncocytic/Hürthle cells appear to be less active than typical follicular cells, demonstrating lower levels of thyroglobulin (Tg) production, and HCCs have been shown to have markedly lower iodine uptake than their follicular counterparts. HCCs do, however, contain high levels of oxidative enzymes [5, 17]. A functional thyroid-stimulating hormone receptor-adenylate cyclase system has been demonstrated in the benign oncocytic adenoma (Hürthle cell adenoma) [20].

The process of mitochondria accumulation in the cytosol of follicular epithelial cells does not occur rapidly. It is believed to occur slowly over time, which explains why Hürthle cells are rarely seen in nonneoplastic and neoplastic lesions in children [11]. In addition, accumulations would be most evident in cells with a low turnover rate such as follicular epithelial cells. Rapidly dividing cells would prevent the accumulation of mitochondria.

Behaviorally, although has been long listed as a subgroup of follicular thyroid carcinoma (FTC) and was classified as such by the World Health Organization (WHO) in 2012 [21], oncocytic/Hürthle cell carcinomas (HCCs) were morphologically, behaviorally, and genetically distinct. For example, FTCs are well known to metastasize in a manner unique to their architecture and morphology, avoiding lymphatic spread and localized neck disease and, instead, favoring more insidious metastatic patterns via a hematogenous route to distant sites, including lungs, bone, and brain [22, 23], whereas papillary thyroid carcinomas (PTCs) are more likely to present, in advanced cases, with localized neck disease with lymph node (LN) metastases [24]. Oncocytic/Hürthle cell carcinomas also follow a lesion-specific pattern of metastasis, employing the aggressive components of both FTCs and PTCs, with advanced disease consisting of both LN metastases to the central and lateral neck, along with vascular spread to distant tissue sites [25]. Differences between oncocytic (Hürthle cell) neoplasms and follicular neoplasms are summarized in Table 4.1.

Table 4.1 Oncocytic (Hürthle cell) neoplasms versus follicular neoplasms

Criteria	Oncocytic (Hürthle cell) neoplasms	Follicular neoplasm
Cellular appearance	Large, polygonal	Small, rounded
Cytoplasm	Eosinophilic, finely granular, low nuclear/cytoplasm ratio	Coarsely granular or nongranular, pale, may be scanty
Mitochondria	Highly dense (up to 5000/cell)	Low to moderate density
Nucleus	Enlarged, hyperchromatic, prominent nucleolus	Round to oval in shape, nucleolus not prominent
Thyroglobulin (Tg)	Lower level (+)	Higher level (++ or +++)
Iodine avidity	Poor (~ 5%)	Good (~ 75%)
Risk of malignancy	15–65%	15–30%
Route of metastasis	Lymphatic/hematogenous	Hematogenous
Prognosis (cancer)	Overall SR similar to FTC, risk factors: Gender, old age, tumor size	10-year SR 85%

SR survival rare, *FTC* follicular thyroid cancer

4.3 Controversy of Clinical Significance

The clinical significance of oncocytic change in thyroid tumors is controversial. Oncocytic thyroid tumors have historically been perceived as carrying a higher risk of malignancy, and in case of malignancy, to carry a worse prognosis than their conventional counterparts [26]. More recent evidence suggests that oncocytic thyroid neoplasms are *not* more aggressive than usual variants [1, 27].

The World Health Organization (WHO) prefers the term "oncocytic" or "oncocyte" to "Hürthle cell" [28]. Oncocytic variants of papillary thyroid cancer (PTC) and follicular thyroid cancer (FTC) have the typical molecular features of their conventional counterparts and, stage for stage, have similar prognoses [1, 3]. They do, however, demonstrate a lesser ability to concentrate iodine and thus are less responsive to radioactive iodine therapy. The WHO has previously classified Hürthle cell adenoma (HCA) and Hürthle cell carcinoma (HCC) as oncocytic variants of follicular adenoma and follicular cell carcinoma, respectively. Despite this, HCC is considered by many to be a distinctly separate entity by virtue of its distinct genetic profile and clinically more aggressive behavior when compared with PTC and FTC [26, 29, 30].

More recently, the fifth edition of the WHO classification of thyroid tumors in 2022, has used the term "oncocytic cells" instead of the famous misnomer "Hürthle cells" and classified oncocytic carcinoma of the thyroid gland (previously called Hürthle cell carcinoma) as a separate entity of differentiated thyroid cancer (DTC) and not a subvariety of follicular thyroid carcinoma (FTC) [31].

References

1. Schwab M. Encyclopedia of cancer. Berlin/Heidelberg (Germany)/New York: Springer; 2011.
2. Asa SL. My approach to oncocytic tumours of the thyroid. J Clin Pathol. 2004;57:225–32.
3. Tsybrovskyy O, Rößmann-Tsybrovskyy M. Oncocytic versus mitochondrion-rich follicular thyroid tumors: should we make a difference? Histopathology. 2009;55:665–82.
4. Máximo V, Sobrinho-Simões M. Mitochondrial DNA "common" deletion in Hürthle cell lesions of the thyroid. J Pathol. 2000;192:561–2.
5. Máximo V, Soares P, Lima J, Cameselle-Teijeiro J, Sobrinho-Simões M. Mitochondrial DNA somatic mutations (point mutations and large deletions) and mitochondrial DNA variants in human thyroid pathology: a study with emphasis on Hürthle cell tumors. Am J Pathol. 2002;160:1857–65.
6. Gasparre G, Porcelli AM, Bonora E, Pennisi LF, Toller M, Iommarini L, et al. Disruptive mitochondrial DNA mutations in complex I subunits are markers of oncocytic phenotype in thyroid tumors. Proc Natl Acad Sci USA. 2007;104:9001–6.
7. Bonora E, Porcelli AM, Gasparre G, Biondi A, Ghelli A, Carelli V, et al. Defective oxidative phosphorylation in thyroid oncocytic carcinoma is associated with pathogenic mitochondrial DNA mutations affecting complexes I and III. Cancer Res. 2006;66:6087–96.
8. Müller-Höcker J, Jacob U, Seibel P. Hashimoto thyreoiditis is associated with defects of cytochrome-c oxidase in oxyphil askanazy cells and with the common deletion (4,977) of mitochondrial DNA. Ultrastruct Pathol. 1998;22:91–100.

9. Mete O, Asa SL. Oncocytes, oxyphils, Hürthle, and Askanazy cells: morphological and molecular features of oncocytic thyroid nodules. Endocr Pathol. 2010;21:16–24.
10. Esapa CT, Johnson SJ, Kendall-Taylor P, Lennard TWJ, Harris PE. Prevalence of Ras mutations in thyroid neoplasia. Clin Endocrinol. 1999;50:529–35.
11. Jeong SH, Hong HS, Kwak JJ, Lee EH. Analysis of RAS mutation and PAX8/PPARγ rearrangements in follicular-derived thyroid neoplasms in a Korean population: frequency and ultrasound findings. J Endocrinol Investig. 2015;38:849–57.
12. Nikiforova MN, Lynch RA, Biddinger PW, Alexander EK, Dorn GW 2nd, Tallini G, et al. RAS point mutations and PAX8-PPARγ rearrangement in thyroid tumors: evidence for distinct molecular pathways in thyroid follicular carcinoma. J Clin Endocrinol Metab. 2003;88:2318–26.
13. Tallini G, Hsueh A, Liu S, Garcia-Rostan G, Speicher MR, Ward DC. Frequent chromosomal DNA unbalance in thyroid oncocytic (Hürthle cell) neoplasms detected by comparative genomic hybridization. Lab Investig. 1999;79:547–55.
14. Ganly I, Filho JR, Eng S, Ghossein R, Morris LG, Liang Y, et al. Genomic dissection of hurthle cell carcinoma reveals a unique class of thyroid malignancy. J Clin Endocrinol Metab. 2013;98:962–72.
15. Ganly I, Makarov V, Deraje S, Dong Y, Reznik E, Seshan V, et al. Integrated genomic analysis of Hürthle cell cancer reveals oncogenic drivers, recurrent mitochondrial mutations, and unique chromosomal landscapes. Cancer Cell. 2018;34(256):e5–270.e5.
16. Armstrong MJ, Yang H, Yip L, Ohori NP, McCoy KL, Stang MT, et al. PAX8/PPARγ rearrangement in thyroid nodules predicts follicular-pattern carcinomas, in particular the encapsulated follicular variant of papillary carcinoma. Thyroid. 2014;24:1369–74.
17. Agrawal N, Akbani R, Aksoy BA, Ally A, Arachchi H, Sylvia L, et al. Integrated genomic characterization of papillary thyroid carcinoma. Cell. 2014;159:676–90.
18. Gopal RK, Kübler K, Calvo SE, Olak P, Livitz D, Rosebrock D, et al. Widespread chromosomal losses and mitochondrial DNA alterations as genetic drivers in Hürthle cell carcinoma. Cancer Cell. 2018;34(242):e5–255.e5.
19. Ganly I, McFadden DG. Short review: genomic alterations in Hürthle cell carcinoma. Thyroid. 2019;29:471–9.
20. McLeod MK, Thompson NW. Hürthle cell neoplasms of the thyroid. Otolaryngol Clin N Am. 1990;23:441–52.
21. Nikiforov YE, Biddinger PW, Thompson LDR. Diagnostic pathology and molecular genetics of the thyroid: a comprehensive guide for practicing thyroid pathology. Philadelphia: Wolters Kluwer Health; 2012.
22. Glomski K, Nose V, Faquin WC, Sadow PM. Metastatic follicular thyroid carcinoma and the primary thyroid gross examination: institutional review of cases from 1990 to 2015. Endocr Pathol. 2017;28:177–85.
23. Parameswaran R, Shulin HJ, Min En N, Tan WB, Yuan NK. Patterns of metastasis in follicular thyroid carcinoma and the difference between early and delayed presentation. Ann R Coll Surg Engl. 2017;99:151–4.
24. Kim SK, Park I, Hur N, Choe JH, Kim JH, Kim JS. Patterns, predictive factors and prognostic impact of multilevel metastasis in N1b papillary thyroid carcinoma. Br J Surg. 2017;104:857–67.
25. Jalaly JB, Baloch ZW. Hurthle-cell neoplasms of the thyroid: an algorithmic approach to pathologic diagnosis in light of molecular advances. Semin Diagn Pathol. 2020;37:234–42.
26. Rosai J, Kuhn E, Carcangiu ML. Pitfalls in thyroid tumour pathology. Histopathology. 2006;49(2):107–20.
27. Carcangiu ML, Bianchi S, Savino D, Voynick IM, Rosai J. Follicular Hürthle cell tumors of the thyroid gland. Cancer. 1991;68:1994–53.
28. Sobrinho-Simones M, Maximo V, Castro IV, Fonseca E, Soares P, Garcia-Rostan G, et al. Hürthle (oncocytic) cell tumors of thyroid: Etiopathogenesis, diagnosis and clinical significance. Int J Surg Pathol. 2005;13:29–35.

29. Baloch ZW, LiVolsi VA, Asa SL, Rosai J, Merino MJ, Randolph G, et al. Diagnostic terminology and morphologic criteria for cytologic diagnosis of thyroid lesions: a synopsis of the National Cancer Institute thyroid fine-needle aspiration state of the science conference. Diagn Cytopathol. 2008;36:425–37.
30. Giorgadze T, Rossi ED, Fadda G, Gupta PK, LiVolsi VA, Baloch Z, et al. Does fine-needle aspiration diagnosis of "Hürthle-cell neoplasm/follicular neoplasm with oncocytic features" denote increased risk of malignancy? Diagn Cytopathol. 2004;31:307–12.
31. Baloch ZW, Asa SL, Barletta JA, Ghossein RA, Juhlin CC, Jung CK, et al. Overview of the 2022 WHO classification of thyroid neoplasms. Endocr Pathol. 2022;33(1):27–63.

5 Oncocytic (Hürthle Cell) Lesions: Controversy of Oncocytic (Hürthle) Cells in Cytology

5.1 Bethesda System for Reporting Thyroid Cytopathology

5.1.1 Introduction

The third edition (2023) of "The Thyroid Bethesda System for Reporting Thyroid Cytopathology (TBSRTC)" [1] offers several key updates of the two earlier editions. The most important is the assignment of a single name for each of the six diagnostic categories based on fine-needle aspiration cytology (FNAC): (I) nondiagnostic, (II) benign, (III) atypia of undetermined significance (AUS), (IV) follicular neoplasm, (V) suspicious for malignancy, and (VI) malignant (Table 5.1). This resolves the confusion resulting from the prior editions, which assigned alternative names for three of the diagnostic categories. Thus, TBRSTC 2023, discontinued the previously used terms of "unsatisfactory," "follicular lesion of undetermined significance (FLUS)," and "suspicious for a follicular neoplasm."

Nomenclature has been updated to align with the 2022 World Health Organization (WHO) Classification of Thyroid Neoplasms. Two new chapters have been added: one that addresses the significant and expanded use of molecular and ancillary testing in thyroid cytopathology, and another that summarizes clinical perspectives and imaging findings in thyroid disease.

5.1.2 Risk of Malignancy (ROM) in Adults

Each of the six categories of TBSRTC 2023 has an implied risk of malignancy (ROM), which has been updated and refined (Table 5.2). The AUS subcategorization has been simplified into two subgroups based on the implied ROM and molecular profiling. Each reporting category has an updated and management algorithm revised, as recommended by the ATA and other professional endocrine organizations.

M. Sakr, *Oncocytic (Hürthle Cell) Thyroid Lesions*,
https://doi.org/10.1007/978-3-032-03115-0_5

Table 5.1 Diagnostic categories of The 2023 bethesda system for reporting thyroid cytopathology

Category	Category name	Description
I	Nondiagnostic	Cyst fluid only Virtually acellular specimen Other (obscuring blood, clotting or drying artifact, etc.)
II	Benign	Follicular nodular disease Chronic lymphocytic (Hashimoto's) thyroiditis Granulomatous (subacute) thyroiditis
III	AUS	Specify if AUS-nuclear atypia or AUS-other
IV	Follicular neoplasm	Specify if oncocytic (formerly Hürthle cell) type
V	Suspicious for malignancy	Suspicious for PTC Suspicious for MTC Suspicious for metastatic carcinoma Suspicious for lymphoma Other
VI	Malignant	PTC High-grade follicular-derived thyroid carcinoma (known as poorly differentiated thyroid carcinoma" MTC Undifferentiated (anaplastic) carcinoma SCC Carcinoma with mixed features (specify) Metastatic malignancy NHL Other

AUS Atypia of unknown significance, *PTC* papillary thyroid carcinoma, *MTC* medullary thyroid carcinoma, *SCC* squamous cell carcinoma, *NHL* non-Hodgkin lymphoma

Table 5.2 TBSRTC 2023: Risk of malignancy (ROM) and recommended management

Diagnostic category	ROM mean % (range)	Recommended management
Nondiagnostic	13% (5–20)	Repeat FNA with US guidance
Benign	4% (2–7)	Clinical and US follow-up
Atypia of unknown significance (AUS)	22% (13–30)	Repeat FNA, molecular testing, diagnostic lobectomy, or surveillance
Follicular neoplasm	30% (23–34)	Molecular testing, diagnostic lobectomy
Suspicious for malignancy	74% (67–83)	Molecular testing, lobectomy or near-total/total thyroidectomy (TT)
Malignant	97% (97–100)	Lobectomy or near-total/TT

ROM risk of malignancy, *FNA* fine-needle aspiration, *US* ultrasound, *TT* total thyroidectomy

5.1.3 Risk of Malignancy (ROM) in Children

A discussion of pediatric thyroid disease has been added to the TBSRTC 2023, and pediatric ROMs, and management algorithms for this age groups were provided according to the commonly practiced guidelines [2, 3] (Table 5.3).

Table 5.3 TBSRTC 2023: Risk of malignancy (ROM) and recommended management in pediatric patients

Diagnostic category	ROM mean (range)	Recommended management
Nondiagnostic	14% (0–33)	Repeat FNA with US guidance
Benign	6% (0–27)	Clinical and US follow-up
Atypia of unknown significance (AUS)	28% (11–54)	Repeat FNA or surgical resection
Follicular neoplasm	50% (28–100)	Surgical resection
Suspicious for malignancy	81% (40–100)	Surgical resection
Malignant	98% (86–100)	Surgical resection

ROM risk of malignancy, *FNA* fine-needle aspiration, *US* ultrasound

5.1.4 Format of the Report

The TBSRTC 2023 continued to recommend that the "names" of the categories (and not just their numerical designations) should be used for reporting results and publishing scientific articles to avoid confusion with the Thyroid Imaging and Reporting System (TIRADS) and other reporting systems that are primarily numeral based. Adding a category "number" after the category name is an acceptable, optional practice (e.g., benign [Bethesda II], atypia of unknown significance [Bethesda III], etc.) [1]. For several reporting categories, some degree of subcategorization is recommended that further clarifies the FNA diagnosis, such as "suspicious for malignancy [SFM] (Bethesda V)—suspicious for papillary thyroid carcinoma." In addition, the revised and updated range and average ROMs of each diagnostic category is provided by TBSRTC 2023.

5.1.5 Nondiagnostic Category (Bethesda I)

TBSRTC 2023 has discontinued the option of using the term "unsatisfactory" for the first category; henceforth, the sole term "nondiagnostic" is recommended. Every thyroid FNA should be evaluated for sample adequacy, which is defined by both the quantity and quality of the cellular (mostly follicular) and colloid components. Application of adequacy criteria ensures a low false-negative rate with fewer repeats, and more accurate interpretation of the FNA. Thus, for sample adequacy, TBSRTC 2023 continues to recommend a minimum of six groups of well-preserved, well-visualized follicular cells, with each group comprising ≥10 cells, for an adequate sample (quantity). Regarding the sample quality, thyroid FNA preparations should show cells that are well-preserved, well-stained, and easily visualized. Certain limiting factors such as abundant obscuring blood or extensive air-drying artifacts could be included in adequacy statements. Aspirates that consist of cyst fluid only with or without macrophages continue to be interpreted as nondiagnostic (Bethesda I) [1].

The ROM for a nondiagnostic FNA is difficult to calculate because most such nodules are not surgically resected. Among surgically excised nodules initially reported as nondiagnostic, the ROM is 5–20% (mean, 13%), which clearly over-represents the incidence of malignancy compared with the entire cohort of nondiagnostic nodules owing to selection bias [1].

A "repeat aspiration with ultrasound (US) guidance" is recommended for cytologically nondiagnostic nodules and will yield diagnostic results in 60–80% of cases, particularly in the nodules with a smaller cystic component [4]. Some studies have clearly depicted lower diagnostic yields if the "repeat FNA" is performed sooner than 3 months [5]. However, the previous approach of waiting for 3 months before a repeat FNA seems to be less crucial [6, 7]. Additionally, the American Thyroid Association (ATA) guidelines now state that there is no need to wait several months before repeating the FNA [8].

5.1.6 Benign Category (Bethesda II)

The success and clinical value of thyroid FNA centers on its ability to reliably identify benign thyroid nodules and, thus, avoid unnecessary surgical resection for most patients with nodular thyroid disease. A benign (Bethesda II) FNA diagnosis is associated with a very low ROM when these nodules undergo surgical resection (mean 4%, range 2–7%). Because relatively few nodules with a benign (Bethesda II) FNA will actually undergo surgery, the best overall ROM estimate based on long-term follow-up studies is approximately 1–2% [1].

In light of the 2022 WHO classification of thyroid tumors, the use of the term "follicular nodular disease" is preferred to refer to the spectrum of changes previously designated as colloid nodule, hyperplastic nodule, adenomatous nodule, or benign follicular nodule [9].

5.1.7 Atypia of Undetermined Significance (AUS) Category (Bethesda III)

TBSRTC 2023 discontinued the term "follicular lesion of undetermined significance—FLUS" to avoid confusion with reporting terminology and management; henceforth, the only term used is "atypia of unknown significance—AUS," which is one of the three "indeterminate" cytopathological interpretations that convey a diagnosis that is *not* definitively benign or malignant [1].

The AUS category (Bethesda III) is reserved for cases with atypia that is insufficient for either of the other two indeterminate categories of "follicular neoplasm—Bethesda IV" and "suspicious for malignancy—Bethesda V." Among the three indeterminate categories, AUS has the lowest ROM (mean 22%, range 20–32%). Specifically, AUS with nuclear atypia has a significantly higher ROM compared with AUS associated with other patterns, particularly those characterized by architectural atypia alone or a predominance of oncocytes [10, 11]. Similarly, AUS subclassification for pediatric patients might provide further risk stratification. Cherella et al. recently (2022) reported that nuclear atypia was associated with an ROM of 59% compared with 6.5% for architectural or oncocytic atypia [12].

In order to improve communication regarding the ROM between cytopathologists and clinicians, TBSRTC 2023 has introduced further simplification of the AUS subcategorization into two groups: "nuclear" (previously "cytologic"), which conveys a relatively higher ROM, and "other", which conveys a relatively lower risk. The latter includes cases with architectural atypia, oncocytic atypia, and lymphocytic atypia, among others. This two-tiered subclassification is also supported partly by molecular studies performed on AUS cases clearly delineating the "nuclear" from the "other" subgroup [13].

5.1.8 Follicular Neoplasm Category (Bethesda IV)

To ensure clear and unambiguous communication, TBSRTC 2023 recommended discontinuing the use of the term "suspicious for a follicular neoplasm," given the potential confusion of this category with a different category that also incorporated "suspicious" in the title ("suspicious for malignancy [Bethesda V]"). As such, only "follicular neoplasm" has been recommended to be used as the sole name for this category [1].

The diagnostic criteria proposed in the second edition are reaffirmed in this third edition. This category is intended for those aspirates that are at least moderately cellular and composed of follicular cells, most of which show significant architectural abnormality in the form of micro-follicles and/or crowding, trabeculae, or single cells. It is reiterated that follicular-patterned aspirates with only "mild nuclear" changes (mild degree of enlargement, contour irregularity, and/or chromatin clearing) are best classified as "follicular neoplasm" if true papillae are absent and intra-nuclear pseudo-inclusions are either absent or very rare. It is noteworthy that 30% of cases diagnosed as follicular neoplasm (Bethesda IV) on FNA turn out to be benign follicular nodular disease on surgical resection. Molecular testing results can be used to supplement the risk assessment in lieu of proceeding directly to surgery [14]. The recommended management of follicular neoplasm is surgical excision of the nodule, most often hemi-thyroidectomy or lobectomy.

Regarding the previous term "follicular neoplasm, Hürthle cell type," TBSRTC 2023 recommended "follicular neoplasm—oncocytic follicular neoplasm" to align with the 2022 WHO Classification of Thyroid Neoplasms. This diagnosis is associated with a significant ROM (range 25–50%). The criteria for this diagnosis are essentially unchanged from those described in the first two editions: a virtually exclusive population of oncocytes, usually scant to absent colloid, rare to absent background lymphocytes, and, often, with the presence of nuclear and cellular size variations. The differential diagnosis includes benign nodules with focal oncocytic hyperplasia and other neoplasms with oncocytic features, most importantly MTC and subtypes of PTC [1].

5.1.9 Suspicious for Malignancy (SFM) Category (Bethesda V)

The diagnostic category of suspicious for malignancy (SFM) (Bethesda V) is used when the cytomorphological features of a thyroid FNA are worrisome for PTC, MTC, lymphoma, or another malignant neoplasm, but are quantitatively and/or qualitatively insufficient for a definitive malignant (Bethesda VI) diagnosis [1]. This category is quite heterogeneous; however, most cases under SFM are classified as "suspicious for PTC." As the usual management is surgical (either lobectomy or near-TT/TT), the diagnosis of SFM should be used judicially. Some, but not all, of the cases in this category raise the possibility of a follicular variant of PTC.

5.1.10 Malignant Category (Bethesda VI)

The TBSRTC category "malignant (Bethesda VI)" is used whenever the cytomorphological features are conclusive for malignancy. The descriptive comments that follow are used to subclassify the malignancy [1]. The diagnostic morphological criteria of common thyroid malignancies have not changed. A few updates included in the 2023 edition are as follows:

- The term "PTC, variants" is now changed to "PTC, subtypes" in accordance with the WHO tumor classification recommendation to avoid confusion with the term "genetic variant(s)," which is based on the molecular classification.
- The previously recognized subtype of PTC, "cribriform morular variant" is now designated as a "separate" tumor entity.
- The new term "high-grade follicular-derived thyroid carcinoma" is now endorsed, which replaces the older nomenclature of "poorly differentiated thyroid carcinoma."

5.2 Oncocytic (Hürthle) Cell Cytology Categories: Overview

Given the broad spectrum of lesions that can demonstrate oncocytic (Hürthle) cell morphology, it is not surprising that oncocytic (Hürthle) cells are frequently encountered in thyroid fine-needle aspiration (FNA) and can pose diagnostic and hence therapeutic challenges to clinicians. Oncocytic/Hürthle cell–predominant FNA results most often fall into one of three diagnostic categories within The Bethesda System for Reporting Thyroid Cytopathology (TBSRTC), namely, benign (B-II), atypia of unknown (undetermined) significance [AUS] (B-III), and follicular neoplasm (B-IV) [15].

5.3 Cytological Features of Benign Disorders (B-II)

5.3.1 Oncocytic (Hürthle) Cell Change in Benign Thyroid Nodules

Oncocytic (Hürthle) cell change is commonly seen in multinodular hyperplasia, and Hürthle cells may be a predominant finding in FNA of benign thyroid nodules **[56]** and in some cases can demonstrate significant anisonucleosis [15]. However, if admixed with normal (non-Hürthle cell) macro-follicles and abundant colloid (Fig. 5.1), TBSRTC recommends that these nodules be diagnosed as benign (B-II) rather than AUS (B-III) or follicular neoplasm (B-IV). Similarly, if there is a spectrum of morphologies, including follicular cells with varying degrees of "Hürthle-oid" change, the FNA can likely be diagnosed as benign.

5.3.2 Hürthle Cells in Chronic Lymphocytic (Hashimoto's) Thyroiditis

A rather common pathology of benign thyroid nodules with extensive oncocytic/ Hürthle cell change is chronic lymphocytic thyroiditis (Hashimoto's thyroiditis) in which oncocytic (Hürthle) cells may be the predominant cell type, occurring in single

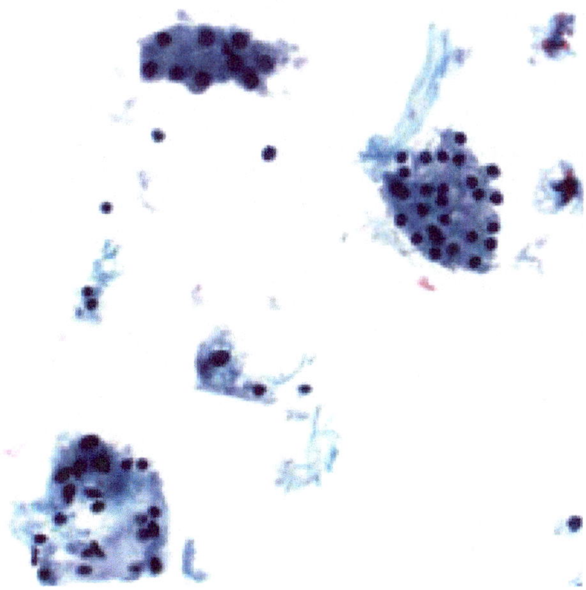

Fig. 5.1 Fine-needle aspirate of a thyroid nodule showing numerous Hürthle cells with abundant colloid and variability in follicular cells with macro-follicular architecture and a spectrum of Hürthle cell change, denoting a benign aspirate

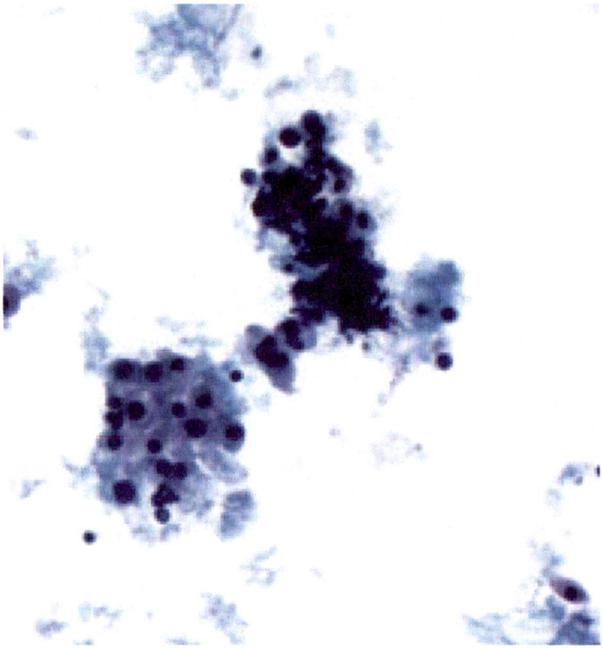

Fig. 5.2 Fine-needle aspirate of a thyroid lesion showing a predominance of Hürthle cells occurring in flat sheets. The scattered lymphocytic aggregates raise the possibility of chronic lymphocytic thyroiditis (Hashimoto's thyroiditis)

cells and sheets (Fig. 5.2). Nuclear atypia, including nuclear clearing and grooves, may be present and suggest PTC rather than oncocytic neoplasia or Hürthle cell neoplasia (HCN). Colloid is also often scant in Hashimoto's thyroiditis, which can further raise the possibility of neoplasia [15, 16]. A background of polymorphous lymphocytes, plasma cells, tingible body macrophages, and lympho-histiocytic aggregates, however, would be suggestive of chronic lymphocytic thyroiditis (Hashimoto's thyroiditis), although it would not necessarily exclude neoplasia/malignancy.

In cases with Hashimoto's thyroiditis where the degree of nuclear atypia is "mild/focal," a diagnosis of "benign" (B-II) may be more appropriate. Similarly, a benign diagnosis may be considered in oncocytic (Hürthle) cell–rich aspirates of Hashimoto's thyroiditis if normal macro-follicles are also present. However, aspirates composed entirely of Hürthle cells or with a less pronounced lymphoid component may warrant a diagnosis of AUS (B-III) or follicular neoplasm (B-IV).

In the absence of Hashimoto's thyroiditis, the situation of a pure population of cohesive flat sheets of oncocytic (Hürthle) cells with scant colloid is very challenging. Some pathologists may opt for AUS (B-III) or follicular neoplasm (B-IV) for such aspirates; however, in the absence of dysplasia, the risk of malignancy is low in such aspirates, and a benign diagnosis is an appropriate alternative, potentially with an explanatory note [15].

The rarity of oncocytic (Hürthle cell) carcinoma of the thyroid among "falsely negative" FNA [17–21] suggests that oncocytic/Hürthle cell–predominant nodules are *not* consistently underdiagnosed, and that the use of the "benign" category for such borderline aspirates is appropriate and hence warranted.

5.4 Cytological Features of Atypia with Unknown Significance (B-III)

The category of AUS (B-III) is heterogeneous and encompasses nodules with (1) architectural atypia (AUS-A), (2) cytological atypia (AUS-C), and (3) a predominance of oncocytic (Hürthle) cells (AUS-HC) [15]. Fine-needle aspirations (FNAs] that fall into the latter subcategory include "sparsely cellular aspirates with minimal colloid" composed exclusively or nearly exclusively of oncocytic (Hürthle) cells (Fig. 5.3).

It has also been suggested in TBSRTC that more cellular samples that would otherwise fulfill the criteria of follicular neoplasm (B-IV) in patients who clinically have chronic lymphatic (Hashimoto's) thyroiditis or multinodular goiter (MNG) could be "down-graded" to AUS (B-III). However, reports in the literature on whether this approach is justified are quite limited. Although some studies have raised the possibility that Hashimoto's thyroiditis may have a modest effect on risk of malignancy (ROM) in patients with Hürthle cell–predominant FNA, the differences in ROM did not reach statistical significance [22, 23]. Likewise, a difference in ROM was not seen in patients with MNG compared to those with solitary thyroid nodules (STNs) [23]. Jeong et al. (2015) reported that very limited available data raise the possibility that multiple oncocytic (Hürthle) cell nodules may represent a low-risk condition, but this observation needs further studies in a larger case series [23]. Generally, incorporation of the clinical findings into cytological diagnoses should thus be performed judiciously.

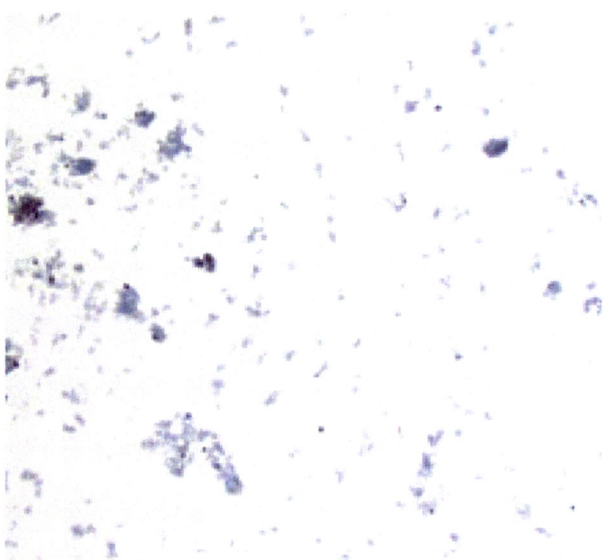

Fig. 5.3 Fine-needle aspirate of a thyroid lesion showing a sparsely cellular sample with nearly all groups consisting of Hürthle cells. A diagnosis of atypia of undetermined significance was therefore provided

5.5 Cytological Features in Follicular Neoplasm (B-IV)

Aspirates that fulfill the criteria of follicular neoplasm (B-IV) are "moderately-to-markedly" cellular samples that are composed exclusively or almost exclusively of oncocytic (Hürthle) cells, present singly (Fig. 5.4) and in clusters (Fig. 5.5). Colloid and lymphocytes are usually scant [15].

The distinction between oncocytic adenoma (Hürthle cell adenoma—HCA) and oncocytic carcinoma of the thyroid (Hürthle cell carcinoma—HCC) is typically deferred to histopathological examination. Although these criteria seem to be straightforward, there are several issues that arise in actual practice. In addition to the situation (mentioned above) of downgrading aspirates diagnosed as follicular neoplasm (B-IV) to AUS (B-III) in the setting of Hashimoto's thyroiditis or MNG, the concept of "atypia" or "dysplasia" required for a diagnosis of follicular neoplasm has generated some controversy.

According to TBSRTC, oncocytic (Hürthle) cells may exhibit two types of dysplasia: (1) small cell dysplasia (Fig. 5.6) or (2) large cell dysplasia (Fig. 5.7). In *small cell dysplasia*, oncocytic (Hürthle) cells are smaller, have less cytoplasm with higher nuclear to cytoplasmic ratios, and are often bland. In contrast, oncocytic (Hürthle) cells with *large cell dysplasia* have abundant cytoplasm and at least two-fold variability in nuclear size [15, 24]. Although many cytopathologists do not require dysplasia to be present to render a diagnosis of follicular neoplasm, a less conservative approach focusing on FNA diagnosis of oncocytic/HCC rather than oncocytic/Hürthle cell neoplasia (HCN) has been advocated by some authors [25] as some studies have reported that HCC almost never occurs in fine-needle aspirates without dysplasia [24, 26, 27].

Fig. 5.4 A cellular fine-needle aspirate of a thyroid lesion showing numerous Hürthle cells, within small clusters and dispersed as single cells. It is thus diagnosed as suspicious of a Hürthle cell neoplasm. Histopathological examination after resection proved to be a Hürthle cell adenoma (HCA)

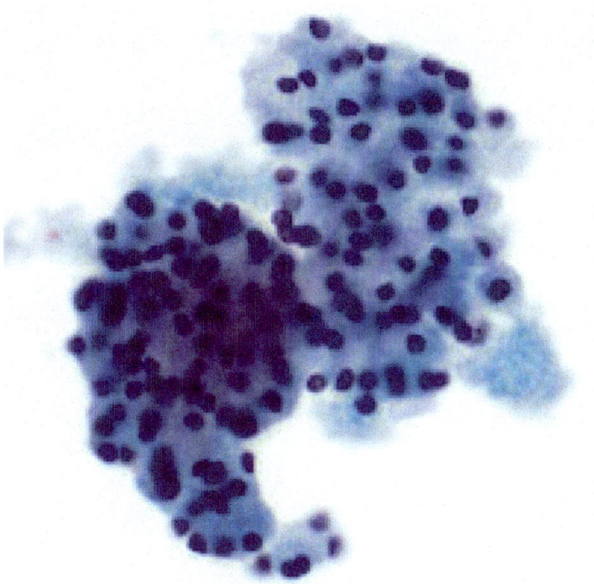

Fig. 5.5 Fine-needle aspirate of a thyroid lesion showing large aggregates (clusters) and syncytial groups of Hürthle. Histopathological examination after resection proved to be a minimally invasive Hürthle cell carcinoma (miHCC)

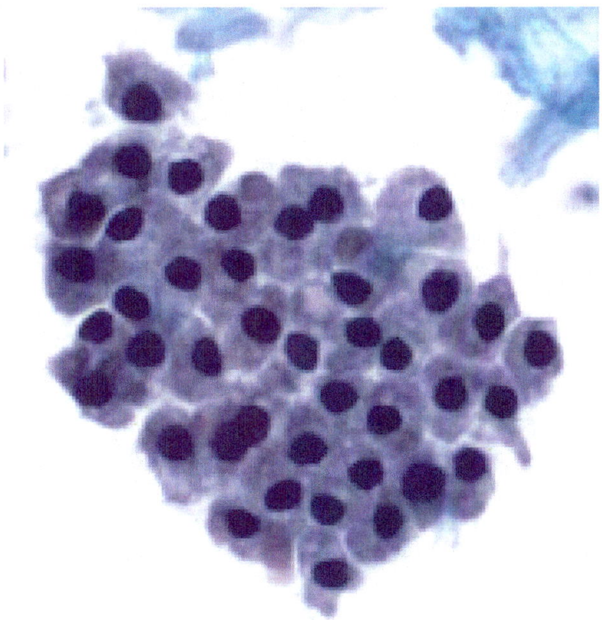

Fig. 5.6 A Hürthle cell–predominant fine-needle aspirate of a thyroid lesion showing small cell dysplasia; characterized by cells with less abundant cytoplasm and a higher nuclear-to-cytoplasmic ratio. Cells are often more uniform in appearance and can demonstrate crowding

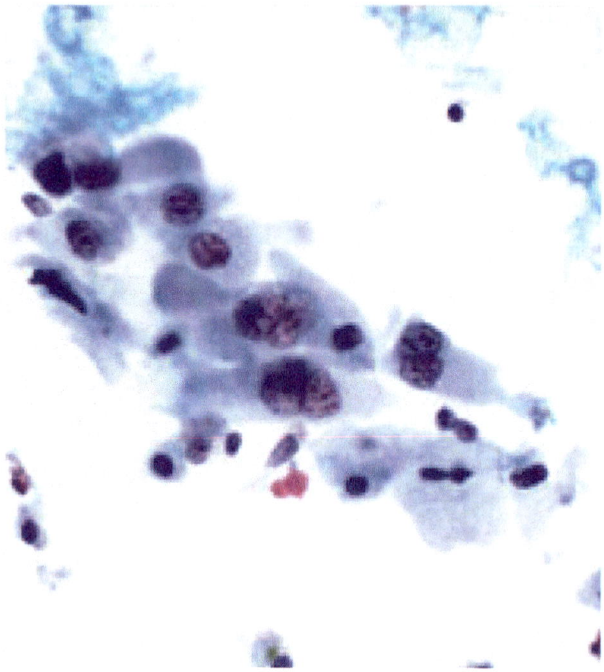

Fig. 5.7 A Hürthle cell–predominant fine-needle aspirate of a thyroid lesion showing cells with large cell dysplasia. Cells demonstrate abundant granular cytoplasm and at least twofold variability in nuclear size, often having prominent nucleoli and more irregular nuclear contours

5.6 Hürthle Cells in Other Pathologies

It is important to recognize other pathologies that may enter in the "differential diagnosis" of oncocytic/Hürthle cell lesions on FNA. These include parathyroid neoplasms, medullary thyroid carcinoma (MTC), non-Hürthle follicular neoplasms, and papillary thyroid carcinoma (PTC).

5.6.1 Neoplasms of the Parathyroid Gland

Differentiating parathyroid from thyroid lesions can be difficult on fine-needle aspiration (FNA) due to overlapping cytomorphological features as shown in Fig. 5.8, where FNA demonstrates clusters of epithelial cells with abundant cytoplasm and small, round, centrally located nuclei, reminiscent of oncocytic (Hürthle) cells. Correlation with clinical findings and imaging is needed to aid in reaching diagnosis. In addition, immunohistochemistry (IHC) for parathyroid hormone (PTH), thyroglobulin(Tg),andthyroidtranscriptionfactor-1(TTF-1)(ahomeodomain-containing nuclear transcription factor, which belongs to the Nkx2 gene family) and GATA-3 (a transcription factor that in humans is encoded by the GATA3 gene) can also be performed to confirm clinical suspicion and reach the final diagnosis.

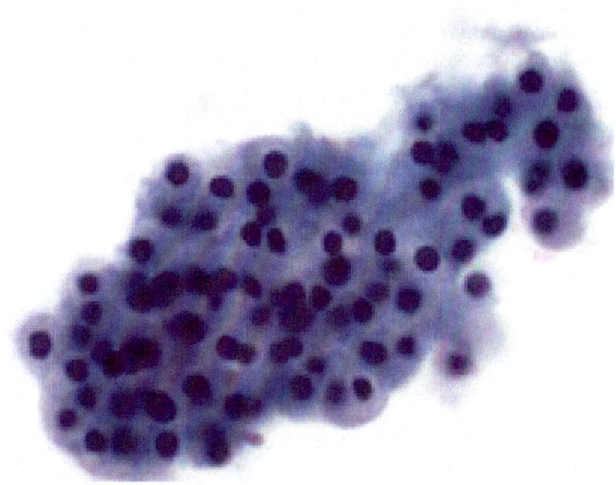

Fig. 5.8 Fine-needle aspirate showing cohesive clusters of epithelial cells with abundant cytoplasm and small, round, centrally located nuclei, reminiscent of Hürthle cells. Chemical analysis of the aspirate demonstrated a parathyroid hormone (PTH) of >3000 pg/mL. The overall findings were consistent with parathyroid tissue

While the traditional parathyroid hormone (PTH) assays can help in the distinction, these tests may be cumbersome, particularly when the lesion is unexpected clinically and a needle wash is not collected at the time of FNA. Application of immunohistochemical staining (IHC) with GATA-3 and TTF-1 on air-dried cytology smears can distinguish parathyroid and thyroid lesions. On air-dried touch preparation slides, GATA 3 expression is observed in all cases of parathyroid origin, but no immunoreactivity is present in thyroid lesions. Moreover, TTF-1 expression is observed in all cases of thyroid origin, but not in parathyroid lesions [28].

5.6.2 Medullary Thyroid Carcinoma (MTC)

Medullary thyroid carcinoma (MTC) can also mimic oncocytic/Hürthle cell tumors and appear on FNA as discohesive cells with moderate to abundant amounts of granular cytoplasm, particularly in the MTCs with epithelioid morphology, which can be especially challenging (Fig. 5.9).

It is well-recognized that MTC can demonstrate a greater variety of morphologies, ranging from plasmacytoid to more spindled cells. Red rather than blue cytoplasmic granules may be seen on Romanowsky stain in MTC [15]. Nuclear pseudo-inclusions may also be seen in MTC, whereas central nucleoli should be absent. Confirmatory IHC for calcitonin (Fig. 5.10) and thyroglobulin (Tg) should be used in challenging cases. Measurement of serum calcitonin levels is often helpful when cytological uncertainty cannot be resolved.

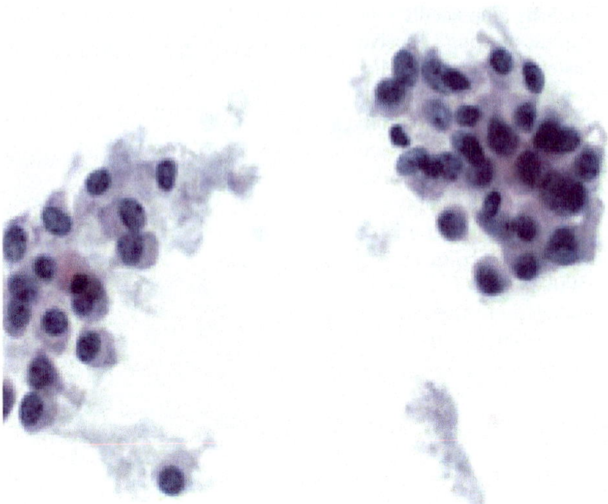

Fig. 5.9 Fine-needle aspirate of a thyroid nodule showing discohesive cells with moderate to abundant amounts of granular cytoplasm

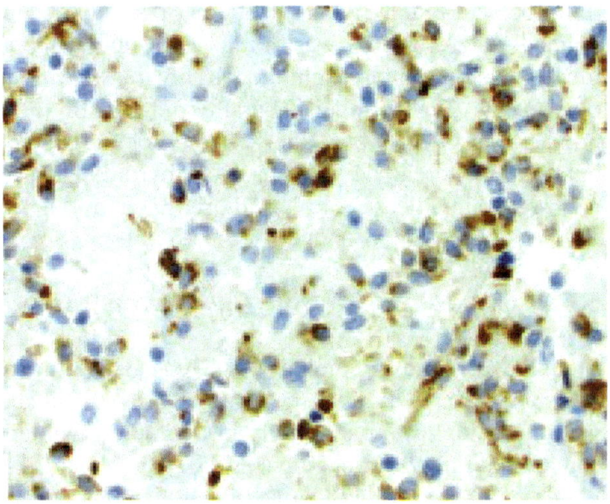

Fig. 5.10 Fine-needle aspirate of a thyroid nodule. Immunohistochemistry for calcitonin is diffusely positive

5.6.3 Non-Hürthle Follicular Cell–Derived Tumors

Non-Hürthle follicular cell–derived tumors of the thyroid gland may pose even greater diagnostic challenges, as IHC and clinical parameters are typically less helpful. Despite the characteristic cytomorphology that is associated with oncocytic/Hürthle cell neoplasms in contrast to non-Hürthle follicular neoplasms, a continuum of cytomorphology may be seen in practice [29].

Follicular-patterned tumors with variably increased amounts of clear to eosinophilic cytoplasm can sometimes be difficult to accurately classify on FNA or resection. If variable or partial (i.e., in <75% of cells) oncocytic/Hürthle cell change is seen on FNA, TBSRTC recommends a diagnosis of follicular neoplasm (B-IV), with a note indicating that some Hürthle cell differentiation is present [15]. To our knowledge, interobserver reproducibility for defining oncocytic (Hürthle) cell morphology has not been established in the literature. Although the clinical implications of this distinction may not necessarily be great, particularly for benign neoplasms, biological behavior and management may differ between oncocytic/HCC and FTC.

5.6.4 Papillary Thyroid Carcinoma (PTC)

Papillary thyroid carcinoma (PTC) can also mimic oncocytic/Hürthle cell lesions on FNA due to the increased amounts of eosinophilic cytoplasm often seen in PTC, including the classical type and its variants such as Warthin-like, tall-cell (Fig. 5.11), and oncocytic variants.

Several researchers reported that PTCs have been found in 25–44% of malignancies on resection of thyroid nodules diagnosed on FNA as follicular neoplasm (B-IV) [22], highlighting the challenges that can occur in interpreting nuclear atypia in oncocytic/Hürthle cell lesions. A potential helpful diagnostic feature of PTC is the heterogeneous morphology that frequently is present. Some or most of the tumor, for example, may have increased cytoplasm and variable or exaggerated nuclear atypia, but foci with more conventional PTC cytomorphology often are seen on both, resection and FNA [29].

Close attention to the characteristic nuclear features of PTC, particularly if cells with less prominent Hürthle-like cytomorphology are admixed, can help differentiate the two PTC from Hürthle cell neoplasms. Cell block preparation may also provide additional information on architecture and stroma that favors one diagnosis over another [29].

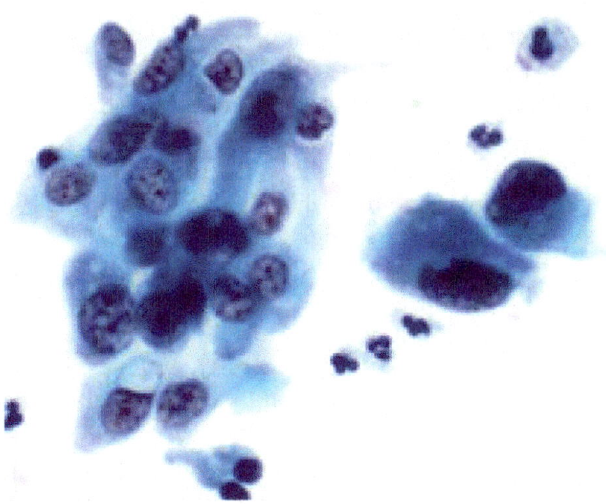

Fig. 5.11 Fine-needle aspirate of a thyroid nodule demonstrating many groups of cells showing abundant cytoplasm and nuclear atypia with variably elongated cells, reminiscent of the large cell dysplasia that may be seen in Hürthle cell lesions

As *BRAF* V600E mutations are common in the classical, tall-cell, Warthin-like, and oncocytic PTC, molecular testing is also a potential consideration. However, in equivocal cases, a diagnosis of suspicious for malignancy (B-V) may be a more appropriate alternative to a diagnosis of follicular neoplasm (B-IV) or malignant (B-VI) [29].

5.7 Cytology Limitations of Oncocytic (Hürthle Cell) Lesions

Although criteria outlined in TBSRTC have been widely adopted by pathologists and incorporated into clinical management algorithms, there have been many efforts to improve risk stratification of indeterminate nodules, including those that are diagnosed as B-III (AUS-HC) and B-IV (follicular neoplasm). While various morphological criteria have been evaluated in the past, interest has largely focused on application of molecular testing in recent years [29].

5.7.1 Risk of Malignancy in Indeterminate Oncocytic/Hürthle Cell Nodules

The risk of malignancy of thyroid nodules diagnosed on FNA as AUS is approximately 10–30% [15], although there is significant variability depending on the type of atypia. Many studies in the literature have demonstrated that the risk of malignancy associated with cytological atypia (AUS-C), whether alone or in combination with architectural atypia (AUS-A), is often significantly higher than AUS-A or AUS-HC [10, 30–39]. The risk of malignancy of AUS-HC is variable, but appears to be toward the lower end of the spectrum for AUS reported by TBSRTC, with a 0% to approximately 30% risk (median, 15%) reported repeatedly in the literature [23, 31–34, 37, 38, 40].

The risk of malignancy of thyroid nodules diagnosed on FNA as follicular neoplasm (B-IV) also has a wide reported range (14–45%; median 23%) [20–24, 41–48] again tending to occur toward the lower bound reported in TBSRTC for follicular neoplasm (25–40%) [15].

The wide ranges reported in the risk of malignancy are probably due in part to interobserver variability, which is known to be high in the indeterminate TBSRTC categories [49]. Interestingly, in a trio of studies, VandenBussche et al., from The Johns Hopkins University, examined in 2015 [50] and 2014 [51, 52] interobserver variability in indeterminate thyroid FNA through comparison of cytotechnologist and cytopathologist diagnoses over a 10-year period. They found that AUS-HC, in comparison with AUS-A and AUS-C, was most likely to be downgraded to benign and least likely to be upgraded to a higher Bethesda category by cytopathologists. Additionally, the ratios of AUS-A to suspicious for follicular neoplasm and AUS-C to suspicious for PTC were approximately 1 and 2, respectively. The ratios were also similar between cytotechnologists and cytopathologists. On the contrary, the ratio of AUS-HC to follicular neoplasm was over 4 for cytopathologists, which was about triple the ratio seen for cytotechnologists. The authors attributed the higher cytopathologist threshold for follicular neoplasm to the presence of chronic lymphocytic thyroiditis (Hashimoto's thyroiditis) in the background of many of the aspirates, although they also acknowledged that cytopathologists seemed to be less willing to dismiss some degree of oncocytic/Hürthle cell atypia as benign in other cases.

5.7.2 Role of Morphological Features in Suggesting Neoplasia or Malignancy

Given the variability in interpretation of Hürthle cell–predominant FNA biopsy specimens, many investigators have attempted to evaluate other cytological features that may predict oncocytic/Hürthle cell neoplasia or even malignancy. Although no single criterion is completely sensitive or specific, features that have suggested neoplasia in some studies include (1) concurrent architectural atypia (including nonmacrofollicular groups or discohesive/single cells) [53, 54], (2) transgressing blood vessels [53, 55], and (3) absence of lymphocytes [53, 54]. Scant colloid has also been associated with neoplasia by some investigators [46, 53], whereas others have found it less helpful [42, 54].

Despite the inclusion of "dysplasia" (small cell dysplasia and large cell dysplasia) as a potential criterion in TBSRTC, the terminology used in the literature has been inconsistent, and the results have been variable. "Nuclear features," including atypia/pleomorphism and prominent nucleoli (which would align with the concept of large cell dysplasia) have been helpful in predicting oncocytic/Hürthle cell neoplasia by some researchers [54], but not by others [46, 53]. While "monotony of cells" has been suggested as an indicator of neoplasia [16], which would seemingly include small cell dysplasia, the ability of the latter to distinguish nonneoplastic from neoplastic oncocytic/Hürthle cell proliferations has *not* been well-characterized in the literature. Instead, the concept of dysplasia (both small and large cell) has been suggested by some to correlate more specifically with malignancy, albeit in relatively small series [24, 26, 27]. In a larger series of 127 cases, however, Yang et al. (2013) [42] did not find that either small or large cell dysplasia could determine malignancy. Of note, none of the other cytological characteristics examined in that study (micro-follicular architecture, discohesive single cells, transgressing blood vessels, or colloid) could reliably distinguish oncocytic/HCC from benign lesions either [42].

References

1. Ali SZ, Baloch ZW, Cochand-Priollet B, Schmitt FC, Vielh P, VanderLann PA. The 2023 Bethesda system for reporting thyroid cytopathology. Thyroid. 2023;23(9):1039–44.
2. Cherella CE, Angell TE, Richman DM, Frates MC, Benson CB, Moore FD, et al. Differences in thyroid nodule cytology and malignancy risk between children and adults. Thyroid. 2019;29:1097–104.

3. Vuong HG, Chung DGB, Ngo LM, Bui TQ, Hassell L, Jung CK, et al. The use of the Bethesda system for reporting thyroid cytopathology in pediatric thyroid nodules: a meta-analysis. Thyroid. 2021;31:1203–11.
4. Ferreira MA, Gerhard R, Schmitt F. Analysis of nondiagnostic results in a large series of thyroid fine-needle aspiration cytology performed over 9 years in a single center. Acta Cytol. 2014;58:229–34.
5. Souteiro P, Polónia A, Eloy C. Repeating thyroid fine-needle aspiration before 3 months may render increased nondiagnostic results. Clin Endocrinol. 2019;91:899–900.
6. Singh RS, Wang HH. Timing of repeat thyroid fine needle aspiration in the management of thyroid nodules. Acta Cytol. 2011;55:544–8.
7. Lee HY, Baek JH, Yoo H, Kim JK, Lim MK, Chu YC, et al. Repeat fine-needle aspiration biopsy within a short interval does not increase the atypical cytologic results for thyroid nodules with previously nondiagnostic results. Acta Cytol. 2014;58:330–4.
8. Cibas ES, Ali SZ. The 2017 Bethesda system for reporting thyroid cytopathology. Thyroid. 2017;27:1341–6.
9. Baloch ZW, Asa SL, Barletta JA, Ghossein RA, Juhlin CC, Jung CK, et al. Overview of the 2022 WHO classification of thyroid neoplasms. Endocr Pathol. 2022;33:27–63.
10. Olson MT, Clark DP, Erozan YS, Ali SZ. Spectrum of risk of malignancy in subcategories of 'atypia of undetermined significance'. Acta Cytol. 2011;55:518–25.
11. VanderLaan PA, Marqusee E, Krane JF. Usefulness of diagnostic qualifiers for thyroid fine-needle aspirations with atypia of undetermined significance. Am J Clin Pathol. 2011;136:572–7.
12. Cherella CE, Hollowell ML, Smith JR, Zendejas B, Modi BP, Cibas ES, et al. Subtype of atypia on cytology and risk of malignancy in pediatric thyroid nodules. Cancer Cytopathol. 2022;130:330–5.
13. Glass RE, Levy JJ, Motanagh SA, Vaickus LJ, Liu X. Atypia of undetermined significance in thyroid cytology: nuclear atypia and architectural atypia are associated with different molecular alterations and risks of malignancy. Cancer Cytopathol. 2021;129:966–72.
14. Carty SE, Ohori NP, Hilko DA, McCoy KL, French EK, Manroa P, et al. The clinical utility of molecular testing in the management of thyroid follicular neoplasms (Bethesda IV nodules). Ann Surg. 2020;272:621–7.
15. Ali SZ, Cibas ES. The Bethesda system for reporting thyroid cytopathology: definitions, criteria, and explanatory notes. Berlin: Springer; 2018.
16. Montone KT, Baloch ZW, LiVolsi VA. The thyroid Hürthle (oncocytic) cell and its associated pathologic conditions: a surgical pathology and cytopathology review. Arch Pathol Lab Med. 2008;132:1241–50.
17. Amrikachi M, Ramzy I, Rubenfeld S, Wheeler TM. Accuracy of fine-needle aspiration of thyroid: a review of 6226 cases and correlation with surgical or clinical outcome. Arch Pathol Lab Med. 2001;125:484–8.
18. Lew JI, Snyder RA, Sanchez YM, Solorzano CC. Fine needle aspiration of the thyroid: correlation with final histopathology in a surgical series of 797 patients. J Am Coll Surg. 2011;213:188–94.
19. Richmond BK, Judhan R, Chong B, Ubert A, AbuRahma Z, Mangano W, et al. False-negative results with the Bethesda system of reporting thyroid cytopathology: predictors of malignancy in thyroid nodules classified as benign by cytopathologic evaluation. Am Surg. 2014;80:811–6.
20. Sclabas GM, Staerkel GA, Shapiro SE, Fornage BD, Sherman SI, Vassillopoulou-Sellin R, et al. Fine-needle aspiration of the thyroid and correlation with histopathology in a contemporary series of 240 patients. Am J Surg. 2003;186:702–9.
21. Sangalli G, Serio G, Zampatti C, Bellotti M, Lomuscio G. Fine needle aspiration cytology of the thyroid: a comparison of 5469 cytological and final histological diagnoses. Cytopathology. 2006;17:245–50.
22. Roh MH, Jo VY, Stelow EB, et al. The predictive value of the fine-needle aspiration diagnosis "suspicious for a follicular neoplasm, Hürthle cell type" in patients with Hashimoto thyroiditis. Am J Clin Pathol. 2011;135:139–45.

23. Wong KS, Jo VY, Lowe AC, Faquin WC, Renshaw AA, Shah AA, et al. Malignancy risk for solitary and multiple nodules in Hürthle cell–predominant thyroid fine-needle aspirations: a multi-institutional study. Cancer Cytopathol. 2020;128:68–75.
24. Renshaw AA. Hürthle cell carcinoma is a better gold standard than Hürthle cell neoplasm for fine-needle aspiration of the thyroid. Cancer. 2002;96:261–6.
25. Renshaw AA. Fine-needle aspiration of hurthle cell lesions: making the best of what consumers want. Diagn Cytopathol. 2003;29:183–4.
26. Wu HH-J, Clouse J, Ren R. Fine-needle aspiration cytology of Hürthle cell carcinoma of the thyroid. Diagn Cytopathol. 2008;36:149–54.
27. Renshaw AA, Gould EW. Impact of specific patterns on the sensitivity for follicular and Hurthle cell carcinoma in thyroid fine-needle aspiration. Cancer Cytopathol. 2016;124:729–36.
28. Shi Y, Brandler TC, Yee-Chang M, Cangiarella J, Wei XJ, Leung A, et al. Application of GATA 3 and TTF-1 in differentiating parathyroid and thyroid nodules on cytology specimens. Diagn Cytopathol. 2020;48(2):128–37.
29. Wong KS, Angell TE, Barletta JA, Krane JF. Hurthle cell lesions of the thyroid: progress made and challenges remaining. Cancer Cytopathol. 2021;129:347–62.
30. Horne M. Thyroid follicular lesion of undetermined significance: evaluation of the risk of malignancy using the two-tier sub-classification. Diagn Cytopathol. 2012;40:410–5.
31. Valderrabano P, Khazai L, Thompson ZJ, Leon ME, Otto KJ, Hallanger-Johnson JE, et al. Cancer risk stratification of indeterminate thyroid nodules: a cytological approach. Thyroid. 2017;27:thy.2017.0221.
32. Renshaw AA. Should "atypical follicular cells" in thyroid fine-needle aspirates be subclassified? Cancer Cytopathol. 2010;118:186–9.
33. Kim SJ, Roh J, Baek JH, Hong SJ, Shong YK, Kim WB, et al. Risk of malignancy according to sub-classification of the atypia of undetermined significance or follicular lesion of undetermined significance (AUS/FLUS) category in the Bethesda system for reporting thyroid cytopathology. Cytopathology. 2017;28:65–73.
34. Wu H, Inman A, Cramer HM. Subclassification of "atypia of undetermined significance" in thyroid fine-needle aspirates. Diagn Cytopathol. 2014;42:23–9.
35. Baca SC, Wong KS, Strickland KC, Heller HT, Kim MI, Barletta JA, et al. Qualifiers of atypia in the cytologic diagnosis of thyroid nodules are associated with different Afirma gene expression classifier results and clinical outcomes. Cancer Cytopathol. 2017;125:313–22.
36. Gan TRX, Nga ME, Lum JHY, Wong WM, Tan WB, Parameswaran R, et al. Thyroid cytology—nuclear versus architectural atypia within the "atypia of undetermined significance/follicular lesion of undetermined significance" Bethesda category have significantly different rates of malignancy. Cancer Cytopathol. 2017;125:245–56.
37. Onder S, Firat P, Ates D. The Bethesda system for reporting thyroid cytopathology: an institutional experience of the outcome of indeterminate categories. Cytopathol. 2014;25:177–84.
38. Park HJ, Moon JH, Yom CK, et al. Thyroid "atypia of undetermined significance" with nuclear atypia has high rates of malignancy and BRAF mutation. Cancer Cytopathol. 2014;122:512–20.
39. Hyeon J, Ahn S, Shin JH, Oh YL. The prediction of malignant risk in the category "atypia of undetermined significance/follicular lesion of undetermined significance" of the Bethesda system for reporting thyroid cytopathology using subcategorization and braf mutation results. Cancer Cytopathol. 2014;122:368–76.
40. Ho AS, Sarti EE, Jain KS, Wang H, Nixon IJ, Shaha AR, et al. Malignancy rate in thyroid nodules classified as Bethesda category III (AUS/FLUS): is there a correct answer? Thyroid. 2014;24:787–8.
41. Sippel RS, Elaraj DM, Khanafshar E, Zarnegar R, Kebebew E, Duh QY, et al. Tumor size predicts malignant potential in Hürthle cell neoplasms of the thyroid. World J Surg. 2008;32:702–7.
42. Yang GCH, Schreiner AM, Sun W. Can abundant colloid exclude oncocytic (Hürthle cell) carcinoma in thyroid fine needle aspiration? Cytohistological correlation of 127 oncocytic (Hürthle cell) lesions. Cytopathology. 2013;24:185–93.

43. Sorrenti S, Trimboli P, Catania A, Ulisse S, De Antoni E, D'Armiento M. Comparison of malignancy rate in thyroid nodules with cytology of indeterminate follicular or indeterminate Hürthle cell neoplasm. Thyroid. 2009;19:355–60.
44. Kauffmann P, Dejax C, de Latour M, Dauplat J. The meaning and predictivity of Hürthle cells in fine needle aspiration cytology for thyroid nodular disease. Eur J Surg Oncol. 2004;30:786–9.
45. Castro MR, Espiritu RP, Bahn RS, Henry MR, Gharib H, Caraballo PJ, et al. Predictors of malignancy in patients with cytologically suspicious thyroid nodules. Thyroid. 2011;21:1191–8.
46. Alaedeen DI, Khiyami A, McHenry CR. Fine-needle aspiration biopsy specimen with a predominance of Hürthle cells: a dilemma in the management of nodular thyroid disease. Surgery. 2005;138:650–7.
47. Deandrea M, Ragazzoni F, Motta M, Torchio B, Mormile A, Garino F, et al. Diagnostic value of a cytomorphological subclassification of follicular patterned thyroid lesions: a study of 927 consecutive cases with histological correlation. Thyroid. 2010;20:1077–83.
48. Raparia K, Min SK, Mody DR, Anton R, Amrikachi M. Clinical outcomes for "suspicious" category in thyroid fine-needle aspiration biopsy: patient's sex and nodule size are possible predictors of malignancy. Arch Pathol Lab Med. 2009;133:787–90.
49. Cibas ES, Baloch ZW, Fellegara G, LiVolsi VA, Raab SS, Rosai J, et al. A prospective assessment defining the limitations of thyroid nodule pathologic evaluation. Ann Intern Med. 2013;159:325–32.
50. VandenBussche CJ, Adams C, Ali SZ, Olson MT. Cytotechnologist performance for screening Hürthle cell atypia in indeterminate thyroid fine-needle aspirates. Acta Cytol. 2015;59:377–83.
51. VandenBussche CJ, Olson MT, Adams C, Ali SZ. Cytotechnologist performance for screening microfollicular atypia in indeterminate thyroid fine-needle aspirates. Acta Cytol. 2014;58:432–8.
52. VandenBussche CJ, Adams C, Ali SZ, Olson MT. Cytotechnologist performance for detecting nuclear atypia in indeterminate thyroid fine needle aspirates. Acta Cytol. 2014;58:239–47.
53. Elliott DD, Pitman MB, Bloom L, Faquin WC. Fine-needle aspiration biopsy of hurthle cell lesions of the thyroid gland: a cytomorphologic study of 139 cases with statistical analysis. Cancer. 2006;108:102–9.
54. Gonzalez JL, Wang HH, Ducatman BS. Fine-needle aspiration of Hürthle cell lesions: a cytomorphologic approach to diagnosis. Am J Clin Pathol. 1993;100:231–5.
55. Yang YJ, Khurana KK. Diagnostic utility of intracytoplasmic lumen and transgressing vessels in evaluation of Hürthle cell lesions by fine-needle aspiration. Arch Pathol Lab Med. 2001;125:1031–5.

Oncocytic (Hürthle Cell) Lesions: Controversy of Diagnosis: Neoplastic or Nonneoplastic

6

6.1 The Challenge of Neoplastic or Nonneoplastic

When approaching thyroid fine-needle aspiration (FNA) samples containing oncocytic (Hürthle) cells (HCs), the traditional aim is to distinguish nonneoplastic from neoplastic lesions, a diagnostic dichotomy that largely guides the ensuing clinical management. Approximately, 15–30% of fine-needle aspiration biopsy (FNAB) specimens are reported as "indeterminate" [1]. For these indeterminate cases in which oncocytic (Hürthle) cells predominate, the more specific term "Hürthle cell lesion" (HCL) is often reported [2]. It encompasses a variety of neoplastic as well as nonneoplastic thyroid follicular lesions.

Nonneoplastic conditions in which oncocytic (Hürthle) cells may be present include autoimmune thyroiditis (Hashimoto's thyroiditis and Graves' disease), multinodular goiter (MNG) (with oncocytic metaplasia), as well as aging, lesions following irradiation to the head and neck or therapy with ^{131}Iodine, and in patients who have had a history of partial thyroidectomy [3–6]. In such "indeterminate cases," FNAB *cannot* reliably diagnose neoplasia versus hyperplasia, and carcinoma versus adenoma.

Alaedeen et al. [7] sought to identify factors, clinical and/or cytopathological, that might distinguish neoplastic from nonneoplastic lesions in patients with FNAB aspirates containing a predominance of oncocytic (Hürthle) cells [7]. They reported that demographic (age and sex), clinical (nodule size), and laboratory (thyroid function) data were unhelpful in differentiating neoplastic from nonneoplastic cases [7]. Many of these pathologies may be managed conservatively if neoplasia can be excluded. Thus, a challenging clinical situation may arise if oncocytic (Hürthle) cells are detected in FNABs. A distinction between neoplastic and nonneoplastic HCLs should be made in order to segregate patients for whom surgery is indicated from those who may be managed conservatively.

Over the years, diverse diagnostic "cytological" criteria have been proposed in the literature to distinguish nonneoplastic from neoplastic lesions in FNAs

M. Sakr, *Oncocytic (Hürthle Cell) Thyroid Lesions*,
https://doi.org/10.1007/978-3-032-03115-0_6

containing oncocytic (Hürthle) cells. Nevertheless, even when the most accepted criteria are applied, it is unrealistic to expect a 100% correct classification into non-neoplastic versus neoplastic. It appears that no cytological feature, whether present or absent, can entirely exclude a neoplastic process; in fact, studies have shown that up to 25% of the cases diagnosed as "neoplastic" on FNAs prove to be, on histological follow-up, simply hyperplastic proliferations (i.e., nonneoplastic lesions), often in the context of nodular goiter or lymphocytic thyroiditis [2, 7–16].

Similar to follicular adenoma, the requirement of a capsule in oncocytic adenoma (Hürthle cell adenoma—HCA) is somewhat arbitrary in that the presence of a capsule does *not* equate to a neoplastic/clonal process. Some pathologists may refer to unencapsulated follicular-patterned proliferations as "adenomatous," "adenomatoid," or "hyperplastic" nodules, although many of these are likely clonal in origin [17, 18]. The distinction of HCA from a nonneoplastic proliferation can be difficult or even impossible to determine in the absence of molecular studies, and the designation is often arbitrary in nodules without "classical" features [19]. It is important to keep this challenge in mind when correlating with FNA findings.

6.2 Oncocytic (Hürthle Cell) Lesion: Is It Nonneoplastic?

6.2.1 Definition of Nonneoplastic Oncocytic (Hürthle Cell) Lesions

An "oncocytic lesions" or "Hürthle cell lesion" (HCL) has been defined as "a discrete lesion composed mainly of oncocytic (Hürthle) cells." However, the percentage of oncocytic (Hürthle) cells required for the lesion to be diagnosed as an oncocytic/HCL has been controversial. The majority of authors in the literature defined the lesion as HCL when oncocytes make 75% or more of follicular cells [20, 21]. Some authors considered it a HCL when oncocytes exceed 50% of follicular cells in fine-needle aspiration biopsy (FNAB) [22–24]. However, most authors used the Figs. 75% [25–30] and 50% [31–35] to refer to neoplastic rather than nonneoplastic HCL. Others required more than 90% oncocytes to define the lesion as oncocytic or Hürthle cell neoplasm [31, 36].

A skilled and experienced cytopathologist is irreplaceable in the interpretation of FNAB results, rendering an opinion as to the presence or absence of "true" oncocytic (Hürthle) cells and whether or not the nodule of interest is sufficiently HC-predominant to raise clinical concern. The Bethesda classification scheme was recently developed in an effort to create a more unified language for reporting the results of thyroid FNABs [37–39]. The Bethesda system appears to be gaining wider acceptance and usage in sound clinical decision-making; however, it is not yet universally employed. The main objective should be to identify clinically relevant nodules that unequivocally require surgery; however, FNAB may be less reliable when "a monotonous population of three-dimensional groups of follicular cells with scarce colloid is aspirated." In such cases, hyperplastic lesions (nonneoplastic) and benign and malignant neoplasms are cytologically indistinct [40].

Fine-needle aspiration biopsy (FNAB) aspirates of nonneoplastic lesions are often comprised of oncocytic (Hürthle) cells, benign follicular cells without oncocytic change, and colloid, as in the case of nodular goiter, or of HCs, aggregates of lymphocytes and dendritic cells, and benign follicular cells, as seen in chronic lymphocytic thyroiditis. In rare circumstances, FNAB of a thyroid nodule may reveal oxyphilic cells from an intrathyroidal parathyroid adenoma. The cells may be indistinguishable from oncocytic (Hürthle) cells with their true identity revealed only on final pathology [41].

6.2.2 Cytological Features of Nonneoplastic Oncocytic (Hürthle Cell) Lesions

The cytological features considered the most useful for nonneoplastic Oncocytic (Hürthle cell) lesions include the following:

- Presence of oncocytic (Hürthle) cells in cohesive flat sheets.
- Polymorphism (i.e., presence of non-Hürthle follicular cells in addition to the oncocytic (Hürthle) cells.
- Presence of inflammatory cells (lymphocytes and plasma cells).
- A honeycomb or macro-follicular arrangement of the oncocytic (Hürthle) cells (Fig. 6.1).
- Absent or inconspicuous nucleolus in the oncocytic (Hürthle) cells (Fig. 6.1).
- Abundant colloid.

Intracytoplasmic lumina and transgressing vessels may also help to differentiate neoplastic from nonneoplastic oncocytic/HCLs where their absence favors the diagnosis of nonneoplastic lesions [22, 26, 37]. However, the presence of macrophages

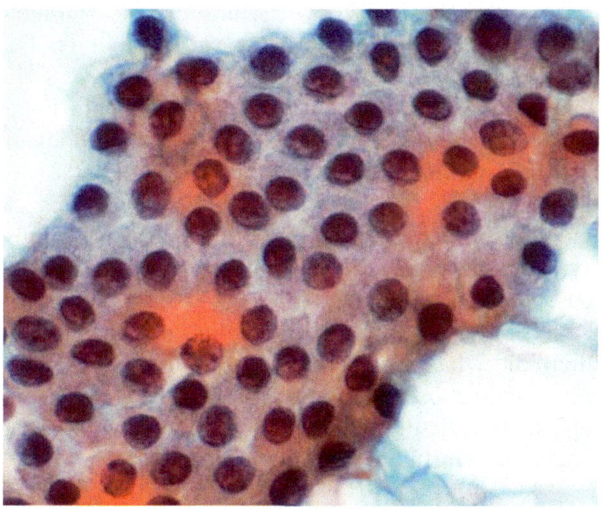

Fig. 6.1 Fine-needle aspirate of the thyroid showing a group of oncocytic (Hürthle) cells in a nonneoplastic lesion (nodular hyperplasia). Note the honeycomb arrangement of the oncocytic (Hürthle) cells and the lack of prominent nucleoli, both features favoring nonneoplastic oncocytic or Hürthle cell lesions. Papanicolaou stain

(with or without cytoplasmic hemosiderin) is controversial. Indeed, some authors consider this feature as favoring nonneoplastic lesions, whereas others deny its usefulness, as it may also be present in neoplastic lesions [42].

Within the nonneoplastic lesions, a sub-categorization (in particular, between benign follicular nodules versus lymphocytic thyroiditis) should be given in the diagnostic interpretation because hyperplastic/adenomatoid nodules in multinodular goiter (MNG) and Hashimoto's thyroiditis can show a preponderance of oncocytic (Hürthle) cells.

6.2.2.1 Hyperplastic Thyroid Nodules

In hyperplastic/adenomatoid nodules in MNG, the background usually shows watery colloid and macrophages; however, of utmost importance is the presence of a second cell population of small follicular cells containing scant cytoplasm and small nuclei with dense chromatin [8, 43]. The oncocytic (Hürthle) cells may demonstrate intranuclear grooves and even focal nuclear chromatin clearing; however, the nuclei are round in shape with prominent nucleoli and other features of papillary thyroid carcinoma (PTC) are *not* seen [8].

In general, fine needle aspirates from a benign follicular nodule exhibiting oncocytic/Hürthle cell metaplasia are characterized by a mixture of follicular cells and oncocytic (Hürthle) cells arranged in macro-follicles, a mixture of macro- and micro-follicles, or in monolayers with a honeycomb arrangement [11, 44, 45]. Although there is usually no significant nuclear atypia in the context of a benign follicular nodule, occasional pleomorphic oncocytic (Hürthle) cells may be seen and can become a cause of concern or of false-positive diagnoses; however, unlike those seen in the context of oncocytic/Hürthle cell neoplasms (HCNs), those cells exhibit either absent or inconspicuous nucleoli [10, 11, 45–47].

6.2.2.2 Lymphocytic Thyroiditis

On the other hand, fine needle aspirates from lymphocytic thyroiditis typically consist of either single oncocytic (Hürthle) cells or fragments of these cells, usually in a honeycomb arrangement, in a background of a polymorphous lymphocytic population (Fig. 6.2); in this particular nonneoplastic setting, oncocytic (Hürthle) cells may exhibit prominent nucleoli. The lymphoid population consists of small and large lymphocytes often admixed with tingible-body macrophages, and plasma cells and rare multinucleated foreign-body giant cells may also be seen [12, 45]. The most important feature is that the lymphocytes are also seen percolating among the majority of cell groups. This is an important feature that distinguishes neoplastic versus nonneoplastic oncocytic/Hürthle cell lesions arising in a background of chronic lymphocytic thyroiditis [48–50].

It is important to keep in mind that chronic lymphocytic thyroiditis (Hashimoto's thyroiditis) has been reported in the literature to be an important cause of false-positive diagnoses in thyroid FNAs [10, 11, 14]. The most problematic FNA cases of lymphocytic thyroiditis are those with a predominance or exclusive presence of oncocytic (Hürthle) cells and a paucity of lymphocytes. A similar situation can also

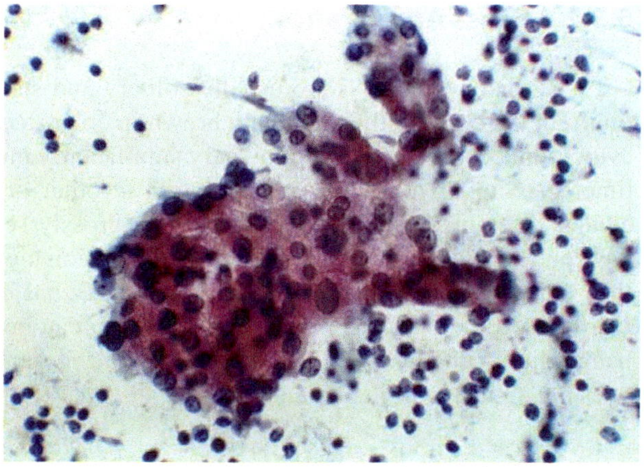

Fig. 6.2 Fine-needle aspiration of the thyroid in lymphocytic thyroiditis. Note the group of oncocytic (Hürthle) cells seen in a background of a polymorphous lymphoid population. Note the occasional pleomorphic oncocytic (Hürthle) cell. Both the honeycomb arrangement and the presence of lymphocytes favor a nonneoplastic oncocytic/Hürthle cell lesion. Papanicolaou stain

occur in the context of any oncocytic (Hürthle) cell hyperplastic proliferations in the context of any benign follicular nodule. Such cases are known causes of pitfalls and are often overinterpreted as oncocytic/HCNs.

It is noteworthy that lymphocytic thyroiditis can also be a cause of false-positive diagnoses of papillary thyroid carcinoma (PTC) because mild nuclear atypia, occasional nuclear clearing with grooves, and rarely intranuclear inclusions may sometimes be encountered [12]. Usually the oncocytic (Hürthle) cells with these atypical nuclei still maintain a round shape with smooth nuclear membrane and prominent nucleoli. Some authors have suggested that immunostains for cytokeratin 19, HBME-1, and galectin-3 can be helpful in solving this diagnostic dilemma; however, others have shown that follicular and oncocytic (Hürthle) cells in Hashimoto's thyroiditis can show positive immunostaining with all the previously mentioned markers [27].

6.3 Oncocytic (Hürthle Cell) Lesion: Is It Neoplastic?

6.3.1 Introduction

Although oncocytic thyroid neoplasms encompass a variety of phenotypes, the lesions that have produced the most debate and controversy are those with a follicular and solid pattern and the ones to which most pathologists refer to as oncocytic/Hürthle cell neoplasms (HCNs) [51]. A variety of thyroid neoplasms are characterized as having oncocytic cytology. These include benign (oncocytic or Hürthle cell adenoma, granular cell tumor) and malignant (oncocytic or Hürthle cell carcinoma) neoplasms, variants of papillary thyroid carcinoma (PTC) (tall-cell variant, oncocytic variant, and Warthin-like variant), and the oncocytic variant of medullary thyroid carcinoma (MTC).

6.3.2 Gross Appearance

Grossly, oncocytic/HCNs are usually solitary and show at least partial encapsulation. They are distinctly mahogany brown in color due the abundant mitochondrial cytochrome content. Lesions may vary significantly in size from one to several centimeters. Similar to oncocytic neoplasms in other organs, a central scar may be evident. Hemorrhage and necrosis may be grossly seen especially in lesions that have undergone preoperative fine-needle aspiration biopsy (FNAB); massive infarction either spontaneously or following FNAB has been reported in oncocytic/ Hürthle cell tumors [9, 52, 53]. The infarction can be extensive, leading to severe hampering of the histological assessment. The presence of spontaneous infarction does *not* equate with malignancy.

6.3.3 Cytological Features of Neoplastic Oncocytic (Hürthle Cell) Lesions

The cytological features mentioned most often in the literature as favoring an oncocytic/Hürthle cell neoplasm (HCN) include the following [22, 54–56]:

- Mono-morphism (i.e., absence of non-Hürthle cells in addition to oncocytic (Hürthle) cells or predominance of oncocytic (Hürthle) cells (at least 75% of cells).
- Micro-follicular/syncytial/ non-macro-follicular or trabecular arrangement (Fig. 6.3).
- Presence of single/dyshesive oncocytic (Hürthle) cells (Fig. 6.3).
- Prominent nucleoli (Fig. 6.4).
- Transgressing blood vessels (Fig. 6.5).
- Absence of a background of chronic inflammation.

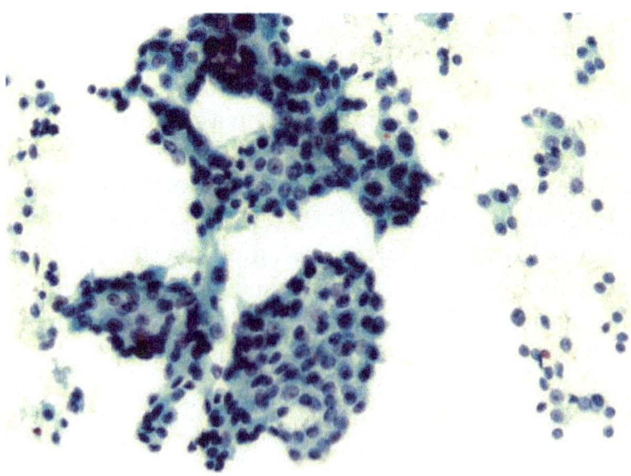

Fig. 6.3 Fine-needle aspiration of the thyroid in an oncocytic/Hürthle cell neoplasm. Note the syncytial/micro-follicular arrangement of oncocytic (Hürthle) cells, the dyshesive oncocytic (Hürthle) cells, and the prominent nucleoli, favoring oncocytic/Hürthle cell neoplasm. Papanicolaou stain

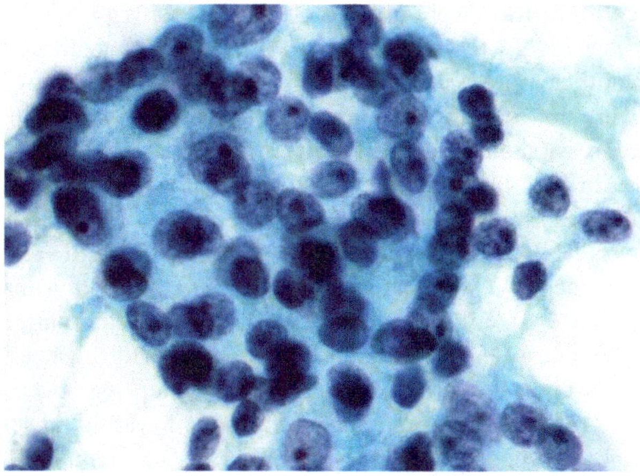

Fig. 6.4 Fine-needle aspiration of the thyroid in a case of oncocytic/Hürthle cell neoplasm Note the prominent nucleoli of the neoplastic oncocytic (Hürthle) cells. Papanicolaou stain

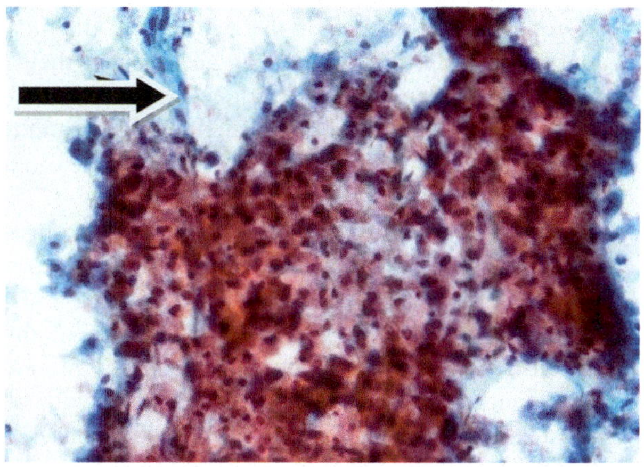

Fig. 6.5 Fine-needle aspiration of the thyroid in the case of oncocytic/Hürthle cell neoplasm. Note the transgressing blood vessel (arrow) within the sheet of oncocytic (Hürthle) cells, which are in a syncytial arrangement. This feature favors oncocytic/Hürthle cell neoplasm. Papanicolaou stain

A lesser-known parameter, the "intra-cytoplasmic vacuole," has been cited by some authors in the literature as favoring oncocytic/HCN [27, 57, 58]. Ultrastructurally, intracytoplasmic vacuoles correspond to intracytoplasmic lumina with villi and secretions [59]. By light microscopy, the intracytoplasmic lumina are best seen in Diff-Quik-stained slides where they appear as vacuoles containing magenta-colored material; the latter stains positively for thyroglobulin (Tg) by immunocytochemistry [27]. In a retrospective study by Yang et al. [26] reviewing 30 FNAs with a cytological diagnosis of nonneoplastic oncocytic/Hürthle cell lesion or oncocytic/HCN, intracytoplasmic lumina were seen predominantly (70%) in HCN, but they were not entirely specific because they could also be identified in 15% of the nonneoplastic oncocytic/Hürthle cell cases [27]. Nevertheless, by adding intracytoplasmic lumina and transgressing blood vessels to their armamentarium of diagnostic criteria (in addition to the evaluation of conventional criteria including abundance of oncocytic or Hürthle cells, lymphocytic component, and colloid), they were able to obtain a sensitivity and specificity of 100% and 85%, respectively (compared with 90% and 65% with conventional criteria alone). In another more recent study by Elliot et al. [22], however, intracytoplasmic lumina were not found to be statistically significant when either univariate or step logistic regression analyses were performed [22].

In fact, in the particular study by Elliot et al. [22] in which 14 cytological features in 139 cases of benign nonneoplastic oncocytic/Hürthle cell lesions and oncocytic/HCNs were evaluated, the only cytological features found to be statistically significantly associated with HCNs were non-macro-follicular arrangement, absence of colloid, absence of chronic inflammation, presence of transgressing blood vessels, more than 90% oncocytic (Hürthle) cells, and more than 10% single cells upon univariate analysis. With a step logistic regression analysis, only non-macrofollicular arrangement, absence of colloid, absence of chronic inflammation, and presence of transgressing blood vessels remained significant, and when all four of these features were present, an oncocytic/HCN was correctly identified 86% of the time [22].

A controversial aspect of the cytological diagnosis of oncocytic/Hürthle cell lesions relates to a few authors suggesting that their cytological diagnosis can be further refined in an attempt to triage the "malignant" oncocytic/Hürthle cell neoplasms from all the other benign (nonneoplastic and neoplastic) oncocytic/Hürthle cell lesions [45]. Kini (2008) identified four cytological criteria characteristic of oncocytic/HCNs: (1) syncytial tumor fragments, (2) small tumor cells with a high nucleocytoplasmic ratio, (3) single or multiple prominent nucleoli, and (4) intranuclear inclusions. Using these criteria, she was able to correctly diagnose 60% of the oncocytic/HCNs [45].

Renshaw [60] has suggested an evaluation of thyroid FNAs containing HCs based on five cytomorphological features seen more often in HCNs, namely (1) a predominant oncocytic/Hürthle cell population with scant colloid, (2) at least one of either small cell dysplasia (cytoplasmic diameter less than twice the nuclear diameter, with often bland cells), (3) large cell dysplasia (greater than twice the variation in nuclear diameter; large cells typically demonstrate prominent nucleoli and irregular nuclear outlines), (4) crowding, and (5) dyshesion [60]. Using this assessment scheme, Renshaw was able to identify the ten HCNs in his study [60]. However, approximately 63% of follicular adenomas, oncocytic (Hürthle cell) type, and 25% of nonneoplastic oncocytic/Hürthle cell lesions also fulfilled those criteria and could not be reliably diagnosed as benign. In the future, investigators may find an optimal combination to better triage the malignant cases from all the other oncocytic/Hürthle cell lesions, possibly combining the proposed cytological criteria of Kini [45] and Renshaw [60], along with other clinical parameters such as size, distribution, and radiographical characteristics of the lesions and gender of the patient, as proposed by some authors; however, at this point, the optimal formula remains elusive [61–64].

Most authors have not found any reliable cytological criteria to diagnose oncocytic/HCNs in FNA specimens; in fact, most believe that nuclear features in nonpapillary follicular lesions are unreliable indicators of malignancy [65]. For example, Yang et al. [66] looked at 127 hypercellular, oncocyte-exclusive, lymphocyte-absent FNAs and looked at 6 cytological features (micro-follicular pattern, dyshesive single cells, small cell dysplasia, large cell dysplasia, transgressing blood vessels, and colloid) and found that *none* of the cytological features could exclude an oncocytic/HCN [66]. In a study by McIvor et al. [67], three cases were correctly predicted to be oncocytic/HCN on the basis of cellular and nuclear atypia, but three oncocytic/HCNs composed of bland cells were incorrectly diagnosed as adenomas, leading the authors to conclude that the differentiation between benign and malignant oncocytic/Hürthle cell lesions is less reliable than the distinction between non-neoplastic and neoplastic [67]. Therefore, the recommended traditional and safest approach, at least to date, is to diagnose an oncocytic/HCN as such and leave the categorization into benign versus malignant to the histological examination of the resected tumor [11, 68]. The significance of a cytological diagnosis of oncocytic/HCN can be derived from the data from many cyto-histological studies published in the literature [2, 7, 8, 15, 16, 50, 66, 69–77]. According to these studies, the reported rates of malignancy on follow-up surgical excision vary from 10% to 45%.

Recently, Yuan et al. [78] reported "a four risk-factor model" for predicting oncocytic/HCN and excluding malignancy in patients with oncocytic (Hürthle) cell-predominant thyroid FNAC [78]. The study included 69 patients with the diagnosis of nonneoplastic lesion (n = 35), oncocytic/HCA (n = 20), and oncocytic/HCC (n = 14). On univariable analysis, significant predictors of "neoplasm" were high cellularity, isolated single cells, absent colloid, nonuniform oncocytic (Hürthle) cell population (anisonucleosis), larger nodule size, and higher ATA (American Thyroid Association) score. Large-cell dysplasia and transgressing blood vessels were *not* found to be significant factors. Multivariable analysis identified a combination of four risk factors; namely, high cellularity, anisonucleosis, absent colloid, and size ≥2.9 cm that was associated with neoplasm in 10/11 patients. None of 15 patients with 0 or 1 out of 4 risk factors had malignancy or neoplasm on follow-up. The authors concluded that in the absence of 4 or 3 risk factors, the model excluded malignancy and neoplasm in all patients. The presence of all 4 factors predicted neoplasm and malignancy in 91% and 46% of cases, respectively.

6.4 Oncocytic (Hürthle Cell) Lesion: Molecular Biology

6.4.1 The Role of Molecular Biology in the Diagnosis of Hürthle Cell Neoplasms

Since cytomorphological criteria for neoplasia or malignancy in oncocytic/Hürthle cell lesions appear to have limited sensitivity and specificity, interest in molecular discriminants has increased as testing has become more accessible [79].

Molecular biology techniques may offer another tool for the diagnosis of oncocytic/Hürthle cell neoplasms (HCNs) since RET/PTC activation was detected in a significant number of neoplastic cases, but *not* in hyperplastic nodules [80]. Chiappetta et al. [80] analyzed specimens from 49 patients with oncocytic cell nodular lesions ($n = 49$) including 20 adenomas, 19 carcinomas, and 10 hyperplasias for RET/PTC (papillary thyroid carcinoma) activation, which is the most frequent genetic alteration in PTCs. RET/PTC activation was detected in a significant number of cases of oncocytic/Hürthle cell adenomas and carcinomas, but in zero of ten patients with hyperplastic nodules. In particular, the RET/PTC1 isoform was found in 7 of 12 adenomas and 4 of 7 carcinomas. These results indicate that RET/PTC is a genetic event common to papillary thyroid carcinoma (PTC) and to oncocytic/Hürthle cell neoplasia (HCN) [80].

de Vries et al. [81] investigated a series of 20 follicular oncocytic/Hürthle cell tumors [17 follicular Hürthle cell carcinomas (FHCCs) and three follicular Hürthle cell adenomas (FHCAs)] for the presence of RET/PTC and PAX8/PPARG rearrangements and BRAF, HRAS, and NRAS mutations. They reported that RET/PTC rearrangements were found in 33% of FHCAs and in 38% of FHCCs. All RET/PTC-positive FHCCs had a solid pattern of growth. PAX8/PPARG rearrangement was present in 27% of the FHCCs, which displayed, in most cases, a follicular architecture. NRAS mutation was detected in only one FHCC. Moreover, an FHCC with a solid/microfollicular growth pattern scored positive for both RET/PTC and PAX8/PPARG rearrangement. In conclusion, this study showed a significant association between RET/PTC rearrangements and FHCCs with a solid growth pattern, thus raising the possibility of using tyrosine kinase inhibitors for the treatment of patients with FHCCs, which are often refractory to radioactive iodine (RAI) treatment [81].

6.4.2 Application of Molecular Testing in Cytologically Indeterminant Oncocytic (Hürthle Cell) Lesions

6.4.2.1 Goal of Molecular Testing

The goal of molecular testing is primarily to differentiate biologically benign nodules from those that are at higher risk and should undergo resection. Most commercially used molecular assays currently involve the interrogation of RNA expression profiles, including messenger RNA or micro-RNA, and/or sequencing for the detection of mutations, gene fusions, and copy number alterations using next-generation sequencing techniques [79].

6.4.2.2 Commercial Platforms in the USA

Two of the commercial platforms most widely used in the USA are Afirma (Veracyte, Inc., South San Francisco, California) and ThyroSeq (University of Pittsburgh Medical Center, Pittsburgh, Pennsylvania, and CBLPath, Inc., Rye Brook, New York) [79].

6.4.2.3 Afirma

Gene Expression Classifier (GEC)

The Afirma Gene Expression Classifier (GEC) is a classification algorithm that categorizes indeterminate FNA as "benign" or "suspicious." In the initial validation study, the GEC demonstrated 92% sensitivity and 52% specificity for malignancy among Bethesda-III (B-III) and Bethesda-IV (B-IV) nodules [82]. However, the performance of the GEC varied by the type of atypia in indeterminate nodules, with lower predictive value for oncocytic/Hürthle cell–predominant FNA [83–86].

Genomic Sequencing Classifier (GSC)
The most recent iteration of Afirma, the Genomic Sequencing Classifier (GSC), uses an updated algorithm incorporating messenger RNA expression, sequencing, and genomic copy number detection. Notable additions to the GSC also include dedicated classification algorithms providing Hürthle cell and Hürthle neoplasm indices to improve the specificity of Hürthle cell lesion classification [87].

The GSC demonstrated, in the validation study, an overall sensitivity similar to that of GEC, but showed a 36% increase in specificity. The most dramatic improvements were in the classification of oncocytic/Hürthle cell lesions. Among oncocytic/Hürthle cell neoplasms (HCA and HCC), the sensitivity and specificity were approximately 89% and 59%, respectively, as compared to approximately 89% and 12% in the GEC) [87]. When accounting for Hürthle/non-Hürthle cell cytology rather than only histological diagnoses of Hürthle cell lesions, Angell et al. [88] demonstrated that the GSC benign call rate (BCR) was significantly higher compared with that of the GEC for both Bethesda-III (100% versus ~ 37%) and Bethesda-IV (64% versus ~ 16%). Similar improvements in the BCR of oncocytic/Hürthle cell–predominant FNA have also been reported by Endo et al. [89] and San Martin et al. [90] in subsequent studies, which found an approximately threefold increase in the BCR of indeterminate Hürthle cell FNA with the GSC compared with the GEC [89, 90]. In these latter studies, follow-up also revealed increased specificity and positive predictive value for the GSC in nodules with preceding oncocytic/Hürthle cell–predominant FNA [89, 90]. San Martin et al. notably observed a significant decrease in the number of surgeries performed for GSC-tested oncocytic (Hürthle) cell FNA as well [90].

ThyroSeq
An updated version of the ThyroSeq assay (v3) was recently validated. ThyroSeq v3, in contrast to Afirma, is primarily a sequencing-based test, using next-generation sequencing to evaluate hotspot mutations and fusions in a large panel of genes. More limited analyses of gene expression and copy number alterations are also performed [91]. Nikiforova et al. [91] reported that unlike Afirma, ThyroSeq v3 routinely reports specific molecular alterations and corresponding probabilities of malignancy. Additionally, a genomic classifier score based on the weighted sum of alterations is provided [91]. Based on this score, results are considered "negative," "currently negative" (i.e., if only a low-risk alteration is detected), or "positive" [91, 92].

Similar to the Afirma GSC, Thyroseq v3 demonstrated notable improvements in the classification of oncocytic (Hürthle) cell nodules compared with its predecessor (ThyroSeq v2) [91] with a sensitivity of 100% and specificity of 67% in the validation study [93]. However, performance in oncocytic/Hürthle cell nodules was based on histological diagnoses rather than preceding FNA diagnoses. There have only been a few studies evaluating the performance of any version of ThyroSeq in oncocytic/Hürthle cell–predominant FNA (with or without comparison with non-Hürthle FNA) [86, 92, 94]. Parajuli et al. [86] evaluated a small cohort of patients with oncocytic/Hürthle cell–predominant FNA (B-III or B-IV) and a ThyroSeq (v1 or v2) result, showing that only 8% had a high-risk mutation compared with 19% in the non-Hürthle group. In a study only evaluating oncocytic/Hürthle cell–predominant FNA, Schatz-Siemers et al. [94] reported that 62% of B-III and 59% of B-IV Hürthle cell FNAs had negative Thyroseq (v2 or v3) results. Finally, Ohori et al. [92] evaluated a cohort of B-IV FNAs and found that 32% of oncocytic/Hürthle aspirates and 51% of non-Hürthle aspirates had negative (excluding currently negative) molecular results (ThyroSeq v3). Given the limited data, differences in methodologies, and variability in test version available, it is difficult to draw conclusions about performance in oncocytic/Hürthle cell–predominant FNAs between ThyroSeq versions or when compared with non-Hürthle FNAs.

References

1. Cooper DS, Doherty GM, Haugen BR, Kloos RT, Lee SL, Mandel SJ, et al. Revised American thyroid association management guidelines for patients with thyroid nodules and differentiated thyroid cancer. Thyroid. 2009;19(11):1167–214.
2. Pu RT, Yang J, Wasserman PG, Bhuiya T, Griffith KA, Michael CW. Does Hurthle cell lesion/neoplasm predict malignancy more than follicular lesion/neoplasm on thyroid fine-needle aspiration? Diagn Cytopathol. 2006;34(5):330–4.
3. Friedman N. Cellular involution in the thyroid gland: significance of Hurthle cells in myxedema, exhaustion atrophy, Hashimoto's disease and the reactions to irradiation, thiouracil therapy and subtotal resection. J Clin Endocrinol Metab. 1949;9:874–82.
4. Harach HR, Zusman SB, Saravia DE. Nodular goiter: a histo-cytological study with some emphasis on pitfalls of fine-needle aspiration cytology. Diagn Cytopathol. 1992;8:409–19.
5. Granter SR, Cibas ES. Cytologic findings in thyroid nodules after 131I treatment of hyperthyroidism. Am J Clin Pathol. 1997;107:20–5.
6. Montone KT, Baloch ZW, LiVolsi VA. The thyroid Hürthle (oncocytic) cell and its associated pathologic conditions: a surgical pathology and cytopathology review. Arch Pathol Lab Med. 2008;132:1241–50.
7. Alaedeen DI, Khiyami A, McHenry CR. Fine-needle aspiration biopsy specimen with a predominance of Hürthle cells: a dilemma in the management of nodular thyroid disease. Surgery. 2005;138(4):650–7.
8. Gonzales JL, Wang HH, Ducatman BS. Fine-needle aspiration of Hurthle cell lesions. A cytomorphologic approach to diagnosis. Am J Clin Pathol. 1993;100:231–5.
9. Kini SR, Miller JM, Hamburger JI. Cytopathology of Hurthle cell lesions of the thyroid gland by fine needle aspiration. Acta Cytol. 1981;25:647–52.
10. Nguyen GK, Ginsberg J, Crockford PM, Villanueva RR. Hashimoto's thyroiditis: cytodiagnostic accuracy and pitfalls. Diagn Cytopathol. 1997;16:531–6.
11. Nguyen GK, Ginsberg J, Crockford PM. Fine needle aspiration biopsy cytology of the thyroid. Its value and limitations in the diagnosis and treatment of solitary thyroid nodules. Pathol Annu. 1991;26(1):63–91.
12. Ali SZ, Cibas ES. The Bethesda system for reporting thyroid cytopathology: definitions, criteria and explanatory notes. Berlin: Springer; 2010. p. 171.
13. Ali SZ. Thyroid cytopathology: Bethesda and beyond. Acta Cytol. 2011;55:4–12.

14. MacDonald L, Yazdi HM. Fine needle aspiration biopsy of Hashimoto's thyroiditis: sources of diagnostic error. Acta Cytol. 1999;43:400–6.
15. Nguyen GK, Husain M, Akin MR. Cytodiagnosis of benign and malignant Hurthle cell lesions of the thyroid by fine-needle aspiration biopsy. Diagn Cytopathol. 1999;20:261–5.
16. Giorgadze T, Rossi ED, Fadda G, Gupta PK, LiVolis VA, Baloch Z. Does the fine-needle aspiration diagnosis of "Hurthle cell neoplasm/follicular neoplasm with oncocytic features" denote increased risk of malignancy? Diagn Cytopathol. 2004;31:307–12.
17. Mete O, Asa SL. Oncocytes, oxyphils, Hürthle, and Askanazy cells: morphological and molecular features of oncocytic thyroid nodules. Endocr Pathol. 2010;21:16–24.
18. Baloch ZW, LiVolsi VA. Our approach to follicular-patterned lesions of the thyroid. J Clin Pathol. 2007;60:244–50.
19. Lloyd RV, Osamura RY, Klöppel GRJ, editors. World Health Organization classification of Tumours of endocrine organs. 4th ed. IARC Press; 2017.
20. Asa S. My approach to oncocytic tumours of the thyroid. J Clin Pathol. 2004;57(3):225–32.
21. Kroeker T, Prisman E, Shah M, , MacMillan C, Freeman JL. Hurthle cell lesions – a retrospective review of final surgical pathology. Thyroid Disord Ther 2014; 3(155): 2.
22. Elliott DD, Pitman MB, Bloom L, Faquin WC. Fine-needle aspiration biopsy of Hurthle cell lesions of the thyroid gland: a cytomorphologic study of 139 cases with statistical analysis. Cancer. 2006;108(2):102–9.
23. Barnabei A, Ferretti E, Baldelli R, Procaccini A, Spriano G, Appetecchia M. Hurthle cell tumours of the thyroid. Personal experience and review of the literature. Acta Otorhinolaryngol Ital. 2009;29(6):305–11.
24. McHenry CR, Thomas SR, Slusarczyk SJ, Khiyami A. Follicular or Hu rthle cell neoplasm of the thyroid: can clinical factors be used to predict carcinoma and determine extent of thyroidectomy? Surgery. 1999;126(4):798–804.
25. Pisanu A, Di Chiara B, Reccia I, Uccheddu A. Oncocytic cell tumors of the thyroid: factors predicting malignancy and influencing prognosis, treatment decisions, and outcomes. World J Surg. 2010;34(4):836–43.
26. Yang YJ, Khurana KK. Diagnostic utility of intracytoplasmic lumen and transgressing vessels in evaluation of Hurthle cell lesions by fine-needle aspiration. Arch Pathol Lab Med. 2001;125(8):1031–5.
27. Lee KH, Shin JH, Ko ES, Hahn SY, Kim JS, Kim JH, et al. Predictive factors of malignancy in patients with cytologically suspicious for Hurthle cell neoplasm of thyroid nodules. Int J Surg. 2013;11(9):898–902.
28. Mills SC, Haq M, Smellie WJ, Harmer C. Hurthle cell carcinoma of the thyroid: retrospective review of 62 patients treated at the Royal Marsden Hospital between 1946 and 2003. Eur J Surg Oncol. 2009;35(3):230–4.
29. Hoos A, Stojadinovic A, Singh B, Dudas ME, Leung DH, Shaha AR, et al. Clinical significance of molecular expression profiles of Hurthle cell tumors of the thyroid gland analyzed via tissue microarrays. Am J Pathol. 2002;160(1):175–83.
30. Maizlin ZV, Wiseman SM, Vora P, Kirby JM, Mason AC, Filipenko D, et al. Hurthle cell neoplasms of the thyroid: sonographic appearance and histologic characteristics. J Ultrasound Med. 2008;27(5):751–7.
31. Cannon J. The significance of Hürthle cells in thyroid disease. Oncologist. 2011;16(10):1380–7.
32. Melck A, Bugis S, Baliski C, Irvine R, Anderson DW, Wilkins G, et al. Hemithyroidectomy: the preferred initial surgical approach for management of Hurthle cell neoplasm. Am J Surg. 2006;191(5):593–7.
33. Chao T-C, Lin J-D, ChenM-F. Surgical treatment of Hurthle cell tumors of the thyroid. World J Surg. 2005;29(2):164–8.
34. Chen H, Nicol TL, Zeiger MA, Dooley WC, Ladenson PW, Cooper DS, et al. Hurthle cell neoplasms of the thyroid: are there factors predictive of malignancy? Ann Surg. 1998;227(4):542–6.
35. Hudak K, Mazeh H, Sippel RS, Chen H. Hürthle cell metaplasia on fine-needle aspiration biopsy is not by itself an indication for thyroid surgery. Am J Surg. 2012;203(3):287–91.

36. Montone KT, Baloch ZW, LiVolsi VA. The thyroid Hurthle (oncocytic) cell and its associated pathologic conditions: a surgical pathology and cytopathology review. Arch Pathol Lab Med. 2008;132(8):1241–50.
37. Baloch ZW, LiVolsi VA, Asa SL, Rosai J, Merino MJ, Randolph G, et al. Diagnostic terminology and morphologic criteria for cytologic diagnosis of thyroid lesions: a synopsis of the National Cancer Institute thyroid fine-needle aspiration state of the science conference. Diagn Cytopathol. 2008;36:425–37.
38. Cibas ES, Ali SZ. The Bethesda system for reporting thyroid cytopathology. Thyroid. 2009;19:1159–65.
39. Layfield LJ, Cibas ES, Baloch Z. Thyroid fine needle aspiration cytology: a review of the National Cancer Institute state of the science symposium. Cytopathology. 2010;21:75–85.
40. Troncone G, Volante M, Iaccarino A, Zeppa P, Cozzolino I, Malapelle U, et al. Cyclin D1 and D3 overexpression predicts malignant behavior in thyroid fine-needle aspirates suspicious for Hürthle cell neoplasms. Cancer. 2009;117:522–9.
41. Wakely PE. Oncocytic and oncocyte-like lesions of the head and neck. Ann Diagn Pathol. 2008;12:222–30.
42. Jaffar R, Mohanty SK, Khan A, Fischer AH. Hemosiderin laden macrophages and hemosiderin within follicular cells distinguish benign follicular lesions from follicular neoplasms. Cytojournal. 2009;6:3–9.
43. Caraway NP, Sneige N, Samaan NA. Diagnostic pitfalls in thyroid fine-needle aspiration: a review of 394 cases. Diagn Cytopathol. 1993;9(3):345–50.
44. DeMay RM. Thyroid gland. Chapter 12. In: In: DeMay RM., editor. The art and science of cytopathology, vol. 2. 2nd ed. Hong Kong: ASCP Press; 2012. p. 863–915.
45. Kini SR. Chapter 8: Hurtle cell lesions. In: Kini SR, editor. Thyroid cytopathology. An atlas and text. Philadelphia: Wolters Kluwer, Lippincott Williams Wilkins; 2008. p. 100–31.
46. Galera-Davidson H. Diagnostic problems in thyroid FNAs. Diagn Cytopathol. 1997;17:422–8.
47. Poropatitch G, Marcus D, Oertel YC. Hashimoto's thyroiditis: fine needle aspiration cytology of 50 asymptomatic cases. Diagn Cytopathol. 1994;11:141–5.
48. Kauffmann PR, Dejax C, de Latour M, Dauplat J. The meaning and predictivity of Hürthle cells in fine needle aspiration cytology for thyroid nodular disease. Eur J Surg Oncol. 2004;30(7):786–9.
49. Kumar N, Ray C, Jain S. Aspiration cytology of Hashimoto's thyroiditis in an endemic area. Cytopathology. 2002;13(1):31–9.
50. Barroeta JE, Baloch ZW, Lal P, Pasha TL, Zhang PJ, LiVolsi VA. Diagnostic value of differential expression of CK19, Galectin-3, HBME-1, ERK, RET, and p16 in benign and malignant follicular-derived lesions of the thyroid: an immunohistochemical tissue microarray analysis. Endocr Pathol. 2006;17(3):225–34.
51. Hedinger C, Williams E, Sobin L. Histological typing of thyroid Tumours. In: World Health Organisation international histological classification of Tumours. 2nd ed. Albany, NY: Springer; 1988.
52. Layfield LJ, Lones MA. Necrosis in thyroid nodules after fine needle aspiration biopsy: report of two cases. Acta Cytol. 1991;35:427–30.
53. Bolat F, Kayaselcuk F, Nursal TZ, Reyhan M, Bal N, Yildirim S, Tuncer I. Histopathological changes in thyroid tissue after fine needle aspiration biopsy. Pathol Res Pract. 2007;203(9):641–5.
54. Galera-Davidson H, González-Cámpora R. Chapter 23: Thyroid. In: Wilbur MB, editor. Comprehensive cytopathology. 3rd ed. Edinburgh: WB Saunders; 2008. p. 633–70.
55. Clark D, Faquin W. Hurthle cell lesions. In: Thyroid cytopathology. US: Springer; 2010. p. 93–107.
56. Kasper K, Stewart J III, Das K. Fine needle aspiration cytology of thyroid nodules with Hürthle cells: cytomorphologic predictors for neoplasms, improving diagnostic accuracy and overcoming pitfalls. J Am Soc Cytopathol. 2012;1(1):S62–3.
57. Hurthle K. Beitrage zur Kenntniss des sekretionsvorgangs in der childdr use. Arch Gesammte Physiolie Menschen Thiere. 1894;56:1–44.

58. Bonilla AJ, Caudill JL, Goellner JR. Neoplastic versus non-neoplastic Hurthle cell lesions: the diagnostic role of transgressing vessels and intracytoplasmic inclusions [abstract]. Acta Cytol. 1999;43:951.
59. Gonzales-Campora R, Herrero-Zapatero A, Lerma E, Sanchez F, Galera H. Hurthle cell and mitochondrion-rich tumors. A clinicpathologic study. Cancer. 1986;57:1154–63.
60. Renshaw AA. Hurthle cell carcinoma is a better gold standard than Hurthle cell neoplasm for fine-needle aspiration of the thyroid. Defining more consistent and specific cytologic criteria. Cancer Cytopathol. 2002;96:261–6.
61. Wu HH, Clouse J, Ren R. Fine-needle aspiration cytology of Hurthle cell carcinoma of the thyroid. Diagn Cytopathol. 2008;36:149–54.
62. Schlinkert RT, van Heerden JA, Goellner JR, Gharib H, Smith SL, Rosales RF, et al. Factors that predict malignant thyroid lesions when fine-needle aspiration is "suspicious for follicular neoplasm". Mayo Clin Proc. 1997;72:913–6.
63. Tyler DS, Winchester DJ, Caraway NP, Hickey RC, Evans DB. Indeterminate fine-needle aspiration biopsy of the thyroid: identification of subgroups at high-risk for invasive carcinoma. Surgery. 1994;116:1054–60.
64. Tuttle RM, Lemar H, Burch HB. Clinical features associated with an increased risk of thyroid malignancy in patients with follicular neoplasia by fine-needle aspiration. Thyroid. 1998;8:377–83.
65. Baloch ZW, LiVolsi VA. Oncocytic lesions of the neuroendocrine system. Semin Diagn Pathol. 1999;16:190–9.
66. Yang GCH, Schreiner AM, Sun W. Can abundant colloid exclude oncocytic (Hurthle cell) carcinoma in thyroid fine needle aspiration? Cytohistological correlation of 127 oncocytic (Hurthle cell) lesions. Cytopathology. 2013;24:185–93.
67. McIvor NP, Freeman JL, Rosen I, Bedard YC. Value of fine needle aspiration in the diagnosis of Hurthle cell neoplasm. Head Neck. 1993;15:335–41.
68. Skoog L, Tani E. Hurthle cell carcinoma: time for a drastic change? Cancer Cytopathol. 2002;96:259–60.
69. Roh MH, Jo VY, Stelow EB, Faquin WC, Zou KH, Alexander EK, et al. The predictive value of the fine-needle aspiration diagnosis suspicious for a "FNHCT" in patients with Hashimoto thyroiditis. Am J Clin Pathol. 2012;120:73–86.
70. Gharib H, Goeller JR, Zinsmeister AR, Grant CS, Heerden JA. Fine-needle aspiration biopsy of the thyroid. The problem of suspicious cytologic findings. Ann Intern Med. 1984;101:25–8.
71. Sorrenti S, Trimboli P, Catanai A, Ulisse S, De Antoni E, D'Armiento M. Comparison of malignancy rate in thyroid nodules with cytology of indeterminate follicular or indeterminate Hurthle cell neoplasm. Thyroid. 2009;19:355–60.
72. Castro MR, Epiritu RP, Bahn RS, et al. Predictors of malignancy in patients with cytologically suspicious thyroid nodules. Thyroid. 2011;21:91–1198.
73. Sangalli G, Serio G, Zampatti C, Bellotti M, Lomuscio G. Fine needle aspiration cytology of the thyroid: a comparison of 5469 cytological and final histological diagnoses. Cytopathology. 2006;17:245–50.
74. Kelman AS, Rathn A, Leibowitz J, Burstein DE, Haber RS. Thyroid cytology and the risk of malignancy in thyroid nodules: importance of nuclear atypia in indeterminate specimens. Thyroid. 2001;11:271–7.
75. Deandra M, Ragazzoni F, Motta M, Torchio B, Mormile A, Garino F, et al. Diagnostic value of a cytomorphological subclassification of follicular patterned thyroid lesions: a study of 927 consecutive cases with histological correlation. Thyroid. 2010;20:1077–83.
76. Renshaw AA. Should "atypical follicular cells" in thyroid fine-needle aspirates be subclassified? Cancer Cytopathol. 2010;118:186–9.
77. Raparia K, Min SK, Mody DR, Anton R, Amrikacki M. Clinical outcomes for "suspicious" category in thyroid fine-needle aspiration biopsy: patient's sex and nodule size are possible predictors of malignancy. Arch Pathol Lab Med. 2009;133:787–90.

78. Yuan L, Nasr C, Bena JF, Elsheikh TM. Hürthle cell-predominant thyroid fine needle aspiration cytology: a four risk-factor model highly accurate in excluding malignancy and predicting neoplasm. Diagn Cytopathol. 2022;50(9):424–35.
79. Wong KS, Angell TE, Barletta JA, Krane JF. Hurthle cell lesions of the thyroid: progress made and challenges remaining. Cancer Cytopathol. 2021;129:347–62.
80. Chiappetta G, Toti P, Cetta F, Giuliano A, Pentimalli F, Amendola I, et al. The RET/PTC oncogene is frequently activated in oncocytic thyroid tumors (Hurthle cell adenomas and carcinomas), but not in oncocytic hyperplastic lesions. J Clin Endocrinol Metab. 2002;87(1):364–9.
81. de Vries MM, Celestino R, Castro P, Eloy C, Máximo V, van der Wal JE, Plukker JT, Links TP, Hofstra RM, Sobrinho-Simões M, Soares P. RET/PTC rearrangement is prevalent in follicular Hürthle cell carcinomas. Histopathology. 2012;61(5):833–43.
82. Alexander EK, Kennedy GC, Baloch ZW, Cibas ES, Chudova D, Diggans J, et al. Preoperative diagnosis of benign thyroid nodules with indeterminate cytology. N Engl J Med. 2012;367:705–15.
83. Lastra RR, Pramick MR, Crammer CJ, LiVolsi VA, Baloch ZW. Implications of a suspicious afirma test result in thyroid fine-needle aspiration cytology: an institutional experience. Cancer Cytopathol. 2014;122:737–44.
84. Brauner E, Holmes BJ, Krane JF, Nishino M, Zurakowski D, Hennessey JV, et al. Performance of the Afirma gene expression classifier in Hürthle cell thyroid nodules differs from other indeterminate thyroid nodules. Thyroid. 2015;25:789–96.
85. Wu JX, Young S, Hung ML, Li N, Yang SE, Cheung DS, et al. Clinical factors influencing the performance of gene expression classifier testing in indeterminate thyroid nodules. Thyroid. 2016;26:916–22.
86. Parajuli S, Jug R, Ahmadi S, Jiang X "Sara." Hurthle cell predominance impacts results of Afirma gene expression classifier and ThyroSeq molecular panel performance in indeterminate thyroid nodules. Diagn Cytopathol 2019; 47: 1177–1183.
87. Patel KN, Angell TE, Babiarz J, Barth NM, Blevins T, Duh QY, et al. Performance of a genomic sequencing classifier for the preoperative diagnosis of cytologically indeterminate thyroid nodules. JAMA Surg. 2018;153:817–24.
88. Angell TE, Heller HT, Cibas ES, Barletta JA, Kim MI, Krane JF, et al. Independent comparison of the Afirma genomic sequencing classifier and gene expression classifier for cytologically indeterminate thyroid nodules. Thyroid. 2019;29:650–6.
89. Endo M, Nabhan F, Porter K, Roll K, Shirley LA, Azaryan I, et al. Afirma gene sequencing classifier compared with gene expression classifier in indeterminate thyroid nodules. Thyroid. 2019;29:1115–24.
90. San Martin VT, Lawrence L, Bena J, Madhun NZ, Berber E, Elsheikh TM, et al. Real-world comparison of Afirma GEC and GSC for the assessment of cytologically indeterminate thyroid nodules. J Clin Endocrinol Metab. 2020;105:428–35.
91. Nikiforova MN, Mercurio S, Wald AI, Barbi de Moura M, Callenberg K, Santana-Santos L, et al. Analytical performance of the ThyroSeq v3 genomic classifier for cancer diagnosis in thyroid nodules. Cancer. 2018;124:1682–90.
92. Ohori NP, Landau MS, Manroa P, Schoedel KE, Seethala RR. Molecular-derived estimation of risk of malignancy for indeterminate thyroid cytology diagnoses. J Am Soc Cytopathol. 2020;9:213–20.
93. Steward DL, Carty SE, Sippel RS, Yang SP, Sosa JA, Sipos JA, et al. Performance of a multigene genomic classifier in thyroid nodules with indeterminate cytology. JAMA Oncol. 2018;15213:1–8.
94. Schatz-Siemers N, Brandler TC, Oweity T, Sun W, Hernandez A, Levine P. Hürthle cell lesions on thyroid fine needle aspiration cytology: molecular and histologic correlation. Diagn Cytopathol. 2019;47:977–85.

7 Oncocytic (Hürthle Cell) Lesions: Controversy of Management

7.1 General Considerations

The management of thyroid nodules with oncocytic/Hürthle cell–predominant cytology is challenging given the wide spectrum of possible etiologies, ranging from benign nonneoplastic conditions to neoplastic conditions that may be benign (oncocytic adenoma/Hürthle cell adenoma—HCA), or malignant (oncocytic carcinoma of the thyroid/Hürthle cell carcinoma—HCC). Clinicians must make thoughtful decisions regarding patients presenting with thyroid nodules and fine-needle aspiration biopsy (FNAB) aspirates containing oncocytic (Hürthle) cells. Being familiar with the expressions commonly used by one's institution and referring laboratories cannot be emphasized enough. Equally important is the histological resultant final pathology based on those FNAB reports. For example, in one institution, an FNAB report of "suspicious for X carcinoma" may carry a $\geq 90\%$ rate of malignancy on final histology, whereas in another, the rate may be closer to 60–70%. This information may greatly influence operative decision and therapeutic plan [1].

It is noteworthy that FNAB specimens consistent with follicular neoplasm (FN) or oncocytic/Hürthle cell neoplasm (HCN) are variously categorized as indeterminate, suspicious, cellular, or, in the Bethesda system, category 4 (B-IV). They represent approximately 20% of all FNAB results in patients with thyroid nodules. Of these, about 10% are HCNs. As previously stated, although referral patterns may affect malignancy rates, historically, 15–30% of patients with a nodule and FNAB results consistent with FN or HCN are subsequently diagnosed with a malignant lesion [1].

It is well known that surgery is an important line for managing thyroid pathologies. For oncocytic/Hürthle cell lesions, however, prudency of surgical decision, appropriateness of surgery extent, and postoperative management are controversial. Although the outcome of oncocytic/HCC has been somewhat variable, accurately

M. Sakr, *Oncocytic (Hürthle Cell) Thyroid Lesions*,
https://doi.org/10.1007/978-3-032-03115-0_7

identifying HCC is nevertheless important due to the potential for more aggressive disease. Oncocytic/HCC may portend a lower 10-year survival compared with other well-differentiated thyroid cancers (DTCs) [2], frequently metastasizes to lymph nodes (LNs) and distant sites, and often responds poorly to radioactive iodine (RAI) therapy [3].

Like other nodules with indeterminate cytology, ultrasonographic features, molecular characteristics, and other clinical findings are considered to improve the clinical evaluation of oncocytic/Hürthle cell–predominant lesions. Validated sonographic features or patterns are now used to select thyroid nodules for FNA and to predict malignancy more accurately [4–7]. Assessment with ultrasonography (US) also improves the risk stratification of B-III and B-IV nodules [8–12]; however, it may be less reliable for identifying oncocytic/HCC, since these neoplasms more often present as solid, isoechoic, or hyper-echoic nodules that lack the high-risk features typical of papillary thyroid carcinoma (PTC), such as marked hypoechogenicity, invasive borders, or frequent involvement of cervical LNs [13, 14].

Evaluation by fluorodeoxyglucose-positron emission tomography (FDG-PET) has been also used to assess thyroid nodules for malignancy, but data reported in the literature also suggest more limited benefit for oncocytic/Hürthle cell nodules [15].

7.2 To Operate or Not to Operate

7.2.1 Whether or Not to Operate

The first controversy in the management of oncocytic/Hürthle cell lesions is to operate or not to operate. Not all lesions with oncocytic (Hürthle) cells on fine needle aspiration biopsy (FNAB) require surgical intervention. The importance of clinical context must be emphasized. Given the high incidence of malignancy in their series, Azidan et al. [16] concluded that the cytological detection of oncocytic (Hürthle) cells in FNAB was an indication for surgery after excluding chronic lymphocytic thyroiditis (Hashimoto's thyroiditis). On the contrary, subsequent studies suggested that the percentage, rather than the mere detection, of oncocytic (Hürthle) cells should guide the operative decision with the detection of more than 50% oncocytic (Hürthle) cells being an adequate criterion for opting surgery [17, 18].

Refined versions of commercially available molecular tests have markedly improved accuracy of diagnosis of oncocytic/Hürthle cell–predominant nodules [19–21] helping identify those that have a high likelihood of benignity and that can be managed with US observation rather than surgical resection. Even if a clinically significant malignancy is present, surgery may, rarely, not be pursued due to a patient's comorbidities or short-life expectancy. More commonly, resection is determined to be necessary even if a molecular test were to indicate a benign process. Very large size, compressive symptoms, or suspicious sonographic features may all indicate a need for resection, and in such situations, molecular testing generally should *not* be performed [15].

7.2.2 Observation and Surveillance

The initial limitations of molecular testing of oncocytic/Hürthle cell lesions led to caution against its use in this context by some clinical guidelines [22]. However, refined versions of commercially available molecular tests have markedly improved accuracy of diagnosis of oncocytic/Hürthle cell–predominant nodules helping identify those lesions that have a high likelihood of benignity and that can be managed with ultrasonography (US) observation rather than surgical resection [19–21].

In general, it is conceivable that aspirates with scattered oncocytic (Hürthle) cells, macro-follicular architecture, or abundant, watery colloid, and those seen in the context of Hashimoto's disease without dominant nodules, as well as those that do not meet the criteria for oncocytic/Hürthle cell neoplasia (HCN) (<75% oncocytic [Hürthle] cells) can generally be observed with surveillance US and a repeat FNAB when indicated.

7.3 How Much to Resect

7.3.1 Whether Hemithyroidectomy or Total Thyroidectomy

A second controversy in the management of oncocytic/Hürthle cell lesions is how much to resect if surgery is indicated. Several issues stand behind such controversy. Firstly, based on the relative rarity of oncocytic/Hürthle cell neoplasms (HCNs) in general [23] and of oncocytic carcinomas (Hürthle cell carcinomas—HCCs) in particular [24], a single institutional experience is usually *not* sufficient to define an ultimate management plan. Secondly, the inability to preoperatively differentiate malignant from benign tumors or even to predict the clinical behavior or outcome usually affect the treatment decision in a way that, given a presumed aggressive nature, more radical surgery is preferable. Thirdly, most studies evaluating the outcome of surgery were retrospective studies confounded by non-matching of variables (age, gender, and tumor size), which also influence the outcome.

7.3.2 Hemithyroidectomy as the Initial Procedure

When surgery is indicated for a nodule diagnosed as Bethesda-III (B-III) or Bethesda-IV (B-IV), thyroid lobectomy is the recommended procedure for diagnostic purposes in the absence of any other considerations [3, 4]. This remains the strategy even for most cases with a positive molecular test, since the positive predictive values of these tests are moderate for these lesions [25, 26]. If the final histopathological diagnosis is "benign," lobectomy would have proved adequate and minimized the risks of surgical complications and postoperative hypothyroidism. For cases in which oncocytic/HCC is confirmed on resection, lobectomy is also considered adequate therapy for minimally invasive, and thus low-risk, oncocytic/HCC [4, 27]. Chindris et al. [28] found no instances of recurrence or disease-specific mortality in a clinical review of 39 cases of minimally invasive HCC (miHCC) over a median follow-up of 70 months. In 2016, Haugen et al. reported that, in contrast, oncocytic/HCCs with gross local invasion or extensive vascular invasion are treated as intermediate- to high-risk for recurrence, and therefore warrant completion thyroidectomy and consideration of radioactive iodine (RAI) therapy [4].

Given the relatively small proportion of oncocytic/HCCs among oncocytic/HCN nodules and the benign course identified in most miHCCs, Kroeker et al. [29], in agreement with previous reports of Parikh et al. in 2013 [30], Melck et al. in 2006 [31], and McHenry et al., in 1999 [32], have also advocated thyroid lobectomy for initial management of oncocytic/HCNs keeping in mind two possibilities. Firstly, proceeding to total thyroidectomy (TT) may be decided immediately if extra-thyroidal extension (ETE) or lymphadenopathy was detected intraoperatively. Secondly, completion thyroidectomy may be planned either a few days of the initial procedure or 3 months later if oncocytic/HCC was revealed on paraffin sections. Additionally, in their large series, Haigh et al. reported that there is no significant association between the extent of thyroidectomy and patient survival [24].

7.3.3 Total Thyroidectomy as the Initial Procedure

7.3.3.1 Justifications of Assertive Resection

Total thyroidectomy (TT), as an initial surgery for oncocytic/HCC, was supported by Mills et al. [33], Paunovic et al. [34], and Khafif et al. [35], as they noticed favorable outcomes associated with assertive resection. A lower threshold for selecting initial radical surgery was advocated by Chen et al. [36], Sippel et al. [37], and Zhang et al. [38] in large size tumors since they detected significant correlation with malignancy. In fact, the latter opinion is fueled by several facts: (1) the aggressive course identified in some reports [39, 40], (2) the low avidity for radioactive iodine (RAI) [41], (3) the low incidence of complications of TT in experienced hands [34, 36], which substantially increase in re-operative surgery, (4) the availability of replacement therapy, (5) the privilege of using thyroglobulin (Tg) as a marker for recurrence, and (6) the potential use of RAI for ablating a possible remnant [42].

7.3.3.2 Indications of Total Thyroidectomy

In some situations, an initial total thyroidectomy (TT) may be preferable as in the following conditions:

- *A history of prior head and/or neck irradiation:* It often predisposes patients to multifocal disease, including a coexisting papillary thyroid carcinoma (PTC). These patients should generally undergo TT as an initial operation because the incidence of carcinoma approaches 40% as reported earlier by McHenry et al. [43].

- *Patients with nodules in the contralateral lobe*: Such patients may be considered for a single-stage TT.
- *Large nodules:* Although size alone cannot be directly correlated with malignancy, large nodules (>4 cm) may be more likely to be carcinomas on final histology. This factor is a "relative" indication, which on an individualized basis may be used to identify those patients who might benefit from a TT at first operation [44–46].
- *High level of anxiety:* Patients who have a high level of concern or anxiety about the possibility of cancer or desire to avoid a second operative procedure are also justifiably served by undergoing a single total procedure at the outset. These patients should be informed that this is a more aggressive approach and will, in 70–80% of cases, be done for a benign process. They should be fully informed of the risks associated with the procedure [43].

7.4 To Use or Not to Use Radiotherapy

7.4.1 Whether or Not to Use Radioactive Iodine (RAI)

A third controversy in managing oncocytic/HCC is whether or not to use RAI postoperatively. Although oncocytic/HCC generally fail to concentrate RAI [47], its controversial role in management is fueled by the varying results published in the literature. In 2003, Lopez-Penabad et al. [48] reported a survival benefit when RAI was used in patients with oncocytic/HCC for remnant ablation, but *not* in metastatic disease.

On the other hand, in their series, Sanders et al. [41] stated that using RAI did *not* improve outcome of patients with oncocytic/HCC. Moreover, Mills et al. [33] reported, in 2009, a worse disease-free survival (DFS) conferred by RAI ablation and therapy. However, the National Comprehensive Cancer Network (NCCN) 2013 Guidelines have considered RAI ablation for suspected or proven thyroid bed uptake, and RAI treatment for suspected or proven RAI responsive residual tumor in postoperative management of the histologically proven oncocytic/HCCs [49].

Malignant HCNs do require aggressive surgery, because they are poorly responsive to chemotherapy, do not concentrate iodine, and are generally not radiosensitive. When metastases are present at the time of diagnosis, aggressive surgical approaches do not appear to have much influence on the long-term outcome and are mainly palliative, underscoring the need to perform timely FNAB of solid thyroid nodules [50]. Some investigators have shown that oncocytic/HCNs demonstrate the ability to synthesize thyroglobulin (Tg) and may stain positive with immunohistochemistry (IHC) techniques; thus, they suggested evaluating each case on an individual basis post-thyroidectomy and treating with a therapeutic dose of ^{131}I, should radioactive iodine uptake be evident [44]. As a general rule, however, only 5–10% of oncocytic/HCCs take up ^{131}I, in contrast to approximately 75% of follicular thyroid carcinomas (FTCs) [43].

7.4.2 Whether or Not to Use External-Beam Radiation Therapy (EBRT)

It is worth mentioning that although external-beam radiation therapy (EBRT) has been used with success in the palliation of bone metastases, it has not been shown to be effective for palliation of residual neck and soft tissue disease as well as metastases [44].

7.5 Conclusion

Oncocytic (Hürthle) cells may be found in different lesions across the wide spectrum of thyroid disorders. The significance of oncocytic (Hürthle) cells in thyroid pathology is currently uncertain. Although surgery may not always be mandatory when an FNAB specimen contains oncocytic (Hürthle) cells, a major concern is that of missing a malignant lesion by abstaining from surgery [18]. Although the mere presence of oncocytic (Hürthle) cells or oncocytic (Hürthle) cell change in an FNAB smear should *not* immediately trigger clinical worry and perhaps an unnecessary surgical referral, clinical context and an appreciation of the variety of findings associated with oncocytes may help guide the clinician to the appropriate management and follow-up [51].

Because oncocytic/Hürthle cell lesions present a particularly challenging component of thyroid pathology, the cornerstone critical to managing oncocytic/Hürthle cell nodules is a highly skilled, experienced pathologist [52]. Although the presence of vascular or capsular invasion on permanent histology may easily be recognized, no unequivocal cytological parameters currently exist that can define carcinoma before or during thyroidectomy. Likewise, there are no specific, reliable clinical factors to distinguish benign from malignant oncocytic/HCN. The safest course of action is for all patients with a diagnosis of oncocytic/HCN, made by a cytopathologist with adequate expertise and using accepted guidelines and criteria, to undergo surgical excision in order to obtain a definitive diagnosis [53].

Standardizing a management plan needs a two-pronged approach. First, starting prospectively designed randomized controlled clinical trials evaluating the efficacy of different management plans on large sample of patients, which given the rarity and long natural history of the disease, would appropriately be multi-institutional. Second, employing molecular biology techniques and advanced imaging tools would resolve much of the diagnostic controversy and subsequently the management debate or controversy; for example, a recently described gene expression classifier has achieved 92% sensitivity in detecting "suspicious" nodules, which were cytologically "indeterminate" [54]. In addition, sonographic elastography scoring may contribute to better characterization of oncocytic/Hürthle cell lesions [55].

References

1. McHenry CR, Thomas SR, Slusarczyk SJ, Khiyami A. Follicular or Hürthle cell neoplasm of the thyroid: can clinical factors be used to predict carcinoma and determine extent of thyroidectomy? Surgery. 1999;126:798–804.
2. Hundahl SA, Fleming ID, Fremgen AM, Menck HR. A national cancer data base report on 53,856 cases of thyroid carcinoma treated in the U.S., 1985-1995. Cancer. 1998;83:2638–48.
3. Ahmadi S, Stang M, Jiang XS, Sosa JA. Hürthle cell carcinoma: current perspectives. Onco Targets Ther. 2016;9:6873–84.
4. Haugen BR, Alexander EK, Bible KC, et al. 2015 American Thyroid Association management guidelines for adult patients with thyroid nodules and differentiated thyroid cancer. Thyroid. 2016;26:1–133.
5. Valderrabano P, Klippenstein DL, Tourtelot JB, et al. New American Thyroid Association sonographic patterns for thyroid nodules perform well in medullary thyroid carcinoma: institutional experience, systematic review, and meta-analysis. Thyroid. 2016;26:1093–100.
6. Ha EJ, Na DG, Moon WJ, Lee YH, Choi N. Diagnostic performance of ultrasound-based risk-stratification systems for thyroid nodules: comparison of the 2015 American Thyroid Association guidelines with the 2016 Korean Thyroid Association/Korean Society of Thyroid Radiology and 2017 American College of Radioology guidelines. Thyroid. 2018;28:1532–7.
7. Castellana M, Castellana C, Treglia G, Giorgino F, Giovanella L, Russ G, et al. Performance of five ultrasound risk stratification systems in selecting thyroid nodules for FNA. J Clin Endocrinol Metab. 2020;105:1659–69.
8. Li F, Pan D, Wu Y, Peng J, Li Q, Gui X, et al. Ultrasound characteristics of thyroid nodules facilitate interpretation of the malignant risk of Bethesda system III/IV thyroid nodules and inform therapeutic schedule. Diagn Cytopathol. 2019;47:881–9.
9. Barbosa TLM, Junior COM, Graf H, Cavalvanti T, Trippia MA, da Silveira Ugino RT, et al. ACR TI-RADS and ATA US scores are helpful for the management of thyroid nodules with indeterminate cytology. BMC Endocr Disord. 2019;19:1–11.
10. Ahmadi S, Herbst R, Oyekunle T, Jiang X, Strickland K, Roman S, et al. Using the ATA and ACR TI-RADS sonographic classifications as adjunctive predictors of malignancy for indeterminate thyroid nodules. Endocr Pract. 2019;25:908–17.
11. Trimboli P, Deandrea M, Mormile A, Ceriani L, Garino F, Limone PP, et al. American Thyroid Association ultrasound system for the initial assessment of thyroid nodules: use in stratifying the risk of malignancy of indeterminate lesions. Head Neck. 2018;40:722–7.
12. Valderrabano P, McGettigan MJ, Lam CA, Khazai L, Thompson ZJ, Chung CH, et al. Thyroid nodules with indeterminate cytology: utility of the American Thyroid Association sonographic patterns for cancer risk stratification. Thyroid. 2018;28:1004–12.
13. Maizlin ZV, Wiseman SM, Vora P, Kirby JM, Mason AC, Filipenko D, et al. Hurthle cell neoplasms of the thyroid: sonographic appearance and histologic characteristics. J Ultrasound Med. 2008;27:751–7.
14. Castellana M, Piccardo A, Virili C, Scappaticcio L, Grani G, Durante C, et al. Can ultrasound systems for risk stratification of thyroid nodules identify follicular carcinoma? Cancer Cytopathol. 2020;128:250–9.
15. Wong KS, Angell TE, Barletta JA, Krane JF. Hurthle cell lesions of the thyroid: progress made and challenges remaining. Cancer Cytopathol. 2021;129:347–62.
16. Azadian A, Rosen IB, Walfish PG, Asa SL. Managemen considerations in Hürthle cell carcinoma. Surgery. 1995;118(4):711–5.
17. Hudak K, Mazeh H, Sippel RS, Chen H. Hürthle cell metaplasia on fine-needle aspiration biopsy is not by itself an indication for thyroid surgery. Am J Surg. 2012;203(3):287–91.

18. Kauffmann PR, Dejax C, de Latour M, Dauplat J. The meaning and predictivity of Hürthle cells in fine needle aspiration cytology for thyroid nodular disease. Eur J Surg Oncol. 2004;30(7):786–9.
19. Wu JX, Young S, Hung ML, Li N, Yang SE, Cheung DS, et al. Clinical factors influencing the performance of Gene Expression Classifier testing in indeterminate thyroid nodules. Thyroid. 2016;26:916–22.
20. Patel KN, Angell TE, Babiarz J, Barth NM, Blevins T, Duh QY, et al. Performance of a genomic sequencing classifier for the preoperative diagnosis of cytologically indeterminate thyroid nodules. JAMA Surg. 2018;153:817–24.
21. Endo M, Nabhan F, Porter K, Roll K, Shirley LA, Azaryan I, et al. Afirma gene sequencing classifier compared with gene expression classifier in indeterminate thyroid nodules. Thyroid. 2019;29:1115–24.
22. Haddad RI, Nasr C, Bischoff L, Busaidy NL, Byrd D, Callender G, et al. NCCN guidelines insights: thyroid carcinoma, version 2.2018 featured updates to the NCCN guidelines. JNCCN J Natl Compr Cancer Netw. 2018;16:1429–40.
23. Chen H, Udelsman R. Chapter 14: Hürthle cell adenoma and carcinoma. In: Kebebew OHC-YD, editor. Textbook of endocrine surgery. 2nd ed. Philadelphia: WB Saunders; 2005. p. 123–8.
24. Haigh PI, Urbach DR. The treatment and prognosis of Hürthle cell follicular thyroid carcinoma compared with its non-Hürthle cell counterpart. Surgery. 2005;138(6):1152–8.
25. Brauner E, Holmes BJ, Krane JF, Ishino M, Zurakowski D, Hennessey JV, et al. Performance of the afirma gene expression classifier in Hürthle cell thyroid nodules differs from other indeterminate thyroid nodules. Thyroid. 2015;25:789–96.
26. San Martin VT, Lawrence L, Bena J, Madhun NZ, Berber E, Elsheikh TM, et al. Real-world comparison of Afirma GEC and GSC for the assessment of cytologically indeterminate thyroid nodules. J Clin Endocrinol Metab. 2020;105:428–35.
27. Haddad RI, Bischoff L, Ball D, Bernet V, Blomain E, Busaidy NL, et al. Thyroid carcinoma, Version 2.2022, NCCN clinical practice guidelines in oncology. J Natl Compr Cancer Netw. 2022;20(8):925–51.
28. Chindris AM, Casler JD, Bernet VJ, Rivera M, Thomas C, Kachergus JM, et al. Clinical and molecular features of Hürthle cell carcinoma of the thyroid. J Clin Endocrinol Metab. 2015;100:55–62.
29. Kroeker T, Prisman E, Shah M, MacMillan C, Freeman JL. Hurthle cell lesions-a retrospective review of final surgical pathology. Thyroid Disord Ther. 2014;3(2):1000155.
30. Parikh PP, Allan BJ, Lew JI. Surgeon-performed ultrasound predictors of malignancy in patients with Hürthle cell neoplasms of the thyroid. J Surg Res. 2013;184(1):247–52.
31. Melck A, Bugis S, Baliski C, Irvine R, Anderson DW, Wilkins G, et al. Hemithyroidectomy: the preferred initial surgical approach for management of Hurthle cell neoplasm. Am J Surg. 2006;191(5):593–7.
32. McHenry CR, Thomas SR, Slusarczyk SJ, Khiyami A. Follicular or Hu rthle cell neoplasm of the thyroid: can clinical factors be used to predict carcinoma and determine extent of thyroidectomy? Surgery. 1999;126(4):798–804.
33. Mills SC, Haq M, Smellie WJ, Harmer C. Hurthle cell carcinoma of the thyroid: retrospective review of 62 patients treated at the Royal Marsden Hospital between 1946 and 2003. Eur J Surg Oncol. 2009;35(3):230–4.
34. Paunovic I, Krgovic K, Tatic S, Diklic A, Zivaljevic V, Kalezic N, et al. Surgery for thyroid Hürthle cell tumours – a single institution experience. Eur J Surg Oncol. 2006;32(4):458–61.
35. Khafif A, Khafif RA, Attie JN. Hürthle cell carcinoma: a malignancy of low-grade potential. Head Neck. 1999;21(6):506–11.
36. Chen H, Nicol TL, Zeiger MA, Ooley WC, Ladenson PW, Cooper DS, et al. Hurthle cell neoplasms of the thyroid: are there factors predictive of malignancy? Ann Surg. 1998;227(4):542–6.
37. Sippel RS, Elaraj DM, Khanafshar E, Zarnegar R, Kebebew E, Duh QY, et al. Tumor size predicts malignant potential in Hurthle cell neoplasms of the thyroid. World J Surg. 2008;32(5):702–7.

38. Zhang Y, Greenblatt D, Repplinger D, Bargren A, Adler JT, Sippel RS, et al. Older age and larger tumor size predict malignancy in Hürthle cell neoplasms of the thyroid. Ann Surg Oncol. 2008;15(10):2842–6.
39. Kushchayeva Y, Duh Q-Y, Kebebew E, D'Avanzo A, Clark OH. Comparison of clinical characteristics at diagnosis and during follow-up in 118 patients with Hurthle cell or follicular thyroid cancer. Am J Surg. 2008;195(4):457–62.
40. Carcangiu ML, Bianchi S, Savino D, Voynick IM, Rosai J. Follicular Hurthle cell tumors of the thyroid gland. Cancer. 1991;68(9):1944–53.
41. Sanders LE, Silverman M. Follicular and Hürthle cell carcinoma: predicting outcome and directing therapy. Surgery. 1998;124(6):967–74.
42. Chao T-C, Lin J-D, Chen M-F. Surgical treatment of Hurthle cell tumors of the thyroid. World J Surg. 2005;29(2):164–8.
43. McHenry CR, Sandoval BA. Management of follicular and Hürthle cell neoplasms of the thyroid gland. Surg Oncol Clin N Am. 1998;7:893–910.
44. McLeod MK, Thompson NW. Hürthle cell neoplasms of the thyroid. Otolaryngol Clin N Am. 1990;23:441–52.
45. Chen H, Nicol TL, Zeiger MA, Dooley WC, Ladenson PW, Cooper DS, et al. Hürthle cell neoplasms of the thyroid: are there factors predictive of malignancy? Ann Surg. 1998;227:542–6.
46. Zhang YW, Greenblatt DY, Repplinger D, Bargren A, Adler JT, Sippel RS, et al. Older age and larger tumor size predict malignancy in Hürthle cell neoplasms of the thyroid. Ann Surg Oncol. 2008;15:2842–6.
47. Yutan E, Clark O. Hürthle cell carcinoma. Curr Treat Options in Oncol. 2001;2(4):331–5.
48. Lopez-Penabad L, Chiu AC, Hoff AO, Schultz P, Gaztambide S, Ordoñez NG, et al. Prognostic factors in patients with Hurthle cell neoplasms of the thyroid. Cancer. 2003;97(5):1186–94.
49. Gallagher L, Hughes M, McMillian L. National Comprehensive Cancer Network (NCCN) clinical practice guidelines in oncology. Thyroid carcinoma, Version 2. 2013
50. Ahmed M, Bin Yousif H, Greer W, Faraz H, Al Sobhi S, Al Zahrani A, et al. Hürthle cell neoplasm of the thyroid gland. ANZ J Surg. 2008;78:139–43.
51. Montone KT, Baloch ZW, LiVolsi VA. The thyroid Hürthle (oncocytic) cell and its associated pathologic conditions: a surgical pathology and cytopathology review. Arch Pathol Lab Med. 2008;132:1241–50.
52. Grant CS, Barr D, Goellner JR, Hay ID. Benign Hürthle cell tumors of the thyroid: a diagnosis to be trusted? World J Surg. 1988;12:488–95.
53. Pisanu A, Sias L, Uccheddu A. Factors predicting malignancy of Hürthle cell tumors of the thyroid: influence on surgical treatment. World J Surg. 2004;28:761–5.
54. Alexander EK, Kennedy GC, Baloch ZW, Cibas ES, Chudova D, Diggans J, et al. Preoperative diagnosis of benign thyroid nodules with indeterminate cytology. N Engl J Med. 2012;67(8):705–15.
55. Tuzun D, Ersoy R, Kilicyazgan A, Kiyak G, Yalcin S, Cakir B. Elastosonography scoring and strain index of thyroid nodules with Hurthle cells. Minerva Endocrinol. 2014;41(2):157–65.

Oncocytic (Hürthle Cell) Neoplasm: Controversy of Pathological Classification

8

8.1 Thyroid Tumors: Classification

8.1.1 Introduction

Thyroid cancer is the most common endocrine malignancy, but represents only 1% of all newly diagnosed malignancies [1]. The wide spectrum of aggressiveness of thyroid cancer is extraordinary, ranging from differentiated malignancies in which most patients live out close to their normal lifespan, to anaplastic varieties that are almost universally lethal. It is crucial to ensure that patients presenting with thyroid nodules are not over or undertreated. Several classifications of thyroid tumors have thus been proposed.

8.1.2 The 2017 World Health Organization (WHO) Classification

The recent classification of thyroid tumors that was published in 2017 by the World Health Organization (WHO) is summarized in Table 8.1. As may be seen, Hürthle cell tumors are no more considered as a variant or subtype of follicular thyroid carcinoma (FTC), instead, it is considered as a separate pathological entity.

8.1.3 THE 2022 World Health Organization (WHO) Classification

General Changes of the Fifth WHO Edition (2022)

The new classification in the fifth edition of the "WHO Classification of Endocrine and Neuro-endocrine Tumors" that relates to the thyroid gland has divided thyroid tumors into several new categories that allow for a clearer understanding of the cell of origin, pathological features (cytopathology and histopathology), molecular

M. Sakr, *Oncocytic (Hürthle Cell) Thyroid Lesions*,
https://doi.org/10.1007/978-3-032-03115-0_8

Table 8.1 The 2017 classification of thyroid tumors by World Health Organization [2]

Tumor class	Description
Primary tumors	*Epithelial tumors* (a) Tumors of follicular cells: Benign (follicular adenoma): conventional—variants Malignant (carcinoma) Differentiated: follicular carcinoma—papillary carcinoma (conventional—variants) Poorly differentiated: insular—others Undifferentiated (anaplastic) (b) Tumors of C- (and related neuroendocrine) cells: Medullary carcinoma Others (c) Tumors of follicular and C-cells *Sarcoma* *Lymphoma* (and related hematopoietic neoplasms) *Miscellaneous neoplasms*
Secondary tumors	
Tumor-like lesions	1. Tumors with oncocytic (Hürthle cell) features: Oncocytic adenoma (Hürthle cell adenoma) Oncocytic carcinoma (Hürthle cell carcinoma) Papillary oncocytic Hürthle cell tumors 2. Tumors with clear cell features 3. Tumors with squamous features 4. Tumors with mucinous features

classification, and biological behavior [3] (Table 8.2). The current classification also emphasizes the value of biomarkers that may aid diagnosis and provide prognostic information. Moreover, additional entities such as thyroid follicular nodular disease, follicular adenoma with papillary architecture, and oncocytic adenoma of the thyroid are included in the benign follicular cell–derived category.

The WHO fifth edition (2022) has refined the spectrum of papillary thyroid carcinoma (PTC) by aligning invasive encapsulated follicular variant PTCs with FTCs. A RAS-like molecular profile is present in most encapsulated/circumscribed thyroid tumors with a predominance of follicular growth [4, 5]. On the other hand, papillary and/or infiltrative growth and florid nuclear atypia characterize the majority of thyroid tumors with a molecular profile of BRAFV600E [4, 5]. Both thyroid tumors that are RAS- and BRAFV600E-like profiles can have further genetic changes and develop into high-grade malignancies [3]. Follicular cell–derived differentiated thyroid carcinomas may also have high-grade features in the absence of morphological dedifferentiation, and hence, differentiated thyroid carcinomas (DTCs) with high-grade features are now recognized as a distinct morphological entity. The Ki-67 proliferation index reporting is required in all medullary thyroid carcinomas (MTCs) for grading [6].

Table 8.2 2022 WHO classification of thyroid tumors compared to 2017 WHO classification

Changes	2022 WHO classification	2017 WHO classification
	Benign tumors	
Follicular cell–derived neoplasms	FND	N/A
	FA	N/A
	FA with papillary architecture	FA with papillary hyperplasia, hyperfunctioning adenoma: variants of FA
	Oncocytic adenoma	Hürthle cell adenoma (HCA)
	Low-risk neoplasms	
	New subtypes: oncocytic NIFTP, sub-centimeter NIFTP	N/A
	Malignant tumors	
Follicular cell–derived neoplasms	Oncocytic cell carcinoma (OCC)	Hürthle cell carcinoma (HCC)
	PTC	PTC
	Papillary micro-carcinoma: does not stand alone as a subtype and should be used with a subtype designation	Papillary micro-carcinoma variant
	Invasive encapsulated follicular variant papillary carcinoma: separated from different PTC subtypes	Invasive encapsulated follicular variant papillary carcinoma: was a subtype of PTC
	High-grade follicular cell–derived non-anaplastic thyroid	Not applicable
	ATC-SCC pattern	SCC
C-cell-derived tumors	MTC: low- and high-grade[a]	MTC: no grading
Embryonal thyroid neoplasm	Thyroblastoma	Malignant teratoma
Thyroid carcinoma of uncertain histogenesis	Cribriform thyroid carcinoma: No longer a subtype of PTC	Cribriform variant of PTC

FND follicular nodular disease, *FA* follicular adenoma, *HCA* Hürthle cell adenoma, *N/A* not applicable, *NIFTP* noninvasive follicular thyroid neoplasm with papillary-like nuclear features, *OCA* oncocytic carcinoma of the thyroid, *HCC* Hürthle cell carcinoma, *PTC* papillary thyroid carcinoma, *ATC* anaplastic thyroid carcinoma, *SCC* squamous cell carcinoma, *MTC* medullary thyroid carcinoma

[a]Based on tumor necrosis, mitosis, and Ki67

Changes in Terminology

The term "Hürthle cell" is a historical misnomer [7]. In the 2022 WHO classification, "oncocytic cell" has replaced "Hürthle cell." Accordingly, oncocytic adenoma and oncocytic carcinoma of the thyroid are the new names for Hürthle cell adenoma (HCA) and Hürthle cell carcinoma (HCC), respectively.

The term "variant" in thyroid pathology has been used to describe the histological subtype of a distinct tumor type, such as the papillary variant of MTC (MTC).

However, "variant" is a term used frequently in genetics. In the fifth edition of the WHO classification (2022), "subtype" is used instead of "variant" to avoid misunderstanding with genetic variants and to maintain consistency in nomenclature. As a result, "histological subtype" has replaced "histological variant."

The recommendation made by the HUGO Gene Nomenclature Committee is to substitute a double colon (::) (PAX8::PPARG) for the hyphen (−) or forward slash (/) when designating genes that are part of gene fusions [8].

8.1.4 Primary Tumors

Changes in Follicular Cell–Derived Tumors

Follicular cell–derived tumors constitute the majority of thyroid neoplasms. In this new classification, they are divided into benign tumors, low-risk neoplasms, and malignant neoplasms (Table 8.3).

A. ***Benign Neoplasms***

Follicular Adenoma (FA) In the fifth edition (2022), benign neoplasms include not only follicular adenoma (FA) (as in the 2017 edition) but also subtypes (variants) of adenoma that are of diagnostic and clinical significance, including the ones with papillary architecture, which are often hyperfunctional, and oncocytic adenomas (Hürthle cell adenomas—HCAs).

Follicular Nodular Disease (FND) For the first time, there is a detailed account of the multifocal hyperplastic/neoplastic lesions that commonly occur in the clinical setting of multinodular goiter (MNG) [9]; the term thyroid follicular nodular disease (FND) achieved consensus as the best to describe this enigmatic entity thus

Table 8.3 Follicular cell–derived neoplasms (tumors) of the 2022 WHO classification

Benign neoplasms	Low-risk neoplasms	Malignant neoplasms
FND FA FA with papillary architecture Oncocytic adenoma	NIFTP Thyroid FT-UMP Thyroid WD-UMP HTT	PTC FTC OCA IEFV-PTC High-grade follicular cell–derived non-anaplastic thyroid carcinoma PDTC ATC

FND follicular nodular disease, *FA* follicular adenoma, *NIFTP* noninvasive follicular thyroid neoplasm with papillary-like nuclear features, *FT-UMP* follicular tumor of uncertain malignant potential, *WD-UMP* well-differentiated tumor of uncertain malignant potential, *HTT* Hyalinizing trabecular tumor, *PTC* papillary thyroid carcinoma, *FTC* follicular thyroid carcinoma, *OCA* oncocytic carcinoma of the thyroid, *IEFVPTC* invasive encapsulated follicular variant papillary thyroid carcinoma, *FT-PDTC* poorly differentiated thyroid carcinoma, *ATC* anaplastic thyroid carcinoma avoiding the diversity of historical terminology underlying the group entity: adenomatous nodule, adenomatous hyperplasia, nodular hyperplasia, and multinodular goiter.

Follicular Adenomas with Papillary Architecture The benign tumors "FAs with papillary architecture" are frequently encapsulated, noninvasive tumors having intrafollicular centripetal papillary growth, and lacking the nuclear characteristics of (PTC) [3, 9]. On a radionuclide thyroid scan, these tumors appear as "hot" or "warm" nodules because they are frequently related to autonomous hyperfunction [9]. The TSHR, GNAS, or EZH1 mutations and changes that activate the protein kinase A (PKA) pathway are the primary causes of these tumors [10, 11]. These may also manifest in the context of the McCune–Albright and Carney complex syndromes, which are PKA pathway-related diseases caused by GNAS and PRKAR1A mutations [12, 13]. Nonfunctional FAs with papillary architecture can include DICER1 mutations, some of which have been linked to DICER1 syndrome [14–16].

Oncocytic Follicular Adenoma (Hürthle Cell Adenomas—HCA) A subset of FA exhibits oncocytic characteristics, and > 75% of the tumor cells are required for an "oncocytic FA" (Hürthle cell adenomas—HCA) to be diagnosed [3]. Oncocytic thyroid tumors are different from other thyroid neoplasms because they may exhibit specific genetic abnormalities, such as mitochondrial DNA (mtDNA) mutations and higher copy number modifications [17–19].

B. ***Low-Risk Neoplasms***

As seen in Table 8.2, low-risk follicular cell–derived neoplasms include noninvasive follicular thyroid neoplasm with papillary-like nuclear features (NIFTP), follicular tumor of uncertain malignant potential (FT-UMP), well-differentiated tumor of uncertain malignant potential (WD-UMP, and hyalinizing trabecular tumor (HTT).

Noninvasive Follicular Thyroid Neoplasm with Papillary-Like Nuclear Features (NIFTP) The NIFTP is a fully follicular-patterned, well-encapsulated, noninvasive neoplasm with PTC-related nuclear atypia without high-grade characteristics (mitoses/necrosis) [20, 21]. Most NIFTPs are RAS-driven or codon 601 BRAF mutations. In the updated WHO classification of thyroid neoplasms, the fewer than 1% true papillae and absence of BRAF V600E mutation remain as criteria for the diagnosis of NIFTP. Gene fusions such as the THADA gene fusion or the PAX8::PPARG may be present in a subgroup of NIFTP [3]. In the fifth edition of the WHO classification (2022), sub-centimeter lesions (<10 mm) and oncocytic lesions (>75% oncocytic cells) meeting the strict diagnostic criteria can be classified as NIFTP [3].

Thyroid Tumors of Uncertain Malignant Potential (UMP) Thyroid tumors of UMP are rare lesions that require a thorough microscopic examination of the entire capsule/tumor interface because a single invasive focus would rule out these diagnoses.

Hyalinizing Trabecular Tumor (HTT) Hyalinizing trabecular tumors (HTTs) are thyroid neoplasms that arise from follicular cells that show nuclear atypia associated with PTC, a trabecular growth pattern, and an extracellular hyaline matrix. It is characterized by GLIS gene rearrangements (PAX8::GLIS1 and PAX8::GLIS3 fusions), which have not been found in other thyroid tumors [22, 23]. These tumors are also devoid of BRAF and RAS mutations [24]. The diagnosis of HTT is confirmed by thyroglobulin (Tg), TTF1, and PAX8 positivity along with membranous staining of Ki67 antibody in the MIB1 clone at room temperature. Antibodies targeting the C-terminus of GLIS3 are used to detect tumor cells with PAX8::GLIS3 fusion that exhibit robust nuclear and cytoplasmic immunostaining [22, 23].

C. ***Malignant Neoplasms***

Papillary Thyroid Carcinoma (PTC) Classical, encapsulated classical, infiltrative follicular, diffuse sclerosing, solid/trabecular, tall cell, columnar cell, hobnail, clear-cell, spindle-cell, Warthin-like, oncocytic, and PTC with fibromatosis/fasciitis-like/desmoid-type stroma are some of the many morphological subtypes of PTC. The macro-follicular and multinodular follicular subtypes are *not* mentioned in the 2022 WHO classification [25]. Tall cells, columnar cells, and hobnail PTCs are examples of aggressive histological PTC subtypes.

Eligibility requirements of "Tall-cell" PTC's have been revisited in the 2022 WHO fifth edition. Tall cells were previously (2017) described as two to three times as tall as wide. A tall cell must have a height ≥ 3 times its breadth, dense eosinophilic cytoplasm, and separate cell membranes to meet the recently established diagnostic criteria. At least 30% of the tumor cells must meet the criteria for the tall cell subtype. However, documentation of even focal tall cell changes (≥10% tall cell features) is recommended in dynamic risk stratification. The "hobnail" subtype of PTC and "solid/trabecular" subtypes of PTC require ≥30% hobnail cell change and ≥ 50% solid/trabecular growth for subtyping, respectively [6].

Based on the fifth edition of the WHO classification (2022), all papillary micro-carcinomas (<1 cm) should be subtyped similar to their counterparts that exceed one cm. Papillary micro-carcinoma does *not* stand alone as a subtype of PTC and should *not* be used alone without a subtype designation as micro-carcinomas can develop from aggressive subtypes [26].

Follicular variant PTCs (FVPTCs) are now separated into two subtypes: infiltrative and encapsulated. The 2022 WHO classification refined the spectrum of PTC subtypes that represent the BRAF-like malignancies, by aligning "invasive encapsulated FVPTCs" with FTCs because these tumors (similar to FTC) represent the morphological spectrum of RAS-like differentiated thyroid carcinomas with exclusive follicular growth [3]. Infiltrative FVPTCs exhibit florid nuclear atypia with invasion of the lymphatic vessels and thyroid parenchyma-like BRAF-driven tumors (thus acting like true PTCs). Cribriform-morular thyroid carcinoma is no longer classified as a subtype of PTC.

Encapsulated Follicular-Derived Thyroid Malignancies Encapsulated follicular-derived thyroid malignancies include (1) FTC (Fig. 8.1), (2) oncocytic carcinoma of the thyroid (Hürthle cell carcinoma—HCC) (Fig. 8.2), and (3) invasive encapsulated follicular variant papillary carcinoma (IEFVPTC) (Fig. 8.3). All of these tumors are categorized into three separate subtypes: minimally invasive, encapsu-

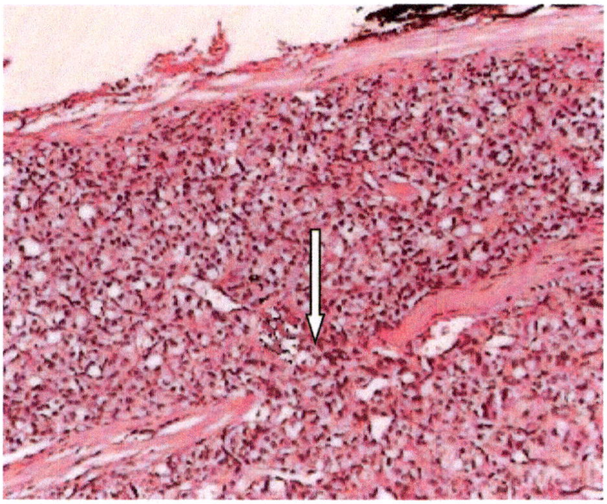

Fig. 8.1 Microscopy of follicular thyroid carcinoma showing capsular invasion (white arrow). H&E × 400

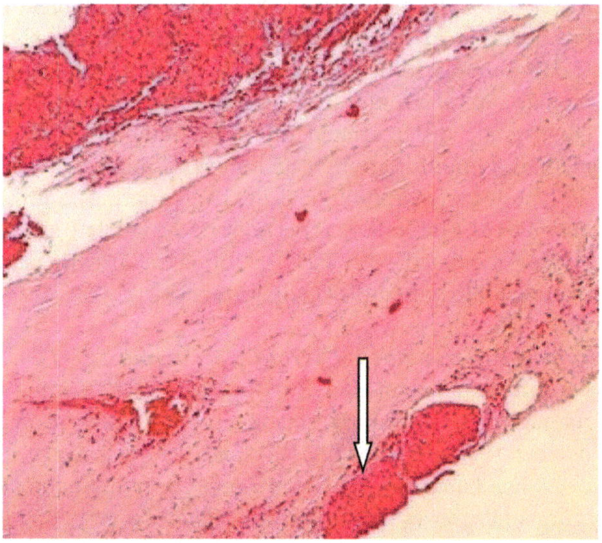

Fig. 8.2 Microscopy of oncocytic carcinoma of thyroid showing capsular invasion (white arrow). H&E × 400

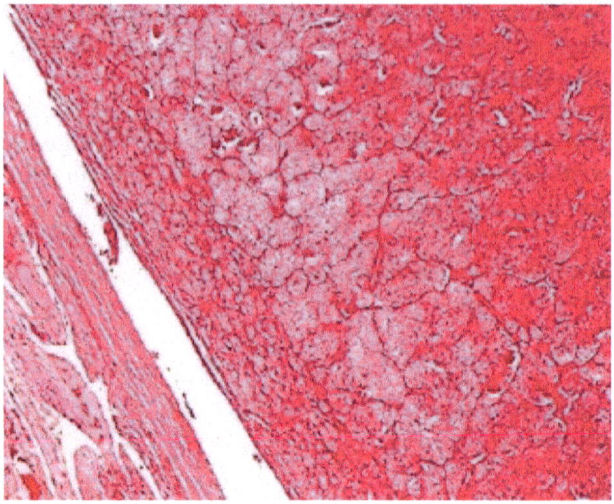

Fig. 8.3 Microscopy of invasive encapsulated follicular variant of papillary thyroid carcinoma. H&E × 100

lated angioinvasive, and widely invasive. The presence of even a single focus of angioinvasion places a tumor into the category of encapsulated angioinvasive subtype [3]. There are two types of encapsulated angioinvasive tumors: those with restricted (four foci) or severe (four or more foci) vascular invasion. However, the fifth edition of the WHO classification questioned the validity of the cutoff point applied for this distinction. For this reason, pathologists are encouraged to document the extent of angioinvasion based on the number of vessels involved.

The term "Hürthle cell" is discouraged in the new classification since it is a misnomer. "Oncocytic carcinoma" is discussed as a distinct entity with the clear recognition that it refers to oncocytic follicular cell–derived neoplasms (composed of >75% oncocytic cells) that lack characteristic nuclear features of PTC (those would be oncocytic PTCs) and high-grade features (necrosis and ≥ 5 mitoses/2 mm^2).

High-grade follicular cell–derived non-anaplastic thyroid malignancies now include both the traditional "poorly differentiated thyroid carcinoma—PDTC" and "high-grade differentiated thyroid carcinomas," since both are characterized by increased mitotic activity (≥5 mitoses/2 mm^2) and tumor necrosis *without* anaplastic histology (morphological dedifferentiation) and clinically behave in a similar manner [3] (Table 8.4). The tumors designated as such may still contain nuclear atypia associated with PTC, a follicular growth pattern, or other characteristics incompatible with a PDTC diagnosis [3].

Poorly Differentiated Thyroid Carcinoma (PDTC) The PDTC diagnostic standards have not been altered in the 2022 WHO edition and are based on Turin criteria, namely (1) a solid, trabecular, or insulating growth pattern, (2) lack of typical nuclear characteristics of PTC, and (3) presence of at least one of the following: convoluted nuclei, ≥3 mitoses/2 mm^2, or tumor necrosis (Fig. 8.4). The microscopic term "high-power field" has been used for a very long period. The square millimeter

Table 8.4 Differences between high-grade follicular cell–derived non-anaplastic carcinoma and poorly differentiated thyroid carcinoma

Histopathological features	High-grade follicular cell–derived non-anaplastic carcinoma	Poorly differentiated thyroid carcinoma
Growth pattern	Papillary, follicular, solid	Solid, trabecular, insular
Nuclear features of PTC	Seen	Not seen
Mitotic count	$>5/2\ mm^2$	$>3/2\ mm^2$
Tumor necrosis	Present	Present
Ki67 index	Not required	Not required

PTC papillary thyroid carcinoma, *PDTC* poorly differentiated thyroid carcinoma

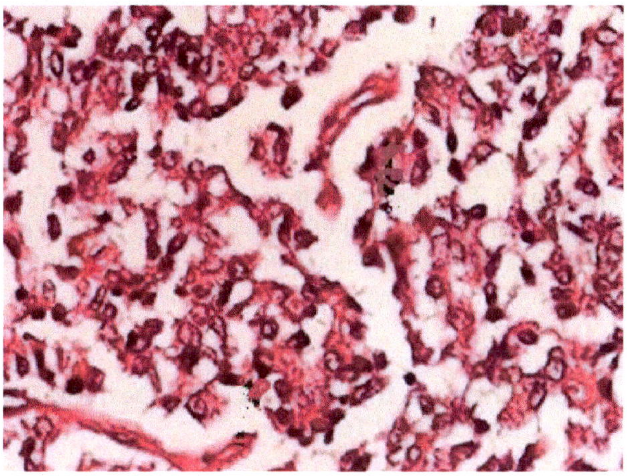

Fig. 8.4 Microscopy of poorly differentiated thyroid carcinoma with increased mitosis and areas of necrosis. H&E × 400

should be used instead of the nonstandard high-power field unit [27]. The Ki-67 labeling index ranges from 10–30% in the majority of PDTCs [3]. A component of DTC can be seen in PDTC, and as little as 10% of a poorly differentiated component is sufficient to confer an aggressive biological behavior.

At the molecular level, high-grade follicular cell–derived non-anaplastic thyroid and PDTCs may be BRAF- or RAS-driven lesions, depending on whether the previous lesion was a PTC or an FTC [3]. Both malignancies can show genetic changes, such as mutations in the TERT promoter and TP53 genes during dedifferentiation [3]. High-grade follicular cell–derived non-anaplastic thyroid is primarily seen with BRAF-driven PTCs [28]. In addition, some PDTC cases in teenagers have been linked to mutations in the DICER1 [29].

Anaplastic Thyroid Carcinoma (ATC) "Anaplastic thyroid carcinoma" (ATC) remains the most undifferentiated form of thyroid carcinoma (Fig. 8.5). "Squamous cell carcinoma" (SCC) of the thyroid is now considered as a morphological subtype of ATC rather than a separate entity as in the fourth edition of the WHO classifica-

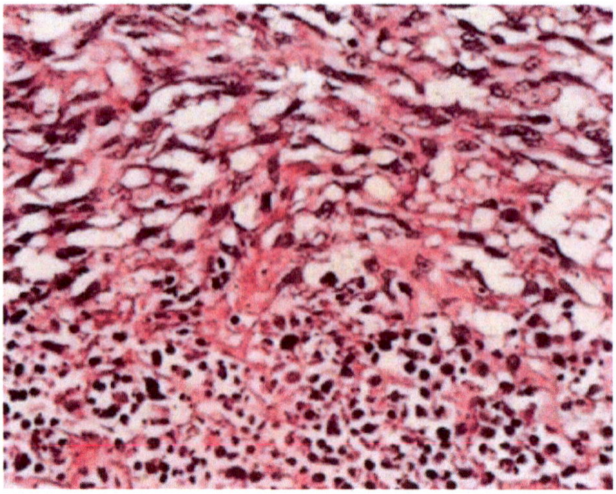

Fig. 8.5 Microscopy of anaplastic thyroid carcinoma showing spindled tumor cells with areas of necrosis. H&E × 400

tion because a large majority of SCC of the thyroid have BRAF p. V600E mutations and exhibit TTF1 and PAX8 immuno-expression, proving the follicular cell origin [30]. Given the potential efficacy of BRAF and MEK inhibitor treatments, the new categorization also promotes the routine use of BRAF p. V600E mutation-specific VE1 immunohistochemistry (IHC) in all patients with ATCA [3].

8.1.5 Changes in Thyroid C-Cell-Derived Tumors and Mixed Tumors

Medullary thyroid carcinomas (MTCs) derived from C-cells retain their distinct section in the new WHO classification (2022), and there is a separate section for mixed tumors composed of both C-cells and any follicular cell–derived malignancy.

A grading system for MTC is also introduced based on high-grade pathological characteristics (mitotic count and tumor necrosis), and Ki67 proliferation index [31, 32]. This method classifies MTCs as high-grade tumors if at least one of the following features is present: tumor necrosis, a mitotic count $\geq 5/2\ mm^2$, and/or a Ki67 proliferation index $\geq 5\%$ (Table 8.5). The percentage of tumor cells that are positively stained out of a total count of 500–2000 tumor cells in hotspots is used to determine the Ki67 proliferation index [31].

8.1.6 Unusual Thyroid Neoplasms

A number of unusual neoplasms that occur in the thyroid have been placed into new sections based on their cytogenesis.

Table 8.5 Grading of medullary thyroid carcinoma—two-tier system

Criteria	Low-grade MTC	High-grade MTC
Tumor necrosis	Absent	Present
Mitotic count	<5/2 mm^2	≥5/2 mm^2
Ki67 index	<5%	≥5%

MTC medullary thyroid carcinoma

8.1.6.1 Salivary Gland–Type Carcinomas of the Thyroid

"Muco-epidermoid carcinoma" (MEC) and "secretory carcinoma" of the salivary gland type are now included in one section in 2022 classified as "salivary gland–type carcinomas of the thyroid." Both tumors exhibit morphologies comparable to those of the salivary gland equivalents. However, they also exhibit various epidemiological, molecular, and prognostic features distinct from those of the salivary gland equivalents. MAML2 gene rearrangements are *not* as common as in their salivary gland counterparts since some manifestations of thyroid MECs have been reported to resemble metaplastic follicular cell–derived thyroid carcinomas [3, 33, 34].

Secretory carcinoma exhibits GATA3, mammaglobin, GCDFP15, and S100 protein positivity, similar to the salivary gland secretory carcinoma, but persistent negativity for TTF1 and Tg [3]. To date, ETV6::NTRK3 fusions have been seen in every thyroid secretory carcinoma [35]. Most salivary gland secretory carcinomas tend to have a milder clinical course; however, thyroid secretory carcinomas tend to be more aggressive and have a later onset.

8.1.6.2 Intrathyroidal Thymic Carcinoma (ITC)

"Thymomas," "thymic carcinomas," and "spindle epithelial tumor with thymus-like elements" are classified as "thymic tumors within the thyroid." To clear confusion regarding the origin of this uncommon malignancy, the tumor formerly described as "thyroid carcinoma showing thymic-like differentiation" has been renamed as ITC. TERT promoter mutations, typically lacking in mediastinal thymic carcinomas, may be present in ITC. The standards for diagnosing these tumors have *not* been changed [6].

8.1.6.3 Embryonal Thyroid Neoplasms

"Malignant teratoma" and "carcino-sarcoma" linked to DICER1 mutations in the thyroid gland are now referred to, in the fifth edition (2022), as "thyroblastoma" [36].

8.1.6.4 Thyroid Carcinomas of Uncertain Histogenesis

The addition of a new group, thyroid tumors of unknown histogenesis (unclear cell lineage), which includes sclerosing MEC with eosinophilia (SMECE) and cribriform morular thyroid carcinoma (CMTC), is a significant change in the 2022 WHO classification. SMECE was categorized as a subtype of thyroid gland carcinomas of the salivary gland in the 2017 WHO classification.

Due to its papillary pattern and similar nuclear characteristics to classic PTC, CMTC was previously categorized by the WHO as a separate subtype of PTC. In contrast to PTC, CMTC has a distinct molecular profile. Genetic changes in the Wnt/beta-catenin pathway have been found in CMTC, including mutations in the APC and CTNNB1 (catenin beta 1) genes [16]. There have not been any BRAF V600E-related CMTC cases. According to IHC, tumor cells exhibit nuclear beta-catenin, estrogen, and progesterone receptor expression. These tumors lack colloid formation and frequently have negative Tg and PAX8 levels, which are indicators of thyroid follicular cell differentiation [16]. TTF1 is positive in the cribriform component, but *not* in the morulae.

8.1.7 Other Primary Tumors

Other primary tumors of the thyroid gland include mesenchymal (and stromal) tumors and thyroid lymphoma as follows:

8.1.7.1 Mesenchymal and Stromal Tumors

Mesenchymal tissues are formed by mesenchymal cells (i.e., cells derived predominantly from embryonic mesoderm and, to a small extent, from embryonic ectoderm), which interact with epithelial tissue to form nearly every organ in the body [37]. A thyroid mesenchymal tumor is defined as a "tumor that arises from the thyroid mesenchymal tissue i.e. the stromal and blood vessel elements of the thyroid gland" [38].

Although robust epidemiological data for the incidence and prevalence of thyroid mesenchymal tumors are currently lacking, these tumors comprise approximately 0•3% of all malignant thyroid tumors [39]. However, over the past few decades, thyroid mesenchymal tumors have been increasingly reported [40, 41]. More than 30 different types of thyroid mesenchymal tumors have been described in the literature.

Benign Thyroid Mesenchymal Tumors Benign mesenchymal tumors of the thyroid include the following [42]:

- Paraganglioma.
- Benign peripheral nerve sheath tumors (Schwannoma, neurofibroma, granular cell tumor).
- Vascular tumors (hemangioma).
- Striated and smooth muscle tumors (rhabdomyoma, leiomyoma).
- Adipose tissue tumors (adeno-lipoma).
- Solitary fibrous tumor.

Malignant Thyroid Mesenchymal Tumors A systematic review of data from 142 patients with primary malignant thyroid mesenchymal tumors between 1990 and 2014 revealed angiosarcomas in 20·4% of patients, epithelioid hemangioendothelioma in 16·3%, undifferentiated pleomorphic sarcoma (previously known as malignant fibrous histiocytoma) in 14·1%, leiomyosarcoma in 11·3%, and fibrosarcoma in 9·2% [30]. However, metastatic mesenchymal tumors into the thyroid (from gastrointestinal stromal tumors, uterine leiomyosarcomas, and malignant breast phyllodes tumor) are more common than primary thyroid mesenchymal tumors [38].

8.1.7.2 Hemato-lymphoid Neoplasms

Thyroid lymphomas comprise 1–5% of thyroid malignancies, and approximately 2% of all lymphomas [43–46]. Determining the exact type of the lymphoma is important for treatment choice and prognosis.

Primary Thyroid Lymphoma Primary thyroid lymphoma can be defined as a "lymphoma that arises from the thyroid gland" [47]. It occurs, in most cases, on a background of Hashimoto's thyroiditis, which is the *only* known risk factor [48, 49], and can increase the risk of developing thyroid lymphoma by up to 60 times [50]. Primary thyroid lymphomas are practically always non-Hodgkin lymphomas (NHLs) of B-cell origin [51, 52], representing approximately 1.2–1.7% of all NHLs [50]. Primary thyroid Hodgkin lymphoma is extremely rare. It represents <5% of thyroid malignancies. NHLs can be divided into aggressive and indolent cell types.

The most common subtype of NHLs that arise primarily from the thyroid gland is "diffuse large-cell lymphoma" (DLBCL). Another subtype that can arise from the thyroid gland is the "mucosa-associated lymphoid tissue [MALT] lymphoma" (MALToma). It usually has a more favorable outcome than DLBCL.

Secondary Involvement by Lymphoma *Secondary involvement* of the thyroid gland by lymphoma can occur in approximately 20% of patients dying from generalized lymphoma [53].

8.1.8 Metastatic Tumors

Given the extensive blood supply to the gland, the low incidence of metastases to the thyroid is surprising [54]. Willis suggested that this is influenced by the glandular micro-environment; the fast arterial blood flow and high concentration of oxygen and iodine could thus prevent the anchorage and secondary growth of circulating tumor cells [54].

While postmortem examination suggests that as many as 24% of patients who die of non-thyroid malignancies have metastases to this gland, these seem rare in clinical practice [55–57]. Although the majority (60–80%) of patients who present with thyroid metastasis are diagnosed in the setting of a known previous malignancy, an "occult" primary tumor accounts for a significant percentage (20–40%) [57, 58]. In addition, some patients with metastases to the thyroid gland are diagnosed during preoperative workup, while others are only diagnosed on histological examination of a thyroidectomy specimen.

Table 8.6 Pathological classification of thyroid neoplasms according to grade (differentiation)

Degree of differentiation	Pathological tumor type
I- Well-differentiated (low-grade malignancy)	Usual papillary thyroid carcinoma (PTC) Micro-carcinoma (< 1 cm) Follicular variant of PTC Usual follicular thyroid carcinoma (FTC) Hürthle cell carcinoma (HCC)
II- Intermediate differentiation	Medullary thyroid carcinoma (MTC) Diffuse sclerosing variant of PTC Columnar-cell variant of PTC Tall-cell variant of PTC Poorly differentiated thyroid carcinoma (PDTC) (insular)
III- Poorly differentiated (high-grade malignancy)	Anaplastic (undifferentiated) thyroid carcinoma (ATC)

Tumors metastasize to the thyroid via (1) direct extension from tumors in adjacent structures, (2) retrograde lymphatic spread, or (3) hematogenously. Hematogenous metastases to the thyroid vary according to the tumor type. Metastases can originate at almost any primary site [59–66]. The most common primary tumors are carcinomas of the kidney (renal cell carcinoma—RCC), lung, colon, and melanoma [67]. Although, in clinical series, RCC is the most common primary neoplasm, the most common in autopsy studies is the lung. Because of the aggressive nature of lung malignancies, patients are often treated with palliative intent from an early stage, and investigation for additional metastases is therefore curtailed. In contrast, RCC is less aggressive, and patients are more likely to be further investigated and treated for metastatic disease [67].

8.1.9 Pathological Classification by Grade (Differentiation)

Most thyroid tumors arise from the follicular cells, and most are well-differentiated. Poorly differentiated and undifferentiated types are rare (Table 8.6). Well-differentiated carcinomas include papillary and follicular carcinomas. Hürthle cell carcinomas in this classification are considered as low-grade malignancy.

8.2 Oncocytic (Hürthle Cell) Neoplasms: Traditional Classifications

8.2.1 Hürthle Cell Adenoma (HCA)/Hürthle Cell Carcinoma (HCC)

Traditionally, Hürthle cell neoplasms (HCNs) (now termed "oncocytic neoplasms" by WHO in 2022) have been classified into benign (Hürthle cell adenoma—HCA) and malignant (Hürthle cell carcinoma—HCC) [68]. Based on histopathological features, Erickson et al. [69] in 2000, added a third category: HCN of uncertain malignant behavior (UMB), characterized by equivocal capsular invasion (CI) with absent vascular invasion (VI).

8.2.2 Hürthle Cell Papillary Carcinoma (HCPC)

In the same year, Cheung et al. [70] classified HCNs into HCA, HCC, and Hürthle cell papillary carcinoma (HCPC) based on data from molecular studies. In fact, demonstration of oncocytic features in certain variants of papillary thyroid cancer (PTC) has long been recognized and reported [71]. However, the diagnosis of this entity is in itself another controversy. Some authors required the demonstration of classic nuclear features of PTC, in addition to the presence of oxyphilic cells with or without papillary growth pattern [72–75]. On the other hand, other investigators necessitated the detection of a papillary architecture, with or without recognizing the diagnostic nuclear features of PTC; as these may be obscured by the nuclear hyperchromasia of Hürthle cells (now called oncocytic cells) [76].

The detection of RET/PTC rearrangement, which was thought to be specific to conventional PTC, in some HCNs, has expanded the diagnosis of HCPC to include a subgroup of cancer that shows this molecular event even without detecting any of the characteristic cyto-architectural features [70, 77, 78].

8.2.3 Encapsulated Papillary Oncocytic Neoplasm (EPON)

Although not as well described as follicular-patterned oncocytic/Hürthle cell tumors (i.e., conventional HCA/HCC), rarely oncocytic neoplasms may demonstrate papillary growth [79–81]. These tumors, which lack nuclear features of PTC, have an oncocytic cytomorphology, but interestingly demonstrate prominent papillary architecture. They were termed "encapsulated papillary oncocytic neoplasm" (EPON) by Woodford et al. [80] and appear to be molecularly distinct from PTC, lacking *BRAF* point mutations and *RET/PTC* rearrangements. Similar to conventional encapsulated Hürthle cell tumors, EPON also may demonstrate capsular and/or vascular invasion, indicating malignancy. Lymph node metastasis has also rarely been reported. Despite this, they appear to demonstrate indolent clinical behavior [80], although published outcome data are limited [82].

8.2.4 Other Aggressive Oncocytic (Hürthle Cell) Tumors

Similar to PTC or FTC, dedifferentiation to poorly differentiated thyroid carcinoma (PDTC) or even anaplastic thyroid carcinoma (ATC) may occur in HCC [83–87]. With progression of HCC to PDTC, it will demonstrate areas with solid, insular, or trabecular growth and tumor necrosis or increased proliferative activity fulfilling the WHO criteria for PDTC [88].

Asioli et al. [85] found that predominant oncocytic features were identified in approximately one-third of PDTC in their validation study of the Turin proposal. Recently, in 2019, Wong et al. found a similar rate of oncocytic tumors among PDTC [89] and have rarely noted anaplastic carcinoma arising from HCC. Although a difference in outcome between non-oncocytic and oncocytic PDTC was not observed in the study by Asioli et al., subsequent studies have found decreased survival in oncocytic PDTC as reported by Dettmer et al. in 2012 [86] and Wong et al. in 2019 [89].

8.3 Oncocytic (Hürthle Cell) Neoplasms: Recent Classifications

Hürthle cell carcinoma (HCC) has been long considered as a subgroup (variant) of follicular thyroid cancer (FTC) and was classified as such by the World Health Organization (WHO) [90] based on similar clinical behavior reported by several authors in the literature [91–94]. However, HCC was reclassified in 2017 in the fourth WHO classification of Tumors of Endocrine Organs as a separate subtype of differentiated thyroid cancer (DTC) [88] different from FTC [68, 95, 96], due to its different genetic (oncogene) expression profile [97], distinct pathological characteristics, specific molecular pathogenesis [98–100], and the aggressive clinical behavior reported by several authors [95]. In the 2022 WHO classification, HCC is a distinct entity referred to as "oncocytic carcinoma" [3].

Higher frequencies of distant metastasis, impaired iodine-avidity, and higher rates of mortality have been reported by many researchers [101, 102]; however, data are still controversial [92, 103, 104]. Moreover, molecular studies [70, 77, 78] have suggested that HCC would be more appropriately subclassified under PTC [105] or at least closer to PTCs than was originally believed. However, more recently and perpetuating the enigma, data by Finely et al. [106] have shown that the molecular signature of oncocytic carcinomas (HCCs) is most similar to FTC.

Based on the degree of capsular invasion and vascular invasion, HCC has been subclassified into two groups: minimally invasive (miHCC) and widely invasive (wiHCC) Hürthle cell carcinoma; however, another controversy exists in the literature concerning definition of miHCC. Stojadinovic et al. [107] defined it as HCC with a single focus of complete capsular invasion (CI) or a single focus of any vascular invasion (VI) or both, while more recently (2014), Chindris et al. [108] defined it as HCC with four or less *foci* of capsular invasion or with less than four foci of vascular invasion. On the other hand, Monotone et al. (2008) stated that vascular invasion should be removed from the definition of miHCC [75]. In their series, Barnabei et al. [109] distinguished HCC as miHCC if only capsular invasion was reported while Sanders et al. [94] included only cases with minimal capsular invasion.

Studies have reported that oncocytic carcinoma (HCC) with focal vascular invasion (<4 foci) can also be associated with less aggressive behavior similar to that of

HCCs with minimal capsular invasion and no vascular invasion. In a retrospective single-institutional study by Xu et al., the experience of 276 patients with encapsulated differentiated thyroid cancers (224 encapsulated PTC, 34 encapsulated FTC, and 16 encapsulated HCCs) showed that extensive vascular invasion (≥4 foci of vascular invasion) is an independent predictor of recurrence in patients with encapsulated differentiated thyroid cancers; indeed, the risk of recurrence was 42% in patients with extensive vascular invasion compared to 1% in patients with no vascular invasion or focal vascular invasion (<4 sites) [110].

In a retrospective, single-institution study of 50 patients with encapsulated HCC, Ghossein et al. also reported that the pathological finding of >4 foci of vascular invasion is the most powerful predictor of recurrence and compromised recurrence-free survival ($P < 0.001$) among patients with encapsulated HCC. In this study, patients with no vascular invasion or < 4 foci of vascular invasion had 100% recurrence-free survival at 5 years compared to only 20% recurrence-free survival among patients with >4 foci of vascular invasion [111].

A recent study (2013) of 27 oncocytic/Hürthle cell tumor samples (8 HCAs, 9 miHCCs, and 10 wiHCCs) used mass spectrometry-based genotyping to interrogate hot spot point mutations in the most common thyroid oncogenes, and real-time polymerase chain reaction (PCR) was used to assess for common oncogenic fusions [112]. Transcriptomes for wiHCC were compared with follicular carcinoma expression array profiles obtained from the "Gene Expression Omnibus." The authors reported only 11% RAS mutations and no Pax8-PPARγ rearrangements in HCC tumor samples; in contrast, follicular carcinomas had a 45% RAS mutation rate and rearrangements of Pax8-PPARγ in 25–60% of cases. This study also showed that the chromosomal copy number profiles of HCCs were distinct from follicular carcinomas, as large regions of gain on chromosomes 5, 7, 12, and 17 are observed in HCC, but not in follicular carcinoma.

Two relevant concepts remain. Initially, although dedifferentiation is well documented in DTC [70], an oncocytic poorly differentiated thyroid cancer has also been described by several investigators [76, 83, 84]. Additionally, oncocytic change can also occur in para-follicular cells and result in oncocytic medullary thyroid carcinoma (MTC) [113]. As a result, Sobrinho et al. [114] stated that with the exception of undifferentiated carcinoma, every type of benign or malignant thyroid tumor has its oncocytic variant. These data support the classification system proposed by Asa [76] in which malignant HCNs are categorized into Hürthle cell papillary carcinoma HCPC, Hürthle cell follicular carcinoma, Hürthle cell poorly differentiated carcinoma, and oncocytic medullary carcinoma.

References

1. British Thyroid Association, Royal College of Physicians: British Thyroid Association. Guidelines for the management of thyroid cancer. 2nd ed; 2007.
2. Cameselle-Teijeiro JM, Sobrinho-Simoes M. New WHO classification of thyroid tumors: a pragmatic categorization of thyroid gland neoplasms. Endocrinol Diabetes Nutr. 2018;65(3):133–5.

3. Baloch ZW, Asa SL, Barletta JA, Ghossein RA, Juhlin CC, Jung CK, et al. Overview of the 2022 WHO classification of thyroid neoplasms. Endocr Pathol. 2022;33(1):27–63.
4. Agrawal N, Akbani R, Aksoy BA, Ally A, Arachchi H, Asa SL, et al. Integrated genomic characterization of papillary thyroid carcinoma. Cell. 2014;159:676–90.
5. Sk Y, Lee S, Sj K, Hg J, Kim BA, Cho H, et al. comprehensive analysis of the transcriptional and mutational landscape of follicular and papillary thyroid cancers. PLoS Genet. 2016;12:e1006239.
6. Sekar MD, Gochhait D, Kamalanathan S. Critical appraisal of the WHO 2022 classification of thyroid cancer. Thyroid Res Pract. 2024;20(1):8–14.
7. Asa SL, Mete O. Oncocytic change in thyroid pathology. Front Endocrinol (Lausanne). 2021;12:678119.
8. Bruford EA, Antonescu CR, Carroll AJ, Chinnaiyan A, Cree IA, Cross NC, et al. Hugo Gene Nomenclature Committee (HGNC) recommendations for the designation of gene fusions. Leukemia. 2021;35:3040–3.
9. Mete O, Asa SL. Pitfalls in the diagnosis of follicular epithelial proliferations of the thyroid. Adv Anat Pathol. 2012;19:363–73.
10. Parma J, Duprez L, Van Sande J, Cochaux P, Gervy C, Mockel J, et al. Somatic mutations in the thyrotropin receptor gene cause hyperfunctioning thyroid adenomas. Nature. 1993;365:649–51.
11. Gozu HI, Lublinghoff J, Bircan R, Paschke R. Genetics and phenomics of inherited and sporadic non-autoimmune hyperthyroidism. Mol Cell Endocrinol. 2010;322:125–34.
12. Kamilaris CD, Faucz FR, Voutetakis A, Stratakis CA. Carney complex. Exp Clin Endocrinol Diabetes. 2019;127:156–64.
13. Nosé V, Gill A, Teijeiro JM, Perren A, Erickson L. Overview of the 2022 WHO classification of familial endocrine tumor syndromes. Endocr Pathol. 2022;33:197–227.
14. Juhlin CC, Stenman A, Zedenius J. Macrofollicular variant follicular thyroid tumors are DICER1 mutated and exhibit distinct histological features. Histopathology. 2021;79:661–6.
15. Wasserman JD, Sabbaghian N, Fahiminiya S, Chami R, Mete O, Acker M, et al. DICER1 mutations are frequent in adolescent-onset papillary thyroid carcinoma. J Clin Endocrinol Metab. 2018;103:2009–15.
16. Cameselle-Teijeiro JM, Mete O, Asa SL, LiVolsi V. Inherited follicular epithelial-derived thyroid carcinomas: from molecular biology to histological correlates. Endocr Pathol. 2021;32:77–101.
17. McFadden DG, Sadow PM. Genetics, diagnosis, and management of Hürthle cell thyroid neoplasms. Front Endocrinol (Lausanne). 2021;12:696386.
18. Gopal RK, Kübler K, Calvo SE, Polak P, Livitz D, Rosebrock D, et al. Widespread chromosomal losses and mitochondrial DNA alterations as genetic drivers in hürthle cell carcinoma. Cancer Cell. 2018;34:242–55.
19. Doerfler WR, Nikitski AV, Morariu EM, Ohori NP, Chiosea SI, Landau MS, et al. Molecular alterations in Hürthle cell nodules and preoperative cancer risk. Endocr Relat Cancer. 2021;28:301–9.
20. Hodak S, Tuttle RM, Maytal G, Nikiforov YE, Randolph G. Changing the cancer diagnosis: the case of follicular variant of papillary thyroid cancer-primum non nocere and NIFTP. Thyroid. 2016;26:869–71.
21. Thompson LD. Ninety-four cases of encapsulated follicular variant of papillary thyroid carcinoma: a name change to noninvasive follicular thyroid neoplasm with papillary-like nuclear features would help prevent overtreatment. Mod Pathol. 2016;29:698–707.
22. Marchiò C, Da Cruz Paula A, Gularte-Merida R, Basili T, Brandes A, da Silva EM, et al. PAX8-GLIS3 gene fusion is a pathognomonic genetic alteration of hyalinizing trabecular tumors of the thyroid. Mod Pathol. 2019;32:1734–43.
23. Nikiforova MN, Nikitski AV, Panebianco F, Kaya C, Yip L, Williams M, et al. GLIS rearrangement is a genomic hallmark of hyalinizing trabecular tumor of the thyroid gland. Thyroid. 2019;29:161–73.

24. Salvatore G, Chiappetta G, Nikiforov YE, Decaussin-Petrucci M, Fusco A, Carney JA, et al. Molecular profile of hyalinizing trabecular tumours of the thyroid: high prevalence of RET/PTC rearrangements and absence of B-raf and N-ras point mutations. Eur J Cancer. 2005;41:816–21.
25. Jung CK, Bychkov A, Kakudo K. Update from the 2022 world health organization classification of thyroid tumors: a standardized diagnostic approach. Endocrinol Metab (Seoul). 2022;37:703–18.
26. Christofer Juhlin C, Mete O, Baloch ZW. The 2022 WHO classification of thyroid tumors: novel concepts in nomenclature and grading. Endocr Relat Cancer. 2023;30:e220293.
27. Cree IA, Tan PH, Travis WD, Wesseling P, Yagi Y, White VA, et al. Counting mitoses: SI (ze) matters! Mod Pathol. 2021;34:1651–7.
28. Wong KS, Dong F, Telatar M, Lorch JH, Alexander EK, Marqusee E, et al. Papillary thyroid carcinoma with high-grade features versus poorly differentiated thyroid carcinoma: an analysis of clinicopathologic and molecular features and outcome. Thyroid. 2021;31:933–40.
29. Chernock RD, Rivera B, Borrelli N, Hill DA, Fahiminiya S, Shah T, et al. Poorly differentiated thyroid carcinoma of childhood and adolescence: a distinct entity characterized by DICER1 mutations. Mod Pathol. 2020;33:1264–74.
30. Xu B, Fuchs T, Dogan S, Landa I, Katabi N, Fagin JA, et al. Dissecting anaplastic thyroid carcinoma: a comprehensive clinical, histologic, immunophenotypic, and molecular study of 360 cases. Thyroid. 2020;30:1505–17.
31. Xu B, Fuchs TL, Ahmadi S, Alghamdi M, Alzumaili B, Bani MA, et al. International medullary thyroid carcinoma grading system: a validated grading system for medullary thyroid carcinoma. J Clin Oncol. 2022;40:96–104.
32. Asa SL, Mete O. Medullary thyroid carcinoma in the IARC/WHO neuroendocrine schema. Endocr Pathol. 2022;33:346–7.
33. Tonon G, Modi S, Wu L, Kubo A, Coxon AB, Komiya T, et al. t (11;19)(q21;p13) translocation in mucoepidermoid carcinoma creates a novel fusion product that disrupts a notch signaling pathway. Nat Genet. 2003;33:208–13.
34. Chambers M, Nosé V, Sadow PM, Tafe LJ, Kerr DA. Salivary-like tumors of the thyroid: a comprehensive review of three rare carcinomas. Head Neck Pathol. 2021;15:212–24.
35. Skálová A, Vanecek T, Sima R, Laco J, Weinreb I, Perez-Ordonez B, et al. Mammary analogue secretory carcinoma of salivary glands, containing the ETV6-NTRK3 fusion gene: a hitherto undescribed salivary gland tumor entity. Am J Surg Pathol. 2010;34:599–608.
36. Tahara I, Oishi N, Mochizuki K, Oyama T, Miyata K, Miyauchi A, et al. Identification of recurrent TERT promoter mutations in intrathyroid thymic carcinomas. Endocr Pathol. 2020;31:274–82.
37. MacCord K. "Mesenchyme" embryo project encyclopedia. Arizona State University; 2012.
38. LiVolsi VA, Montone KT, Baloch ZW. Pathology of the thyroid: a review. In: Luster M, Duntas LH, Wartofsky L, editors. The thyroid and its diseases: a comprehensive guide for the clinician. Cham: Springer; 2019. p. 455–92.
39. Bula G, Waler J, Niemiec A, Trompeta J, Steplewska K, Gawrychowski J. Unusual malignant thyroid tumours – a clinical study of 20 cases. Acta Chir Belg. 2008;108:702–7.
40. Thompson LD, Wei C, Rooper LM, Lau SK. Thyroid gland solitary fibrous tumor: report of 3 cases and a comprehensive review of the literature. Head Neck Pathol. 2019;13:597–605.
41. Mishra P, Padhi S, Behera G. Thyroid paraganglioma: a case-based systematic review of literature. J Cancer Res Ther. 2020;16(Supplement):S11–21.
42. Gubbi S, Thakur S, Avadhanula S, Araque KA, Filie AC, Raffeld M, et al. Comprehensive guidance on the diagnosis and management of primary mesenchymal tumours of the thyroid gland. Lancet Oncol. 2020;21(11):e528–37.
43. Surov A, Gottschling S, Wienke A, Meyer HJ, Spielmann RP, Dralle H. Primary thyroid sarcoma: a systematic review. Anticancer Res. 2015;35:5185–91.
44. Doria R, Jekel JF, Cooper DL, Thyroid lymphoma. The case for combined modality therapy. Cancer. 1994;73:200–6.

45. Compagno J, Oertel JE. Malignant lymphoma and other lymphoproliferative disorders of the thyroid gland. A clinicopathologic study of 245 cases. Am J Clin Pathol. 1980;74:1–11.
46. Samaan NA, Ordonez NG. Uncommon types of thyroid cancer. Endocrinol Metab Clin N Am. 1990;19:637–48.
47. Kesireddy M, Lasrado S. Thyroid Lymphoma. 2024 Feb 26. In: StatPearls [Internet]. Treasure Island: StatPearls; 2024. PMID: 31335002.
48. Pasieka JL. Hashimoto's disease and thyroid lymphoma: role of the surgeon. World J Surg. 2000;24:966–70.
49. Thieblemont C, Mayer A, Dumontet C, Barbier Y, Callet- Bauchu E, Felman P, Berger F, Ducottet X, Martin C, Salles G, Orgiazzi J, Coiffier B. Primary thyroid lymphoma is a heterogeneous disease. J Clin Endocrinol Metab. 2002;87:105–11.
50. Holm LE, Blomgren H, Lowhagen T. Cancer risks in patients with chronic lymphocytic thyroiditis. N Engl J Med. 1985;312:601–4.
51. Derringer GA, Thompson LD, Frommelt RA, Bijwaard KE, Heffess CS, Abbondanzo SL. Malignant lymphoma of the thyroid gland: a clinicopathologic study of 108 cases. Am J Surg Pathol. 2000;24:623–39.
52. Ansell SM, Grant CS, Habermann TM. Primary thyroid lymphoma. Semin Oncol. 1999;26:316–23.
53. Kossev P, Livolsi V. Lymphoid lesions of the thyroid: review in light of the revised European-American lymphoma classification and upcoming World Health Organization classification. Thyroid. 1999;9(12):1273–80.
54. Willis RA. Metastatic tumours in the thyreoid gland. Am J Pathol. 1931;7:187–208.
55. Cordes M, Kuwert T. Metastases of non-thyroidal tumors to the thyroid gland: a regional survey in Middle Franconia. Exp Clin Endocrinol Diabetes. 2014;122:273–6.
56. Stevens TM, Richards AT, Bewtra C, Sharma P. Tumors metastatic to thyroid neoplasms: a case report and review of the literature. Pathol Res Int. 2011;23:86–93.
57. Nixon IJ, Whitcher M, Glick J, et al. Surgical management of metastases to the thyroid gland. Ann Surg Oncol. 2011;18:800–4.
58. Chung AY, Tran TB, Brumund KT, Weisman RA, Bouvet M. Metastases to the thyroid: a review of the literature from the last decade. Thyroid. 2012;22:258–68.
59. Chiumento C, Fiorentino A, Castaldo G, Fusco V. A case of thyroid metastasis of nasopharyngeal cancer. Tumori. 2011;97:24e–6e.
60. Rosen IB, Walfish PG, Bain J, Bedard YC. Secondary malignancy of the thyroid gland and its management. Ann Surg Oncol. 1995;2:252–6.
61. Bae WK, Shim HJ, Choi YD, et al. Severe hypothyroidism induced by thyroid metastasis of cholangiocarcinoma. Cancer Res Treat. 2009;41:56–8.
62. Basu S, Alavi A. Metastatic malignant melanoma to the thyroid gland detected by FDG-PET imaging. Clin Nucl Med. 2007;32:388–9.
63. Delitala AP, Vidili G, Manca A, Dial U, Delitala G, Fanciulli G. A case of thyroid metastasis from pancreatic cancer: case report and literature review. BMC Endocr Disord. 2014;14:6–9.
64. Gherardi G, Scherini P, Ambrosi S. Occult thyroid metastasis from untreated uveal melanoma. Arch Ophthalmol. 1985;103:689–91.
65. De Ridder M, Sermeus AB, Urbain D, Storme GA. Metastases to the thyroid gland – a report of six cases. Eur J Intern Med. 2003;14:377–9.
66. Demir L, Erten C, Somali I, et al. Metastases of renal cell carcinoma to the larynx and thyroid: two case reports on metastasis developing years after nephrectomy. Can Urol Assoc J. 2012;6:E209–12.
67. Lam KY, Lo CY. Metastatic tumors of the thyroid gland: a study of 79 cases in Chinese patients. Arch Pathol Lab Med. 1998;122(1):37–41.
68. Mills SC, Haq M, Smellie WJ, Harmer C. Hurthle cell carcinoma of the thyroid: retrospective review of 62 patients treated at the Royal Marsden Hospital between 1946 and 2003. Eur J Surg Oncol. 2009;35(3):230–4.

69. Erickson LA, Jin L, Goellner JR, Lohse C, Pankratz VS, Zukerberg LR, et al. Pathologic features, proliferative activity, and cyclin D1 expression in Hurthle cell neoplasms of the thyroid. Mod Pathol. 2000;13(2):186–92.
70. Cheung CC, Ezzat S, Ramyar L, Freeman JL, Asa SL. Molecular basis of Hurthle cell papillary thyroid carcinoma. J Clin Endocrinol Metab. 2000;85(2):878–82.
71. Scopa CD. Histopathology of thyroid tumors. An overview. Hormones. 2004;3(2):100–10.
72. Berho M, Suster S. The oncocytic variant of papillary carcinoma of the thyroid: a clinicopathologic study of 15 cases. Hum Pathol. 1997;28(1):47–53.
73. Sabino de Matos P. Thyroid epithelial tumours. Diagn Histopathol. 2008;14(5):236–46.
74. Lloyd RV, Buehler D, Khanafshar E. Papillary thyroid carcinoma variants. Head Neck Pathol. 2011;5(1):51–6.
75. Montone KT, Baloch ZW, LiVolsi VA. The thyroid Hurthle (oncocytic) cell and its associated pathologic conditions: a surgical pathology and cytopathology review. Arch Pathol Lab Med. 2008;132(8):1241–50.
76. Asa S. My approach to oncocytic tumours of the thyroid. J Clin Pathol. 2004;57(3):225–32.
77. Belchetz G, Cheung CC, Freeman J, Rosen IB, Witterick IJ, Asa SL. Hürthle cell tumors: using molecular techniques to define a novel classification system. Arch Otolaryngol Head Neck Surg. 2002;128(3):237–40.
78. Musholt PB, Imkamp F, von Wasielewski R, Schmid KW, Musholt TJ. RET rearrangements in archival oxyphilic thyroid tumors: new insights in tumorigenesis and classification of Hürthle cell carcinomas? Surgery. 2003;134(6):881–9.
79. Mai KT, Elmontaser G, Perkins DG, Thomas J, Stinson WA. Benign hürthle cell adenoma with papillary architecture: a benign lesion mimicking oncocytic papillary carcinoma. Int J Surg Pathol. 2005;13:37–41.
80. Woodford RL, Nikiforov YE, Hunt JL, Bellizzi AM, Zhang X, Mills SE, et al. Encapsulated papillary oncocytic neoplasms of the thyroid: morphologic, immunohistochemical, and molecular analysis of 18 cases. Am J Surg Pathol. 2010;34:1582–90.
81. Bellevicine C, Malapelle U, Docimo G, Ciancia G, Mossetti G, Pettinato G, et al. Multicentric encapsulated papillary oncocytic neoplasm of the thyroid: a case diagnosed by a combined cytological, histological, immunohistochemical, and molecular approach. Diagn Cytopathol. 2012;40:450–4.
82. Wong KS, Angell TE, Barletta JA, Krane JF. Hurthle cell lesions of the thyroid: progress made and challenges remaining. Cancer Cytopathol. 2021;129:347–62.
83. Mete O, Asa SL. Oncocytes, oxyphils, Hürthle, and Askanazy cells: morphological and molecular features of oncocytic thyroid nodules. Endocr Pathol. 2010;21:16–24.
84. Papotti M, Torchio B, Grassi L, Favero A, Bussolati G. Poorly differentiated oxyphilic (Hurthle cell) carcinomas of the thyroid. Am J Surg Pathol. 1996;20:686–94.
85. Asioli S, Erickson LA, Righi A, Jin L, Volante M, Jenkins S, et al. Poorly differentiated carcinoma of the thyroid: validation of the Turin proposal and analysis of IMP3 expression. Mod Pathol. 2010;23:1269–78.
86. Dettmer M, Schmitt A, Steinert H, Moch H, Komminoth P, Perren A. Poorly differentiated oncocytic thyroid carcinoma – diagnostic implications and outcome. Histopathology. 2012;60:1045–51.
87. Hunt JL, Tometsko M, LiVolsi VA, Swalsky P, Finkelstein SD, Barnes EL. Molecular evidence of anaplastic transformation in coexisting well-differentiated and anaplastic carcinomas of the thyroid. Am J Surg Pathol. 2003;27:1559–64.
88. Lloyd RV, Osamura RY, Klöppel GRJ, editors. World Health Organization classification of tumours of endocrine organs. 4th ed. IARC Press; 2017.
89. Wong KS, Lorch JH, Alexander EK, Marqusee E, Cho NL, Nehs MA, et al. Prognostic significance of extent of invasion in poorly differentiated thyroid carcinoma. Thyroid. 2019;29:1255–61.

90. Nikiforov YE, Biddinger PW, Thompson LDR. Diagnostic pathology and molecular genetics of the thyroid: a comprehensive guide for practicing thyroid pathology. Philadelphia: Wolters Kluwer Health; 2012.
91. Haigh PI, Urbach DR. The treatment and prognosis of Hürthle cell follicular thyroid carcinoma compared with its non-Hürthle cell counterpart. Surgery. 2005;138(6):1152–8.
92. Khafif A, Khafif RA, Attie JN. Hürthle cell carcinoma: a malignancy of low-grade potential. Head Neck. 1999;21(6):506–11.
93. Evans HL, Vassilopoulou-Sellin R. Follicular and Hurthle cell carcinomas of the thyroid: a comparative study. Am J Surg Pathol. 1998;22(12):1512–20.
94. Sanders LE, Silverman M. Follicular and Hürthle cell carcinoma: predicting outcome and directing therapy. Surgery. 1998;124(6):967–74.
95. Kushchayeva Y, Duh Q-Y, Kebebew E, D'Avanzo A, Clark OH. Comparison of clinical characteristics at diagnosis and during follow-up in 118 patients with Hurthle cell or follicular thyroid cancer. Am J Surg. 2008;195(4):457–62.
96. Carcangiu ML, Bianchi S, Savino D, Voynick IM, Rosai J. Follicular Hurthle cell tumors of the thyroid gland. Cancer. 1991;68(9):1944–53.
97. Masood S, Auguste L-J, Westerband A, Belluco C, Valderama E, Attie J. Differential oncogenic expression in thyroid follicular and Hürthle cell carcinomas. Am J Surg. 1993;166(4):366–8.
98. Dettori T, Frau DV, Lai ML, Mariotti S, Uccheddu A, Daniele GM, et al. Aneuploidy in oncocytic lesions of the thyroid gland: diffuse accumulation of mitochondria within the cell is associated with trisomy 7 and progressive numerical chromosomal alterations. Genes Chromosom Cancer. 2003;38(1):22–31.
99. Wada N, Duh QY, Miura D, Brunaud L, Wong MG, Clark OH. Chromosomal aberrations by comparative genomic hybridization in Hurthle cell thyroid carcinomas are associated with tumor recurrence. J Clin Endocrinol Metab. 2002;87(10):4595–601.
100. Máximo V, Soares P, Lima J, Cameselle-Teijeiro J, Sobrinho-Simões M. Mitochondrial DNA somatic mutations (point mutations and large deletions) and mitochondrial DNA variants in human thyroid pathology: a study with emphasis on Hürthle cell tumors. Am J Pathol. 2002;160(5):1857–65.
101. Phitayakorn R, McHenry CR. Follicular and Hürthle cell carcinoma of the thyroid gland. Surg Oncol Clin N Am. 2006;15(3):603–23.
102. Khokar AM, Holoubek SA, Kuchta KM, Winchester DJ, Prinz RA, Moo-Young TA. Survival with follicular and hurthle cell microcarcinoma compared to papillary thyroid microcarcinoma: a population study of 84,532 patients. World J Surg. 2020;44(2):469–78.
103. Nagar S, Aschebrook-Kilfoy B, Kaplan EL, Angelos P, Grogan RH. Hurthle cell carcinoma: an update on survival over the last 35 years. Surgery. 2013;154(6):1263–71.
104. Bhattacharyya N. Survival and prognosis in hürthle cell carcinoma of the thyroid gland. Arch Otolaryngol Head Neck Surg. 2003;129(2):207–10.
105. Melck A, Bugis S, Baliski C, Irvine R, Anderson DW, Wilkins G, et al. Hemithyroidectomy: the preferred initial surgical approach for management of Hurthle cell neoplasm. Am J Surg. 2006;191(5):593–7.
106. Finley DJ, Zhu B, Fahey Iii TJ. Molecular analysis of Hurthle cell neoplasms by gene profiling. Surgery. 2004;136(6):1160–8.
107. Stojadinovic A, Ghossein RA, Hoos A, Urist MJ, Spiro RH, Shah JP, et al. Hurthle cell carcinoma: a critical histopathologic appraisal. J Clin Oncol. 2001;19(10):2616–25.
108. Chindris A-M, Casler JD, Bernet VJ, Rivera M, Thomas C, Kachergus JM, et al. Clinical and molecular features of Hürthle cell carcinoma of the thyroid. J Clin Endocrinol Metab. 2014;110(1):55–62.
109. Barnabei A, Ferretti E, Baldelli R, Procaccini A, Spriano G, Appetecchia M. Hurthle cell tumours of the thyroid. Personal experience and review of the literature. Acta Otorhinolaryngol Ital. 2009;29(6):305–11.

110. Xu B, Wang L, Tuttle RM, Ganly I, Ghossein R. Prognostic impact of extent of vascular invasion in low-grade encapsulated follicular cell-derived thyroid carcinomas: a clinicopathologic study of 276 cases. Hum Pathol. 2015;46(12):1789–98.
111. Ghossein RA, Hiltzik DH, Carlson DL, Patel S, Shaha A, Shah JP, et al. Prognostic factors of recurrence in encapsulated Hurthle cell carcinoma of the thyroid gland: a clinicopathologic study of 50 cases. Cancer. 2006;106(8):1669–76.
112. Ganly I, Ricarte Filho J, Eng S, Ghossein R, Morris LG, Liang Y, et al. Genomic dissection of Hurthle cell carcinoma reveals a unique class of thyroid malignancy. J Clin Endocrinol Metab. 2013;98(5):E962–72.
113. Dedivitis RA, Di Giovanni JH, Silva GF, Marinho LC, Guimarães AV. Oncocytic variant of medullary thyroid carcinoma: case report. Arq Bras Endocrinol Metabol. 2004;48(2):315–7.
114. Sobrinho-Simões M, Magalhães J, Fonseca E, Amendoeira I. Diagnostic pitfalls of thyroid pathology. Curr Diagn Pathol. 2005;11(1):52–9.

Oncocytic (Hürthle Cell) Neoplasm: Controversy of Nature: Benign or Malignant?

9

9.1 The Challenge of Benign or Malignant

9.1.1 Introduction

One of the most difficult aspects of examining oncocytic/Hürthle cell neoplasms is to determine whether the lesion is benign or malignant. Investigators have thus tried to employ demographic (age, gender, race, ethnicity), clinicopathological criteria (tumor size, radiation history, family history, multifocality, and coexisting thyroid pathology) to better predict the risk of malignancy in oncocytic neoplasms (Hürthle cell neoplasms—HCN). However, examination of factors related specifically to the likelihood of oncocytic (Hürthle cell) carcinoma is limited.

In the past, it was believed by some authors that every Hürthle cell neoplasm (HCN) carried malignant potential and thus warranted total thyroidectomy (TT) [1]. Later studies found that the histological diagnosis was consistent with the clinical behavior of the tumors and the long-term risk of recurrence [2–4]. The current definition of a malignant oncocytic/HCN depends on capsular and/or vascular invasion, and the presence of metastasis. This cannot be determined by cytological evaluation and relies on histological examination of a surgically resected specimen. Frozen-section evaluation has been shown to be of little use in the intraoperative evaluation of these lesions. Among its limitations, frozen-section evaluation is compromised by sampling error, variable thickness, irregularity of the capsule, and freezing artifacts [5, 6].

9.1.2 Incidence

The incidence of oncocytic/Hürthle cell neoplasms (HCNs) has been reported to vary between 3% and 10% in all thyroid nodules [7–9]. These neoplasms have been classified into oncocytic adenoma (Hürthle cell adenoma—HCA) and oncocytic

M. Sakr, *Oncocytic (Hürthle Cell) Thyroid Lesions*,
https://doi.org/10.1007/978-3-032-03115-0_9

carcinoma of the thyroid (Hürthle cell carcinoma—HCC) [10]. One of the fundamental obstacles to expedited treatment is the inability to establish the diagnosis of HCC preoperatively, either radiologically or with cytology based on fine needle aspiration (FNA). In the absence of metastasis, a controversy arises regarding the nature of an oncocytic/HCN as whether it is benign or malignant since cytological criteria diagnostic of malignancy, like cellular atypia and architectural distortion, may be found in benign oncocytic/HCNs [11]. In this context, FNAB usually reports "benign Hürthle cell lesion/Hürthle cell neoplasm" (BHCL/HCN) [12].

There was a significant debate in the early endocrine and surgery literature on the incidence of malignancy in oncocytic/HCNs [4, 13–17]. Some authors cite that 80% or more of these lesions are benign, whereas others considered all oncocytic/HCNs as malignant. The latter finding was proposed because the initial studies on Hürthle cell tumors showed that even lesions that were initially diagnosed as benign acted in a malignant fashion. Throughout the years though, with good follow-up studies and refinement of criteria of malignancy in encapsulated thyroid neoplasms such as capsular and/or vascular invasion as well as the establishment of molecular techniques that have identified oncocytic follicular variants of papillary thyroid carcinoma (PTC), it has been clearly established that there are oncocytic/HCNs that act in a benign fashion as well as those that act in a malignant fashion [2, 3, 18–22].

Studies that included multiple oncocytic/Hürthle cell nodules that were found in the background of goiter or chronic lymphocytic thyroiditis (Hashimoto's thyroiditis) reported that more than 80% of oncocytic/HCNs are benign [17, 23, 24]. However, other studies that excluded these unencapsulated oncocytic/Hürthle cell nodules have shown that the rate of malignancy is higher in oncocytic/Hürthle cell neoplasms than classical follicular neoplasms (2–3% *versus* 30–45%) [3, 18–22].

9.1.3 Cytology and Histopathology

Flow cytometry and the assessment of cytological atypia have been examined as well in oncocytic/Hürthle cell neoplasms (HCNs). Cytological atypia may include necrosis, nuclear pleomorphism/crowding, greater mitoses, and/or irregular nuclei with hyperchromasia [25]. Cytomorphological criteria alone have *not* been widely shown to be helpful in distinguishing between benign and malignant oncocytic/HCNs; nuclear atypia, multi-nucleation, mitoses, and cellular pleomorphism are not sufficient and reliable determinants of malignant behavior [26–29]. Benign oncocytic nodules found in Graves' disease, long-standing nodular goiter, and chronic lymphocytic thyroiditis (Hashimoto's disease) frequently show cellular atypia and marked nuclear pleomorphism. Flow cytometry has been shown, in some studies, to provide prognostic information in histologically confirmed cancers; those with aneuploid DNA appear to behave more aggressively than those that are diploid. However, benign adenomas may demonstrate aneuploidy and cancers may be diploid. Neither flow cytometry nor analysis of cellular atypia has been proven to be able to discriminate between benign and malignant oncocytic/HCNs [6, 27, 30, 31].

Diagnosis of an oncocytic/HCN by FNA has been typically classified as a follicular lesion of undetermined significance (FLUS) or atypia of undetermined significance (AUS) with Hürthle cell features (AUS/FLUS/Hürthle cell lesion of undetermined significance [HLUS], Bethesda III). Both benign and malignant oncocytic lesions can demonstrate marked cytological atypia, complicating the process of diagnosis on biopsy alone (Fig. 9.1). Overall, the projected risk of malignancy for this diagnostic category is 5–15%. A cytological diagnosis of suspicious for HCN (Bethesda IV) carries a projected 15–30% risk of malignancy [32]. However, the true risk of malignancy for each Bethesda diagnostic cytological category varies by institution, and such institutional data should be examined regularly and made available to clinicians [33, 34].

Recently, the third edition (2023) of The Thyroid Bethesda System for Reporting Thyroid Cytopathology (TBSRTC) [35] assigned a single name for each of the six diagnostic categories based on fine-needle aspiration cytology (FNAC): (I) nondiagnostic, (II) benign, (III) atypia of undetermined significance (AUS), (IV) follicular neoplasm, (V) suspicious for malignancy, and (VI) malignant. This resolves the confusion resulting from the prior editions, which assigned alternative names for three of the diagnostic categories. Thus, TBRSTC 2023 discontinued the previously used terms of "unsatisfactory," "follicular lesion of undetermined significance (FLUS)," and "suspicious for a follicular neoplasm."

In patients with a cytological finding of a Bethesda III (B-III) category, possible management strategies include repeat ultrasound-guided FNA (potentially paired with molecular testing) and close surveillance if the molecular testing is reassuring, or surgical excision for the purpose of definitive diagnosis. The diagnostic category "AUS" (B-III)-0 should be reserved for thyroid FNAs containing cells with architectural and/or nuclear atypia that is not sufficient to classify as follicular neoplasm

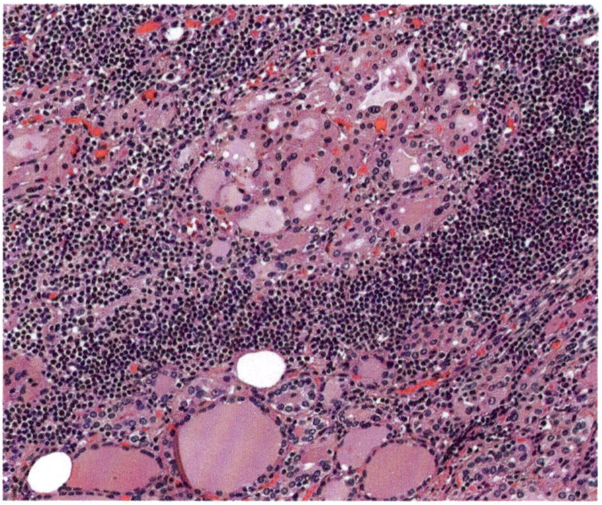

Fig. 9.1 Oncocytic change in chronic lymphocytic thyroiditis, which is characterized by a diffuse lymphoplasmacytic infiltrate that forms lymphoid follicles with germinal centers and is associated with oncocytic change of follicular epithelial cells that develop large, granular eosinophilic cytoplasm

(B-IV), suspicious for malignancy (B-V), or malignancy (B-VI); however, the atypia is more marked than can be designated as benign (B-II) [35–37]. Thus, AUS is a heterogeneous category with different cytological scenarios.

It is suggested to use the AUS category for cases in which there is a predominance of oncocytic (Hürthle) cells in a sparsely cellular FNA with scant colloid, or when there is a moderately or markedly cellular sample composed of a virtually exclusive population of oncocytic (Hürthle) cells yet the clinical setting suggests a benign oncocytic (Hürthle cell) nodule, especially chronic lymphocytic thyroiditis (Hashimoto's thyroiditis) and multinodular goiter (MNG) [38].

Some authors have suggested subclassification of AUS cases because it is likely that different malignant risks are associated with the different cytological presentations. In addition, accrual of data related to the specific cytological subtypes is desirable to better understand this equivocal diagnostic category [39, 40]. At this point, there are only limited data related specifically to the AUS, Hürthle cell type, subcategorization. According to Renshaw [39], the AUS pattern with the highest risk of malignancy (37%) is the AUS with focal nuclear atypia (i.e., AUS, cannot rule out papillary thyroid carcinoma).

Unfortunately, intraoperative frozen-section examination was consistently reported to be unhelpful in discriminating benign from malignant oncocytic/Hürthle cell neoplasms [41–44]. Thus, the sole distinction is based on presence or absence of capsular invasion (CI) (Fig. 9.2) and vascular invasion (VI) (Fig. 9.3), which can only be reliably identified in paraffin section. Therefore, in patients with fine-needle aspiration cytology (FNAC) demonstrating an oncocytic/Hürthle cell neoplasms, diagnostic surgical excision should be performed if molecular testing is not done or if it is inconclusive [45].

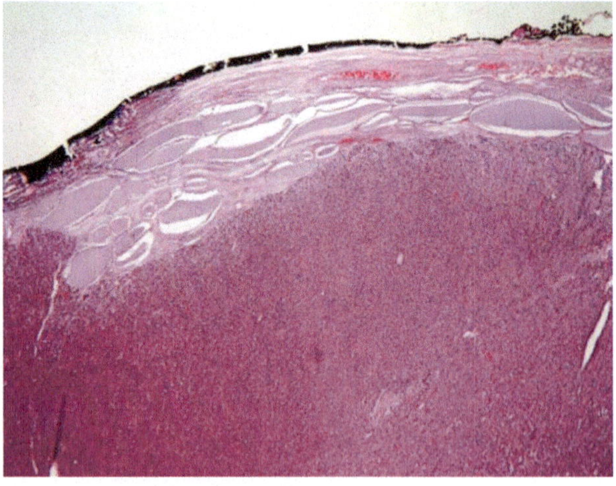

Fig. 9.2 Photomicrograph showing capsular invasion by the tumor on the left portion. H&E × 40

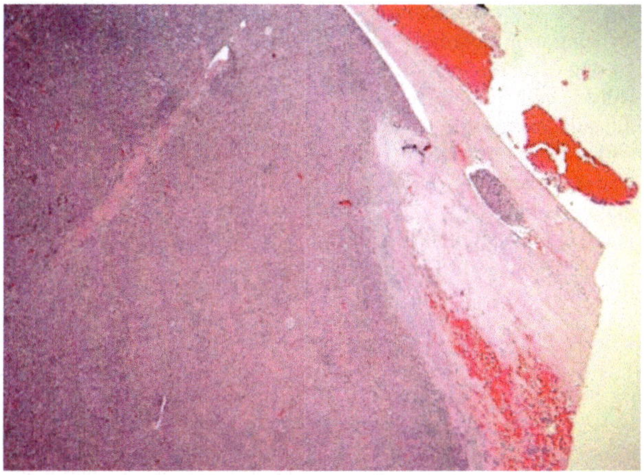

Fig. 9.3 Photomicrograph showing on the right the presence of tumor cells within a vein, indicative of vascular invasion. H&E × 40

Given the aggressive behavior of histologically proven malignant oncocytic/HCN reported by some investigators, such indeterminate findings impose a challenging situation in which clinicians tend to follow a more aggressive surgical approach. However, the incidence of malignancy among nodules, cytologically suspicious oncocytic HCN, was found, by histopathology, to range from 5% to 35% only [8, 42, 46]. Thus, a considerable proportion of these patients are unnecessarily exposed to the risk of surgical complications.

Like follicular carcinomas, oncocytic/HCCs can be classified as (1) minimally invasive, (2) angioinvasive (invasion of vessels in and/or beyond the lesional capsule), and (3) widely invasive. Minimally invasive Hürthle cell carcinomas (miHCCs) show invasion into and/or though the lesional capsule focally. These tumors should *not* have evidence of angioinvasion. Using this strict definition, the prognosis of miHCC should be excellent. Tumors with minimal capsular invasion, but evidence of vascular invasion should be classified as angioinvasive and the number of foci of vascular invasion quantified if possible.

Widely invasive Hürthle cell carcinomas (wiHCCs) are typically not a challenge, in terms of diagnosis, since they may show (1) multinodular growth into adjacent thyroid tissue with no circumscription (Fig. 9.4), (2) irregularly shaped nuclei with hyper-eosinophilic colloid or incipient necrosis (Fig. 9.5), (3) frequent mitoses and variably retained prominent nucleoli (Fig. 9.6), and (4) tumor metastasis to lateral cervical lymph nodes (LNs) (Fig. 9.7), following a typical pattern of metastasis in Hürthle cell malignancies. The presence of a solid, insular, or trabecular growth pattern, not infrequent in oncocytic/Hürthle cell tumors, raises the possibility for transformation to poorly differentiated thyroid carcinoma (PDTC) [47].

The original Turin criteria excluded oncocytic/Hürthle cell lesions [48], but this diagnostic line has become blurred more recently as reported by several

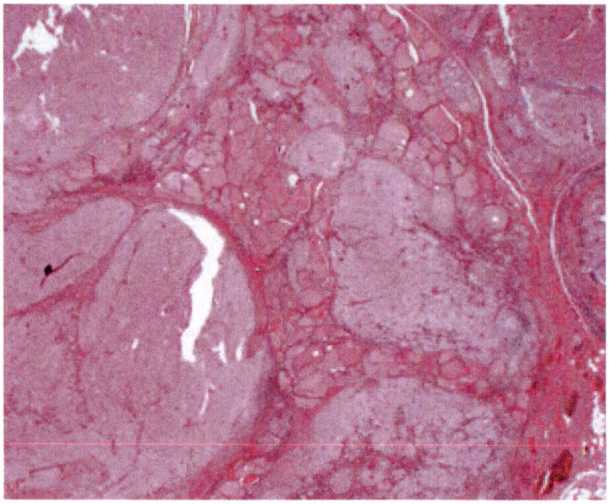

Fig. 9.4 Photomicrograph showing multinodular growth of an oncocytic/Hürthle cell carcinoma into the adjacent thyroid tissue with no circumscription, leading to noncontroversial diagnosis of widely invasive oncocytic/Hürthle cell carcinoma. H&E × 40

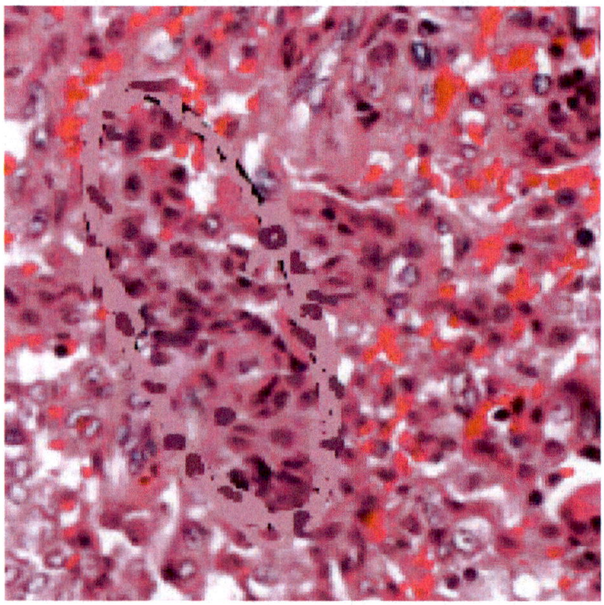

Fig. 9.5 Photomicrograph showing collections of hyper-chromatic, irregularly shaped nuclei with hyper-eosinophilic colloid (called burgeoning) or incipient necrosis indicating a widely invasive oncocytic/Hürthle cell carcinoma. H&E × 400

investigators in the literature [49–52], a line that warrants molecular testing rather than subjective histological review, especially where outcomes and treatment modalities would be modified. These are often widely invasive tumors, with necrosis and mitotic activity, but while the cytoplasm may retain Hürthle cell features, the nuclei may be pleomorphic and lack the distinct prominent, centrally located nucleolus.

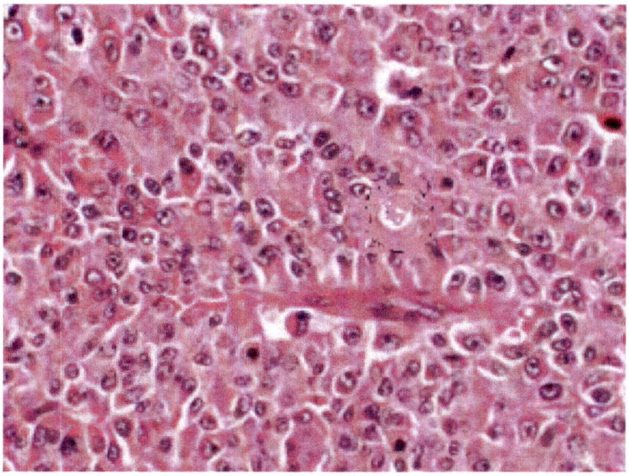

Fig. 9.6 Photomicrograph showing frequent mitoses, scattered irregular (tripolar) mitoses, and variably retained prominent nucleoli. H&E × 400

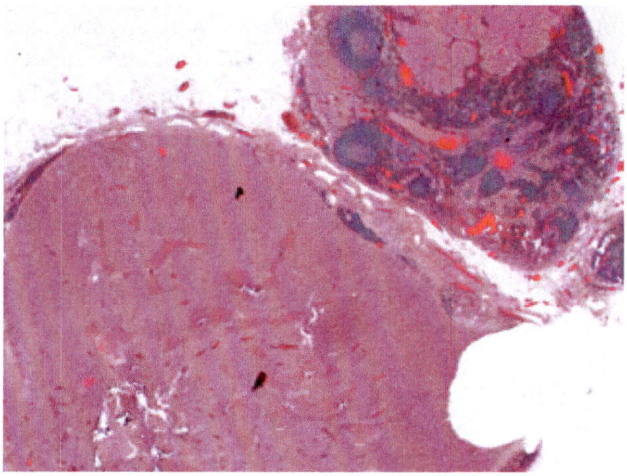

Fig. 9.7 Photomicrograph showing Hürthle cell tumor metastasis to lateral cervical lymph nodes reflecting a widely invasive oncocytic/Hürthle cell carcinoma. H&E × 20

Moreover, oncocytic/Hürthle cell tumors may have variable growth patterns that can correspond with other follicular tumors, including macro- and micro-follicular lesions. However, being hypoxia-sensitive, due to the unique mitochondria-rich nature of these tumors, they are liable to various changes including cystic degeneration, papillary cystic architecture, hyalinization, ossification, and fibrosis [47].

9.1.4 Body Mass Index (BMI) and Fine-Needle Aspiration (FNA)

In continuing trials to resolve this challenge, Arduc et al. [53] reported, in 2014, that larger body mass index (BMI) $\geq$30 kg/m^2 and waist circumference $\geq$ 88 cm were associated with higher malignancy risk in patients with FNAB diagnosis of oncocytic/Hürthle cell neoplasms (HCN). In addition, pathologists tried to refine the FNAB results by finding specific microscopical features; a micro-follicular pattern with marked nuclear atypia in a background of oncocytic (Hürthle) cells was found to be a significant predictor of malignancy [7].

9.1.5 Demographic Data

Several investigators have tried to employ demographic criteria (age, gender, race, ethnicity), and clinicopathological criteria (tumor size, radiation history, family history, multifocality, and coexisting thyroid pathology) to better predict the risk of malignancy in HCN. However, examination of factors related specifically to the likelihood of HCC is limited, as many of the studies examining this question have been small, single-institution, retrospective reviews.

Older age was found to be significantly associated with malignancy in some studies [54, 55], but not by others [56–58]. Lopez-Penbad et al. [54] reviewed the medical records of patients who were treated for oncocytic/Hürthle cell carcinoma (HCC) and oncocytic adenoma (Hürthle cell adenoma—HCA) at The University of Texas MD Anderson Cancer Center from March 1944 to February 1995. They identified 127 patients with oncocytic/Hürthle cell neoplasms, 89 patients with oncocytic/HCC, and 38 patients with oncocytic adenoma (Hürthle cell adenoma—HCA). Compared with the HCA group, the HCC group was significantly older (age 51.8 years *versus* age 43.1. years) and had larger tumors (4.3 cm *versus* 2.9 cm). Giorgadze et al. [59] reported that the risk of malignancy was higher in older patients, as 82% of nodules among patients more than 40 years of age represented a thyroid cancer *versus* 18% in those less than 40 years of age ($p < 0.0001$). Again, the specificity of these findings for oncocytic/HCC is limited, as this study included 53 cases of oncocytic/HCC, 19 cases of papillary thyroid carcinoma (PTC), 3 follicular thyroid carcinomas (FTC), and 1 medullary thyroid carcinoma (MTC).

Similarly, contradictory findings were reported concerning the association between gender and oncocytic/HCC [7, 42, 60, 61]. In the study of Lopes-Penabad et al. [54], no differences between HCA and HCC were seen regarding gender (or previous radiation exposure). In general, male gender has been reported by several authors to be more highly associated with malignancy; however, this too has been inconsistent [25, 28, 55, 62].

9.1.6 Clinical Features

Clinical criteria to guide surgeons' preoperative decision-making and determining the extent of surgery have been sought by numerous investigators [28, 55, 62]. Among the clinical parameters evaluated, the most commonly identified factors predicting malignancy have been older age and size of tumor, yet these are not consistent across series, particularly size [1, 3, 25, 26, 28, 44, 63].

Older age and tumor size were found, by some authors, to be associated with higher malignancy rates [7, 43, 64]. A 1988 study reported that an oncocytic (Hürthle cell) tumor that is 4 cm or larger has an 80% chance of histological evidence of malignancy [65]. This was confirmed 10 years later in a 1998 study by Chen et al. [43] who found that nodule size is the most significant predictor of malignancy. Of 57 patients studied, 20 had oncocytic/HCC, and their tumors were significantly larger (4.0 ± 0.4 cm) than those with oncocytic adenomas (Hürthle cell adenomas – HCAs) (2.4 ± 0.2 cm). In another more recent study (2004) by Pisanu et al. [44], in a series of 23 patients, the mean tumor size was significantly greater for carcinomas than adenomas (3.1 cm *versus* 1.9 cm).

In a 2010 retrospective single-institution study, Kim et al. [66] reviewed clinical features, preoperative imaging, and pathology reports of 57 patients with an FNAC consistent with oncocytic/HCN who underwent thyroidectomy. This study reported that on multi-logistic regression, patients with nodules more than 1.5 cm in size have a higher risk of being associated with a thyroid malignancy compared to those with nodules less than 1.5 cm. This is even more pronounced in older patients, as the predicted probability of malignancy in patients above 45 years of age with a tumor more than 1.5 cm reached 65% in this study. It should be noted that this study examined the risk of any thyroid malignancy and included nine papillary carcinomas and seven follicular carcinomas in addition to ten oncocytic/HCCs.

A similar retrospective single-institution study by Giorgadze and colleagues [59] reviewed 169 FNAs that were associated with a cytological diagnosis of an oncocytic/HCN and reported that the overall risk of thyroid malignancy was 55% for nodules ≥2 cm compared to 45% for nodules less than 2 cm ($p < 0.0001$). Tumor size has consistently been shown to be associated with the increased probability that an oncocytic/HCN on FNA will prove to be malignant. It should be noted that most of these studies were done prior to formalization of FNAC criteria according to the Bethesda scheme, and it is unclear as to how these findings would translate into the current Bethesda lexicon. More robust data are needed before clear criteria can be defined for establishing the likelihood of oncocytic/HCC in the preoperative setting.

On the other hand, several authors reported that tumor size in and of itself is *not* predictive of clinical behavior and that there is no significant correlation between malignancy and tumor size [67, 68].

9.1.7 Laboratory Data

Laboratory data, such as preoperative thyroglobulin (Tg) concentration, were also investigated; some authors found no significant difference between malignant and benign oncocytic/Hürthle cell neoplasms (HCNs), while others reported that preoperative Tg concentration was a predicting factor for malignancy in oncocytic/HCNs [57, 60].

9.1.8 Ultrasonographic Findings

Ultrasound (US) has become a widely recognized tool in the diagnosis and management of nodular thyroid disease. A number of sonographic characteristics have been reported to be more frequently associated with malignant nodules. Among these are hypo-echogenicity, micro-calcifications, ill-defined borders, internal vascularity, and nodules that are taller than wide. Although no single feature has a high degree of accuracy in predicting malignancy, the combined presence of hypo-echogenicity, micro-calcifications, and irregular borders in the same nodule has been shown to correlate with a 30-fold higher risk for malignancy in well-differentiated thyroid cancer (WDTC) [69–71]. Maizlin et al. [72] attempted to apply these criteria to lesions reported as HCNs using FNAB. The sonographic appearance of Hürthle cell neoplasms varied from hypo- to iso- and hyper-echoic regardless of their pathology. Final histological evaluation revealed that there was no characteristic sonographic appearance that could readily distinguish a benign from a malignant tumor [72]. On the other hand, hypo-echogenicity [8, 58] and hyper-echogenicity were reported to be significantly associated with malignancy while iso-echogenicity could significantly predict benignity [58].

Ultrasound may be most useful in oncocytic/HCN diagnosis when sonographically abnormal lymph nodes (LNs) are identified, suggesting metastatic disease, as reported by Pisanu et al. in 2004 [44]. Lew and Solorzano reported that preoperative FNAB of these nodes accompanied by measurement of the thyroglobulin (Tg) level of the specimen can increase the accuracy of a malignant diagnosis and greatly aid preoperative planning [71].

In conclusion, ultrasound (US) "alone" seems to be unable to distinguish oncocytic/HCC from other histological variants, as it can demonstrate a spectrum of sonographic findings from hypo-echogenicity to hyper-echogenicity [72] as shown in Fig. 9.8.

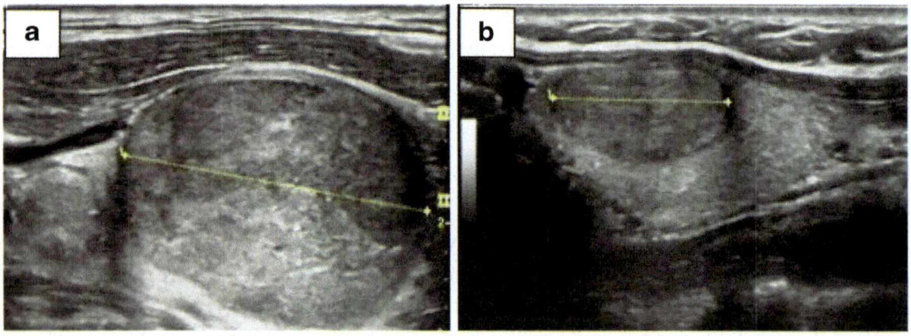

Fig. 9.8 Ultrasonography of the thyroid gland showing (**a**) Hürthle cell carcinoma. (**b**) Hürthle cell adenoma. Both nodules have similar ultrasound characteristics

9.1.9 Other Imaging Modalities

Other imaging modalities, including computed tomography (CT) scan, magnetic resonance imaging (MRI), 18-fluorodeoxyglucose-positron emission tomography (FDG-PET), and ^{99}Tc-sestamibi (MIBI) scan are often the means by which thyroid "incidentalomas" are initially detected.

There are few studies directly investigating the accuracy of FDG-PET for determining malignancy specifically in oncocytic/Hürthle cell lesions. Both adenoma (HCA) and carcinoma (HCC) often demonstrate increased FDG avidity, perhaps related to the genomic changes that lead to accumulation of abundant mitochondria [73–80]. Kim et al. reported that in a study of 36 patients who underwent thyroid surgery for a nodule diagnosed as follicular neoplasm on FNA (pre-TBSRTC), FDG-avidity did not correlate with malignancy [81]. In a later study evaluating FDG-avidity in nodules with indeterminate FNA, Deandreis et al. [82] found that the presence of Hürthle cells was independently associated with high FDG avidity, but was not correlated with malignancy. These results are explained by the fact that Hürthle cell nodules readily take up FDG regardless of their histopathological nature (benign or malignant) [83].

Oncocytic/Hürthle cell lesions often appear especially bright on MIBI scans because of their high mitochondrial content [30]. Pisanu et al. reported that a positive MIBI scan was strongly associated with oncocytic/HCN, but was of no utility in discriminating benign from malignant lesions [44]. The 2009 American Thyroid Association Guidelines for Management of Thyroid Nodules suggest that nodules that are positive on PET scan may demonstrate a higher rate of malignancy and should undergo FNAB, regardless of size [84]. Although not recommended for routine investigation in the initial evaluation of thyroid nodules, these modalities may be useful in identifying metastases associated with lesions that do not concentrate iodine, as in the case of most oncocytic/HCCs [6].

9.1.10 Studies Evaluating Oncocytic (Hürthle Cell) Neoplasm Criteria

As may be seen in Table 9.1, the discrepancy in the results of the literature published in the last three decades about studies evaluating demographic, clinicopathological, sonographic, and laboratory criteria in oncocytic Hürthle cell neoplasms (HCNs) is so obvious since no single factor has maintained consistency throughout all studies. This may be attributed to the retrospective and single institutional nature in all studies. This subsequently calls for the need of prospective multi-institutional studies to better evaluate these factors for preoperative sorting of malignant from benign cases.

Table 9.1 Studies evaluating demographic, clinicopathological, sonographic, and laboratory criteria in oncocytic/Hürthle cell neoplasms

			Significant association with malignancy	
Year	Authors	N	Yes	No
1998	Chen et al. [43]	57	Larger tumor size (4.0 ± 0.4 cm HCC vs. 2.4 ± 0.2 cm benign; $p < 0.005$). Malignancy rate for >4 cm: 65%	Age, gender, and radiation history
1999	McHenry et al. [67]	75		Age, gender, radiation history, and tumor size
2001	Sugino et al. [60]	188	Male gender	Age, tumor size, and Tg concentration
2002	Stojadinovic et al. [85]	56	Tumor size and invasion (22% of miHCC tumors >4 cm vs. 75% of wiHCC tumors >4 cm)	
2003	Lopez-Penabard et al. [54]	127	Older age and larger tumor size	Gender and radiation history
2004	Giorgadze et al. [59]	169	*Size*: (55% cancer for HCN ≥2 cm vs. 45% for HCN <2 cm ($p < 0.0001$) and *age* (82% cancer for HCN ≥40 years vs. 18% for HCN <40 years) ($p < 0.0001$)	Gender (Difference was not statistically significant)
2005	Chao et al. [68]	163		Age, gender, tumor size, and location
2006	Paunovic et al. [64]	199	Larger tumor size	Age
2006	Melck et al. [42]	27	Male gender and larger tumor size	Age and gland nodularity
2008	Sippel et al. [61]	57	Larger tumor size. Mean 5.1 cm HCC vs. 2.7 cm HCA ($p < 0.001$) Malignancy rate 55% for >4 cm & 100% for >6 cm	Age, gender, radiation history, family history, and thyroiditis
2008	Zhang et al. [55]	55	Older age and larger tumor size. *Age*: 66 ± 6 years HCC vs. 53 ± 2 years benign ($p = 0.001$) *Size*: 4.5 ± 0.7 cm HCC vs. 2.5 ± 0.2 cm benign ($p < 0.001$) *Malignancy rate* for >4 cm: 44%	Gender and gland nodularity
2010	Pisanu et al. [7]	57	Larger tumor size and multifocality. Mean 3 cm HCC vs. 1.8 cm benign ($p = 0.003$). Malignancy rate for >3 cm: 83%	Age and gender

(continued)

Table 9.1 (continued)

Year	Authors	N	Significant association with malignancy	
			Yes	No
2010	Kim et al. [66]	57	*Size*: For any thyroid cancer in HCN nodules >1.5 cm *Age* (>45 years)	
2010	Suh et al. [57]	39		Age, gender, tumor size, radiation history, family history, and Tg concentration
2013	Parikh et al. [58]	84	Hypo- or hyper-echogeniciy in US	Age, gender, race, ethnicity, presence of thyroiditis, and other sonographic criteria
2013	Lee at al [8].	75	Larger tumor size and hypo-echogenicity in US	Age, gender, and other sonographic criteria
2014	Kroeker et al. [56]	78		Age, gender, tumor size, history of head and neck radiation, family history of thyroid cancer, and calcifications in US
2014	Petric et al. [86]	244	Male gender and higher preoperative Tg level	Age and tumor size
2015	Chindris et al. [87]	173	*Size*: mean 4.0 cm wiHCC vs. 2.7 cm miHCC (44.9% of wiHCC tumors were > 4 cm vs. 7% of miHCC tumors)	Age and gender
2020	Wong et al. [88]	576	*Size*: mean 2.8 cm (malignant) vs. 2.2 cm (benign)	Age, gender, solitary or multiple nodules, lymphocytic thyroiditis
2024	Sulaiman et al. [89]	32	*Male gender:* 80% of males had HCC vs. 30% of females *Size*: 60% had HCC vs. 13% if <2 cm	Age, family history, Tg level

HCA Hürthle cell adenoma, *HCC* Hürthle cell carcinoma, *WI* widely invasive, *MI* minimally invasive, *PTC* papillary thyroid carcinoma, *FCC* follicular cell carcinoma, *HCN* Hürthle cell neoplasm, *OR* odds ratio, *CI* confidence interval, *PD* poorly differentiated

9.2 Molecular Tests and Immunohistochemistry (IHC)

9.2.1 Molecular Markers/Immunohistochemistry (IHC)

Molecular markers and immunohistochemistry (IHC) are promising tools in the preoperative diagnosis of oncocytic/HCC. *Ki67*, a marker of cell proliferation [90, 91], and *cyclin D1* [91], a cell cycle promoter, are expressed at higher levels in

HCCs than in HCAs. *Bcl-2*, on the other hand, is an antiapoptotic protein that is downregulated in HCC [3]. In 2009, Troncone et al. [29] evaluated the usefulness of a panel of IHC markers, *D-type cyclins D1* and *D3*, to determine their diagnostic performance in the assessment of FNAB samples suspicious of HCN. D-type cyclin upregulation, particularly of D3, was found to be a consistent feature of malignant lesions (HCC). The rate of false-positive diagnosis was lower when both markers were used. Using these methods in the context of a multidisciplinary assessment may improve the diagnostic accuracy [29]. Other markers examined by investigators include *MIB1, p53, galectin, topoisomerase II,* and *laminin*; as yet, none is definitive for discrimination between benign and malignant HCNs.

In 2009, Tsybrovskyy and Röβmann-Tsybrovskyy [92] proposed a theory that oncocytic change is not just an accumulation of mitochondria, but rather a complex, special reorganization of "all" major cell organelles potentially associated with malignancy pathways. They found that significantly greater endoplasmic reticulum (ER), which also stains deeply eosinophilic, was strongly associated with inflammatory processes, whereas neoplasia was characterized by significantly more mitochondria. Their findings suggest that IHC for mitochondria and ER may alter the significance of what is traditionally thought of as "oncocytic change." This merits further investigation and should be considered in the context of tumor stage, invasion, and other validated factors.

MicroRNA (miRNA) analysis is yet another emerging tool that may be helpful in differentiating benign from malignant tumors. Kitano et al. [93] investigated the role of these small, noncoding RNAs that typically serve as regulatory molecules. Microarray analysis was used to perform miRNA profiling on thyroid tissue samples in order to identify those miRNAs that were dysregulated between benign and malignant histologies, focusing on those histologies difficult to distinguish on FNAB. The group included hyperplastic nodules/multinodular goiter (MNG), oncocytic adenoma (Hürthle cell adenoma—HCA), follicular adenoma (FA), oncocytic carcinoma of the thyroid (Hürthle cell carcinoma—HCC), follicular thyroid carcinoma (FTC), papillary thyroid carcinoma (PTC), and follicular variant of PTC in their analysis, as well as normal thyroid tissue. Thirty-four miRNAs were found to be differentially expressed between benign and malignant samples. This was statistically significant ($p < 0.05$) and validated in 25 of 34 miRNAs via quantitative real-time polymerase chain reaction (PCR). Further studies, particularly, validation in additional tumor samples with FNAB samples suggesting an "indeterminant" lesion, such as follicular neoplasia (FN) or oncocytic/Hürthle cell neoplasia (HCN), are warranted [93].

Molecular marker analysis in thyroid cytology has been studied predominantly in thyroid nodules with indeterminate cytology. The three commercial tests for which the most data are available in validation trials are the Afirma Gene Expression Classifier (GEC, mRNA expression of 167 genes) [94], a seven-gene panel of genetic mutation and rearrangement testing [95], and a newer multiplexed next-generation sequencing (NGS) panel examining more than 400 known drivers of oncogenesis in thyroid cancer (ThyroSeq) [45].

Alexander et al. employed the "Gene Expression Classifier" (GEC) to evaluate 265 nodules with Bethesda III, IV, and V cytology results over 19 months in a prospective, multicenter blinded study. All thyroid nodules were ≥ 1 cm, and all study subjects had corresponding histological specimens along with fine needle biopsies. The negative predictive value (NPV) and positive predictive value (PPV) of the GEC were 95% and 38%, respectively, for aspirates classified as Bethesda III (AUS), and 94% and 37% for aspirates classified as Bethesda IV (follicular neoplasm). However, of the 21 patients with oncocytic/Hürthle cell adenomas in this study, 17 (81%) were classified as "suspicious" on the GEC. In this setting, use of the GEC in oncocytic/Hürthle cell lesions may well be associated with a relatively high false-positive result rate [94]. McIver et al. employed the GEC to evaluate 60 nodules that were reported to be either "follicular neoplasm/HCN" (B-IV) or AUS (B-III) in patients who were not at high risk for malignancy (no history of head and neck irradiation, no family history of thyroid cancer, no prior history of thyroid cancer, and no worrisome imaging characteristics). There were 31 patients with cytology suspicious for follicular neoplasm/HCN who underwent surgery; 27 of these patients had suspicious GEC results, and 4 were found to be malignant. The PPV and NPV of the GEC were 15% and 75%, respectively, for aspirates classified as suspicious for follicular neoplasm/Hürthle call neoplasm [95].

In another study, Brauner et al. studied 72 patients with cytologies B-III or B-IV with a predominance of oncocytic (Hürthle) cells who underwent GEC testing between 2010 and 2014. Forty-five (63%) GEC results were classified as suspicious for malignancy; 43 (96%) of these patients underwent surgery, and 6 (14%) were found to be malignant [96]. Similarly, Lastra et al. found that only 15% (2 of 13) of patients with a cytology suspicious for HCN and suspicious GEC harbored a malignancy [97]. Wu et al. also found an increased rate of "suspicious" GEC results in nodules with Hürthle cell predominance (77.4% vs. 50.5% for nodules without oncocytic (Hürthle) cell predominance, $p < 0.01$), but there was no difference in the rate of malignancy (25.8% *versus* 25.3%) [98]. Together, these data raise concern that there is an increased rate of suspicious GEC results in oncocytic/Hürthle cell lesions despite there being a relatively low risk of malignancy on surgical histology.

9.2.2 Genetic Alterations in Oncocytic/Hürthle Cell Neoplasms

Several recent studies using "next generation DNA sequencing methods" have comprehensively characterized the somatic genomes of oncocytic/HCC. Cumulatively, these studies have built upon foundations established by prior focused studies of the nuclear and mitochondrial genomes to unveil unique features of the oncocytic/Hürthle cell neoplasm (HCN) somatic genome compared to other forms of neoplasia [47].

Nikiforov et al. [99] applied the "next-generation sequencing" (NGS) technology to greatly expand the simultaneous testing of thyroid cancer-related genetic markers (ThyroSeq V2) in thyroid FNA samples. In a series of 143 nodules (39 malignant) with the cytological diagnosis of follicular neoplasm/suspicious for follicular neoplasm, the test performance yielded a 90% sensitivity, 93% specificity, 96% NPV, and 83% PPV for detection of any thyroid malignancy based on final surgical pathology. The study included only three oncocytic/HCC cases, of which two had a mutation detected, and the lesion with a false-negative result was reported as a minimally invasive HCC (miHCC). Therefore, the use of molecular testing in the evaluation of thyroid nodules with Hürthle cell cytological features should be understood to have limitations, as oncocytic/HCC has had a limited representation in most clinical studies. Molecular testing should *not* replace clinical judgment and consideration should be given to the pretest probability of malignancy based on clinical risk factors, ultrasound imaging, and cytological findings in interpreting the results of any molecular marker testing of FNA specimens.

9.2.3 Low Frequency of Canonical FDTC Driver Mutations

All forms of thyroid neoplasia most likely have an oncocytic component. This has been shown by several different studies. *BRAF* FV600E mutations are seen in many usual-type papillary thyroid carcinomas (PTCs) and oncocytic variants of PTC, whereas oncocytic follicular variants of PTC do not show this abnormality [100, 101]. In addition, ret. proto-oncogene/papillary thyroid carcinoma (*RET/PTC*) rearrangements have been demonstrated in oncocytic PTCs, but not always in oncocytic follicular variants of PTC [102, 103]. However, Cheung et al. [104] and Belchetz et al. [105] reclassified follicular lesions that would have been interpreted as oncocytic/Hürthle cell adenomas (HCAs) as oncocytic follicular variants of PTC based on nuclear features and the presence of *RET/PTC* rearrangements. Belchetz et al. [105] also observed that some of their lesions with the *RET/PTC* rearrangements showed lymph node (LN) metastases and behaved more like PTCs. None of the oncocytic/Hürthle cell carcinomas (HCCs) or oncocytic/HCAs included in their study contained *RET/PTC* rearrangements. Several investigators examined whether known thyroid oncogenes and tumor suppressor genes were recurrently mutated in oncocytic/HCC. Two studies reported recurrent *RET-PTC* translocations in oncocytic/HCCs using FISH and PCR methods [102, 106]. However, in larger cohorts using DNA-sequencing based methods, RET-PTC (*CCDC6-RET and NCOA4-RET*) translocations were *not* detected, nor were RET-PTC translocations recurrently identified in molecular testing of FNA specimens with Hürthle cell cytology [88, 107–112].

Oncocytic/Hürthle cell carcinomas (HCCs) harbor mutations in known thyroid cancer oncogenes including *RAS*, *TSHR*, *EIF1AX*, *TP53*, *PTEN*, *BRAF*, *PAX8-PPARγ*, and *MEN1* [107–117]. However, mutations in these genes occur in a small fraction of oncocytic/HCC. Mutations in chromatin regulatory proteins were also reported at low frequency, similar to other clinically aggressive thyroid cancers [109, 111, 118, 119]. Overall, these studies were consistent with the notion that oncocytic/HCC represented a molecularly distinct form of thyroid cancer.

Nikiforov et al. studied a panel of common thyroid cancer mutations, including *BRAFV600E, NRAS, HRAS*, and *KRAS*, as well as *RET/PTC* and *Pax8/PPARγ* rearrangements, in 1056 consecutive thyroid FNA samples with Bethesda III, IV, and V cytology results and reported a PPV of 87–95%. The NPV of the same mutational panel was 86% for Bethesda IV cytology and 94% for Bethesda III cytology [120]. However, there were only 11 follicular carcinomas in the study cohort, and the published results did not specify whether any of these were oncocytic in nature and consistent with a HCC. Mutations were detected in only 5 of 11 follicular carcinoma samples (*4 RAS* and *1 Pax8-PPARγ*), yielding a sensitivity of 45% for this histology subgroup. As *RAS* mutations are less common (and *Pax8-PPARγ* mutations nonexistent) in oncocytic/HCC compared to follicular carcinoma [121], it would follow that this limited mutation panel testing is less reliable in detecting oncocytic/HCC.

9.2.4 Identification of Mitochondrial Genome (mtDNA) Alterations in Oncocytic/HCC

The accumulation of structurally abnormal mitochondria is a defining feature of HCN and other oncocytic neoplasms. The mitochondrial genome (mtDNA) is a small circular, bacterial-like genome that originated in the bacterial symbiont, which evolved into the mitochondrion organelle. The mtDNA encodes a total of 37 genes, including 13 components of the mitochondrial "electron transport chain" (ETC). Deleterious germline mutations in the mtDNA, which are maternally inherited, result in variable impairment of the ETC and lead to an array of congenital diseases [122]. In models of severe ETC impairment, morphologically abnormal mitochondria accumulate, which is thought to represent a compensatory response to impaired mitochondrial function [123].

In 2007, Sheu et al. [124] reported that carriers of the C allele of the common C825T polymorphism in guanine nucleotide binding protein 3 gene appear to have an increased risk of developing oncocytic thyroid tumors. They proposed that this polymorphism may be a factor favoring the development of oncocytic thyroid tumors, although the biological mechanism remains obscure. They believe that there may be a genetic predisposition of patients to develop oncocytic thyroid neoplasms. Whether this is somehow related to the mitochondrial DNA (mtDNA) alterations seen in oncocytic thyroid tumors remains to be demonstrated. Gasparre et al. [125] reported that disruptive mutations in mtDNA were found in complex I subunit genes in oncocytic/Hürthle cell neoplasms and this finding appears to be a marker for thyroid oncocytic tumors.

Several groups have examined electron transport chain function and mtDNA in oncocytic/HCC and other thyroid cancers. A study of mtDNA mutations in a "panel of thyroid cancers" revealed frequent mtDNA mutations that clustered in genes encoding subunits of complex I of the ETC [126]. A study of ATP levels and oxygen consumption in a panel of oncocytic/HCNs was also consistent with impaired ETC function [127]. A key development in the field was the derivation of a cancer cell line from an oncocytic/HCC breast metastasis, *XTC.UC1* [128]. The *XTC.UC1* cells were subsequently found to exhibit impaired ETC function and harbor disruptive mtDNA mutations in complex I and complex III [79]. Gasparre et al. then reported a complete mtDNA sequencing study of 45 oncocytic neoplasms [125]. The majority of oncocytic tumors harbored mutations in the mtDNA that clustered within genes encoding subunits of complex I. Approximately 50% (12/25) of the complex I mutations were predicted to be functionally disruptive (frame-shift or nonsense mutations). This study established that mutations in mtDNA-encoded complex I subunits were highly recurrent in oncocytic/HCNs.

Mitochondrial DNA (mtDNA) exists at up to thousands of copies per cell. Therefore, mtDNA mutations can exist in a fraction (heteroplasmy) or all (homoplasmy) of the mtDNA copies. The relative fraction of deleterious mutants can impact the degree of ETC impairment, as well as phenotypes associated with individual mtDNA mutations [122]. Recently (2018), Gopal et al. extended analysis of mtDNA to a cohort of oncocytic/HCC that included sequentially resected primary and metastatic lesions from individual patients [111]. In their study, mtDNA mutations were identified in 60% of oncocytic/HCC patients (24/40).

The depth of sequencing coverage provided by exome sequencing also enabled the investigators to estimate mtDNA heteroplasmy in the samples. According to pan-cancer sequencing data analyzed by Gopal et al., deleterious mutations in complex-I subunits most frequently existed at low fraction across all cancer types (only a small fraction of mtDNA in the tumor carried the disruptive mutation) [111]. This finding suggested that most tumors select against mutations that compromise complex-I function. Interestingly, the opposite trend was observed in oncocytic/HCC: deleterious complex-I mtDNA mutations existed in a very high fraction of mtDNA sequencing reads. This observation suggested that, unlike other forms of cancer, mutations that impaired complex-I function were under positive selection in HCC and therefor possibly advantageous for tumor growth. Additionally, when the deleterious complex-I mtDNA mutation was homoplasmic in the primary tumor, metastases derived from these primary tumors that maintained the mtDNA mutation at similar levels.

The results of this study supported the notion that loss of mitochondrial respiration, specifically through complex-I impairment, was advantageous to oncocytic/HCC tumorigenesis, and might therefore act as a driver alteration in oncocytic neoplasms. Interestingly, similar findings were reported in renal oncocytoma, which also harbored frequent mtDNA mutations in complex-I subunits [129]. Those studies suggested that impairment of complex-I function was an important early driver of oncocytic tumors arising in multiple tissues (common biology). Consistent with this notion, in a recent pan-cancer analysis of nuclear and mitochondrial genomes in over 2600 tumors, the combination of a non-silent mtDNA mutation without another known cancer driver gene mutation was most prevalent in thyroid and chromophobe kidney cancers [130].

9.2.5 Chromosome Gains and Losses in Oncocytic/HCC

Chromosomal aberrations are well-established drivers of cancer initiation and progression. Early studies of overall DNA content in oncocytic/HCN suggested high frequency of aneuploidy [131]. A study by Mazzuchelli et al. systemically assessed individual chromosomes using fluorescence in situ hybridization (FISH) methods [132]. Chromosome losses were observed more frequently compared to chromosomal gains in HCN. Specifically, monosomies of chromosomes *8, 22*, and *2* were and gains of chromosome *7, 12,* and *17* were observed. Another study using FISH by Erickson et al. reported also found that tumors with a greater number of chromosome losses exhibited poorer outcomes by retrospective analysis [133].

Cover et al. utilized genome-wide DNA microarrays to more comprehensively evaluate chromosomal gains and losses in oncocytic/HCN [134]. Whole chromosome losses were widespread leading to near haploidization of the genome in oncocytic/HCC. This finding was validated using single nucleus flow cytometry and FISH, and these alterations were unique in oncocytic/HCN compared to other thyroid cancers. Consistent with the earlier studies, Chr *7* was never haploid, and losses of Chrs *5, 12, 17,* and *20* were infrequent.

Maximo et al. [135] have identified somatic missense mutations in *GRIM19* in approximately 11% of sporadic HCCs. *GRIM19* is believed to promote apoptosis as part of the interferon-β and retinoic acid induced pathway of cell death, is a negative regulator of cell growth, is involved in mitochondrial metabolism, and is linked in part to mitochondrial complex I assembly. Interestingly, *GRIM19* is located at 19p13.2. The *TCO* gene locus, which has been linked to familial Hürthle cell neoplasms, has also been mapped to this locus [136, 137]. Baris et al. [138] reported that oncocytic follicular neoplasms show distinct differences in gene expression as compared with usual-type PTC. For one thing, HCCs more commonly express genes associated with mitochondrial and cellular metabolism. In addition, this group observed that overexpression of the respiratory chain complexes III and IV seems to be specific to the development of oncocytic follicular carcinomas. Bonora et al. [139] reported that there are variations in the inner mitochondrial membrane transporter *TIMM44* in patients with oncocytic thyroid tumors.

Two recent exome sequencing studies of oncocytic/HCC reported similar findings and confirmed prior associations between widespread chromosome gains and losses and clinical outcomes. Ganly et al. reported that miHCC were frequently diploid or harbored a few chromosomal losses or duplications. In contrast, widely invasive HCC (wiHCC) more frequently harbored evidence of chromosomal amplifications, always involving chromosome *7* [109]. Gopal et al. reported a high frequency of near-haploid HCC exhibiting widespread chromosomal losses [111]. A subset of near-haploid oncocytic/HCC underwent whole genome duplication (WGD) that led to amplification of chromosome *7* and uniparental disomy of much of the genome. Interestingly, comparison of the ploidy state of related primary and metastatic tumors suggested that WGD was not a prerequisite for metastatic progression. Near-haploid primary tumors seeded metastases that generally maintained the near-haploid state. However, in a few patients, near-haploid primary tumors seeded metastases that exhibited WGD. Primary tumors that exhibited WGD also maintained this state in metastases.

The underlying basis of chromosomal loss remains unclear, although several hypotheses have been proposed [140, 141]. Specific chromosomes appear to undergo gains or losses more frequently than others, suggesting that unique selective pressures are exerted on individual chromosomes. *Chrs 1, 2, 3, 4, 6, 8, 9, 11, 14, 15, 21, 22* exhibited whole chromosome *LOH* in most cases reported by Gopal et al. In contrast, *Chrs 5, 7, 12,* and *20* exhibited increased copy number relative to other chromosomes. However, it is not clear whether duplication of *Chrs 5, 7, 12,* and *20* stemmed from positive selection for increased DNA copy number of these chromosomes, or rather originated because these Chrs rarely underwent chromosomal loss prior to WGD. Nonetheless, the fact that Chr *5, 7, 12,* and *20* were infrequently lost suggested that genes encoded on these chromosomes contribute to oncocytic/HCC or growth or survival.

Together, these studies suggest an advantage for progressive chromosomal losses during the outgrowth of oncocytic/HCC. Widespread chromosomal loss, as seen in oncocytic/HCC, is observed infrequently in cancer. However, cases of germ cell tumors, leukemia, renal oncocytoma, giant cell glioblastoma, mesothelioma, parathyroid, and adrenocortical carcinoma harbor near-haploid genomes, typically in a much smaller fraction of tumors compared to HCC [129, 142–149]. This observation suggests the near-haploid state can contribute to tumor growth, at least in some cancers.

All of these studies seem to indicate that there is a genetic predisposition to develop oncocytic thyroid tumors.

9.3 Stratification of Hürthle Cell Carcinoma Risk

In the past, oncocytic/Hürthle cell carcinoma (HCC) was designated by the World Health Organization (WHO) as a histopathological variant of follicular thyroid carcinoma (FTC), and this was echoed in the American Thyroid Association (ATA) and National Comprehensive Cancer Network (NCCN) treatment guidelines, with oncocytic/HCC following the same risk stratification as that of follicular carcinoma. The fifth edition of the WHO classification of thyroid tumors published recently (2022) considered Hürthle cell carcinoma (now called by the WHO "oncocytic carcinoma") as a separate pathological entity of well-differentiated thyroid carcinoma (WDC) and not a subtype of follicular thyroid carcinoma (FTC) [150]. For the American Thyroid Association (ATA), intrathyroidal encapsulated tumors with minor capsular or vascular invasion (< 4 foci) or ≤ 5 metastatic lymph nodes (LNs) where the foci of metastases are less than 0.2 cm are considered to be "low risk." The "intermediate risk" is defined by minimal extra-thyroidal extension, or > 5 metastatic LNs (0.2–3 cm). On the other hand, "high-risk" patients include those with *macroscopic extra-thyroidal extension, incomplete tumor resection, metastatic*

Table 9.2 Stratification of Hürthle carcinoma risk

Low risk	Intermediate risk	High risk
Intrathyroidal encapsulated tumors Minor capsular invasion Minor vascular invasion Metastatic LNs (≤5) where metastatic foci are <0.2 cm	Minimal extra-thyroidal extension Vascular invasion Metastatic LNs (>5) where metastatic foci are 0.2–3 cm	Macroscopic extra-thyroidal extension Incomplete tumor resection Metastatic LNs >3 cm Distant metastases

LNs > 3 cm, or distant metastases [45] [Table 9.2]. The NCCN guidelines for HCC (Version 1.2016) describe minimal vascular invasion as a few microscopic foci (≤4) of invasion in an intrathyroidal HCC. The NCCN guidelines assign these patients to a low-risk group [151].

References

1. Gundry SR, Burney RE, Thompson NW, Lloyd R. Total thyroidectomy for Hürthle cell neoplasm of the thyroid. Arch Surg. 1983;118:529–32.
2. Carcangiu ML, Bianchi S, Savino D, Voynick IM, Rosai J. Follicular Hürthle cell tumors of the thyroid gland. Cancer. 1991;68:1994–53.
3. Gosain AK, Clark OH. Hürthle cell neoplasms: Malignant potential. Arch Surg. 1984;119:515–9.
4. Grant CS, Barr D, Goellner JR, Hay ID. Benign Hürthle cell tumors of the thyroid: a diagnosis to be trusted? World J Surg. 1988;12:488–95.
5. LiVolsi VA, Baloch ZW. Use and abuse of frozen section in the diagnosis of follicular thyroid lesions. Endocr Pathol. 2005;16:285–93.
6. McHenry CR, Sandoval BA. Management of follicular and Hürthle cell neoplasms of the thyroid gland. Surg Oncol Clin N Am. 1998;7:893–910.
7. Pisanu A, Di Chiara B, Reccia I, UcchedduA. Oncocytic cell tumors of the thyroid: factors predicting malignancy and influencing prognosis, treatment decisions, and outcomes. World J Surg. 2010;34(4):836–43.
8. Lee KH, Shin JH, Ko ES, Hahn SY, Kim JS, Kim JH, et al. Predictive factors of malignancy in patients with cytologically suspicious for Hurthle cell neoplasm of thyroid nodules. Int J Surg. 2013;11(9):898–902.
9. Zhang YW, Greenblatt DY, Repplinger D, Bargren A, Adler J, Chen H, et al. Factors that predict malignancy in Hürthle cell neoplasms of the thyroid. J Surg Res. 2008;144(2):371–2.
10. Mills SC, Haq M, Smellie WJ, Harmer C. Hurthle cell carcinoma of the thyroid: retrospective review of 62 patients treated at the Royal Marsden Hospital between 1946 and 2003. Eur J Surg Oncol. 2009;35(3):230–4.
11. Stojadinovic A, Ghossein RA, Hoos A, Urist MJ, Spiro RH, Shah JP, et al. Hurthle cell carcinoma: a critical histopathologic appraisal. J Clin Oncol. 2001;19(10):2616–25.
12. Wakely PE Jr. Oncocytic and oncocyte-like lesions of the head and neck. Ann Diagn Pathol. 2008;12(3):222–30.
13. Tallini G, Carcangiu ML, Rosai J. Oncocytic neoplasms of the thyroid gland. Acta Pathol Jpn. 1992;42:305–15.
14. Thompson NW, Dunn EL, Batsakin JG. Hürthle cell lesions of the thyroid gland. Surg Gynecol Obstet. 1974;139:555–60.
15. Bondeson L, Azavedo E, Bondeson AG, Caspersson T, Ljungberg O. Nuclear DNA content and behavior of oxyphil thyroid tumors. Cancer. 1986;58:672–5.

16. Bondeson L, Bondeson AG, Ljungberg O. Treatment of Hürthle cell neoplasms of the thyroid. Arch Surg. 1983;118:1453.
17. Bondeson L, Bondeson AG, Ljungberg O, Tibblin S. Oxyphil tumors of the thyroid: follow-up of 42 surgical cases. Ann Surg. 1981;194:677–80.
18. Har-El G, Hadar T, Segal K, Levy R, Sidi J. Hürthle cell carcinoma of the thyroid gland: a tumor of moderate malignancy. Cancer. 1986;57:1613–7.
19. Bronner M, LiVolsi VA. Oxyphilic (Askenasy/Hürthle cell) tumors of the thyroid: microscopic features predict biologic behavior. Surg Pathol. 1988;1:137–50.
20. Johnson TL, Lloyd RV, Burney RE, Thompson NW. Hürthle cell thyroid tumors: an immunohistochemical study. Cancer. 1987;59:107–12.
21. Arganini M, Behar R, Wu TC, Straus F 2nd, McCormick M, DeGroot LJ, et al. Hürthle cell tumors: a twenty-five-year experience. Surgery. 1986;100:1108–15.
22. Carcangiu ML. Hürthle cell carcinoma: clinic-pathological and biological aspects. Tumori. 2003;89:529–32.
23. Gardner LW. Hürthle-cell tumors of the thyroid. Arch Pathol. 1955;59:372–81.
24. Saull SC, Kimmelman CP. Hürthle cell tumors of the thyroid gland. Otolaryngol Head Neck Surg. 1985;93:58–62.
25. McHenry CR, Thomas SR, Slusarczyk SJ, Khiyami A. Follicular or Hürthle cell neoplasm of the thyroid: can clinical factors be used to predict carcinoma and determine extent of thyroidectomy? Surgery. 1999;126:798–804.
26. McLeod MK, Thompson NW. Hürthle cell neoplasms of the thyroid. Otolaryngol Clin N Am. 1990;23:441–52.
27. Montone KT, Baloch ZW, LiVolsi VA. The thyroid Hürthle (oncocytic) cell and its associated pathologic conditions: a surgical pathology and cytopathology review. Arch Pathol Lab Med. 2008;132:1241–50.
28. Na HY, Moon JH, Choi JY, Yu HW, Jeong WJ, Kim YK, et al. Preoperative diagnostic categories of fine needle aspiration cytology for histologically proven thyroid follicular adenoma and carcinoma, and Hurthle cell adenoma and carcinoma: analysis of cause of under- or misdiagnoses. PLoS One. 2020;15(11):e0241597.
29. Troncone G, Volante M, Iaccarino A, Zeppa P, Cozzolino I, Malapelle U, et al. Cyclin D1 and D3 overexpression predicts malignant behavior in thyroid fine-needle aspirates suspicious for Hürthle cell neoplasms. Cancer. 2009;117:522–9.
30. Layfield LJ, Cibas ES, Baloch Z. Thyroid fine needle aspiration cytology: a review of the National Cancer Institute state of the science symposium. Cytopathology. 2010;21:75–85.
31. Nguyen GK, Husain M, Akin MR. Cytodiagnosis of benign and malignant Hürthle cell lesions of the thyroid by fine-needle aspiration biopsy. Diagn Cytopathol. 1999;20:261–5.
32. Cibas ES, Ali SZ. The Bethesda system for reporting thyroid cytopathology. Thyroid. 2009;19(11):1159–65.
33. Bernstein JM, Shah M, MacMillan C, Freeman JL. Institution-specific risk of papillary thyroid carcinoma in atypia/follicular lesion of undetermined significance. Head Neck. 2016;38(Suppl 1):E1210–5.
34. Wang CC, Friedman L, Kennedy GC, Wang H, Kebebew E, Steward DL, et al. A large multicenter correlation study of thyroid nodule cytopathology and histopathology. Thyroid. 2011;21(3):243–51.
35. Ali SZ, Baloch ZW, Cochand-Priollet B, Schmitt FC, Vielh P, VanderLann PA. The 2023 Bethesda system for reporting thyroid cytopathology. Thyroid. 2023;23(9):1039–44.
36. Nguyen GK, Ginsberg J, Crockford PM. Fine needle aspiration biopsy cytology of the thyroid. Its value and limitations in the diagnosis and treatment of solitary thyroid nodules. Pathol Annu. 1991;26(1):63–91.
37. Gharib H, Goeller JR, Zinsmeister AR, Grant CS, Heerden JA. Fine-needle aspiration biopsy of the thyroid. The problem of suspicious cytologic findings. Ann Intern Med. 1984;101:25–8.
38. Roh MH, Jo VY, Stelow EB, et al. The predictive value of the fine-needle aspiration diagnosis "suspicious for a FNHCT" in patients with Hashimoto thyroiditis. Am J Clin Pathol. 2012;120:73–86.

39. Renshaw AA. Should "atypical follicular cells" in thyroid fine-needle aspirates be subclassified? Cancer Cytopathol. 2010;118:186–9.
40. VanderLaan P, Marqusee E, Krane JF. Clinical outcome for atypia of undetermined significance in thyroid fine-needle aspirations. Should repeated FNA be the preferred initial approach? Am J Clin Pathol. 2011;135:770–5.
41. Stankov K, Romeo G. Oxyphilic carcinoma of the thyroid gland. Arch Oncol. 2003;11(2):81–9.
42. Melck A, Bugis S, Baliski C, et al. Hemithyroidectomy: the preferred initial surgical approach for management of Hurthle cell neoplasm. Am J Surg. 2006;191(5):593–7.
43. Chen H, Nicol TL, Zeiger MA, Dooley WC, Ladenson PW, Cooper DS, et al. Hurthle cell neoplasms of the thyroid: are there factors predictive of malignancy? Ann Surg. 1998;227(4):542–6.
44. Pisanu A, Sias L, Uccheddu A. Factors predicting malignancy of Hürthle cell tumors of the thyroid: influence on surgical treatment. World J Surg. 2004;28(8):761–5.
45. Haugen BR, Alexander EK, Bible KC, Doherty GM, Mandel SJ, Nikiforov YE, et al. 2015 American Thyroid Association management guidelines for adult patients with thyroid nodules and differentiated thyroid cancer: the American Thyroid Association Guidelines Task Force on Thyroid Nodules and Differentiated Thyroid Cancer. Thyroid. 2016;26(1):1–133.
46. Pu RT, Yang J, Wasserman PG, Bhuiya T, Griffith KA, Michael CW. Does Hurthle cell lesion/neoplasm predict malignancy more than follicular lesion/neoplasm on thyroid fine-needle aspiration? Diagn Cytopathol. 2006;34(5):330–4.
47. McFadden DG, Sadow PM. Genetics, diagnosis, and management of hürthle cell thyroid neoplasms. Front Endocrinol (Lausanne). 2021;12:696386.
48. Volante M, Collini P, Nikiforov YE, Sakamoto A, Kakudo K, Katoh R, et al. Poorly differentiated thyroid carcinoma: the turin proposal for the use of uniform diagnostic criteria and an algorithmic diagnostic approach. Am J Surg Pathol. 2007;31:1256–64.
49. Bai S, Baloch ZW, Samulski TD, Montone KT, LiVolsi VA. Poorly differentiated oncocytic (Hurthle cell) follicular carcinoma: an institutional experience. Endocr Pathol. 2015;26:164–9.
50. Dettmer M, Schmitt A, Steinert H, Moch H, Komminoth P, Perren A. Poorly differentiated oncocytic thyroid carcinoma–diagnostic implications and outcome. Histopathology. 2012;60:1045–51.
51. Dettmer MS, Schmitt A, Komminoth P, Perren A. Poorly differentiated thyroid carcinoma : an underdiagnosed entity. Pathologe. 2020;41:1–8.
52. Metovic J, Vignale C, Annaratone L, Osella-Abate S, Maletta F, Rapa I, et al. The oncocytic variant of poorly differentiated thyroid carcinoma shows a specific immune-related gene expression profile. J Clin Endocrinol Metab. 2020;105(12):e4577–92.
53. Arduc A, Dogan BA, Tuna MM, Tutuncu Y, Isik S, Berker D, et al. Higher body mass index and larger waist circumference may be predictors of thyroid carcinoma in patients with Hurthle-cell lesion/neoplasm fine-needle aspiration diagnosis. Clin Endocrinol. 2015;83(3):405–11.
54. Lopez-Penabad L, Chiu AC, Hoff AO, Chultz P, Gaztambide S, Ordoñez NG, et al. Prognostic factors in patients with Hurthle cell neoplasms of the thyroid. Cancer. 2003;97(5):1186–94.
55. Zhang Y, Greenblatt D, Repplinger D, Bargren A, Adler JT, Sippel RS, et al. Older age and larger tumor size predict malignancy in Hürthle cell neoplasms of the thyroid. Ann Surg Oncol. 2008;15(10):2842–6.
56. Kroeker T, Prisman E, Shah M, MacMillan C, Freeman JL. Hurthle cell lesions-a retrospective review of final surgical pathology. Thyroid Disord Ther. 2014;3(2):155.
57. Suh I, Vriens MR, Guerrero MA, Griffin A, Shen WT, Duh QY, et al. Serum thyroglobulin is a poor diagnostic biomarker of malignancy in follicular and Ḧurthle-cell neoplasms of the thyroid. Am J Surg. 2010;200(1):41–6.
58. Parikh PP, Allan BJ, Lew JI. Surgeon-performed ultrasound predictors of malignancy in patients with Hürthle cell neoplasms of the thyroid. J Surg Res. 2013;184(1):247–52.
59. Giorgadze T, Rossi ED, Fadda G, Gupta PK, Livolsi VA, Baloch Z. Does the fine-needle aspiration diagnosis of "Hurthle-cell neoplasm/follicular neoplasm with oncocytic features" denote increased risk of malignancy? Diagn Cytopathol. 2004;31(5):307–12.

60. Sugino K, Ito K, Mimura T, et al. Hürthle cell tumor of the thyroid: analysis of 188 cases. World J Surg. 2001;25(9):1160–3.
61. Sippel RS, Elaraj DM, Khanafshar E, Zarnegar R, Kebebew E, Duh QY, et al. Tumor size predicts malignant potential in Hurthle cell neoplasms of the thyroid. World J Surg. 2008;32(5):702–7.
62. Chen H, Nicol TL, Zeiger MA, Dooley WC, Ladenson PW, Cooper DS, et al. Hürthle cell neoplasms of the thyroid: are there factors predictive of malignancy? Ann Surg. 1998;227:542–6.
63. Wu HH, Clouse J, Ren R. Fine-needle aspiration cytology of Hürthle cell carcinoma of the thyroid. Diagn Cytopathol. 2008;36:149–54.
64. Paunovic I, Krgovic K, Tatic S, Diklic A, Zivaljevic V, Kalezic N, et al. Surgery for thyroid Hürthle cell tumours – a single institution experience. Eur J Surg Oncol. 2006;32(4):458–61.
65. Bronner MP, Clevenger CV, Edmonds PR, Lowell DM, McFarland MM, LiVolsi VA. Flow cytometric analysis of DNA content in Hürthle cell adenomas and carcinomas of the thyroid. Am J Clin Pathol. 1988;89(6):764–9.
66. Kim TH, Lim JA, Ahn HY, Lee EK, Min HS, Won Kim K, et al. Tumor size and age predict the risk of malignancy in Hurthle cell neoplasm of the thyroid and can therefore guide the extent of initial thyroid surgery. Thyroid. 2010;20(11):1229–34.
67. McHenry CR, Thomas SR, Slusarczyk SJ, Khiyami A. Follicular or Hurthle cell neoplasm of the thyroid: can clinical factors be used to predict carcinoma and determine extent of thyroidectomy? Surgery. 1999;126(4):798–804.
68. Chao T-C, Lin J-D, ChenM-F. Surgical treatment of Hurthle cell tumors of the thyroid. World J Surg. 2005;29(2):164–8.
69. Kim EK, Park CS, Chung WY, Oh KK, Kim DI, Lee JT, et al. New sonographic criteria for recommending fine-needle aspiration biopsy of nonpalpable solid nodules of the thyroid. AJR Am J Roentgenol. 2002;178:687–91.
70. Lew JI, Rodgers SE, Solorzano CC. Developments in the use of ultrasound for thyroid cancer. Curr Opin Oncol. 2010;22:11–6.
71. Lew JI, Solσrzano CC. Use of ultrasound in the management of thyroid cancer. Oncologist. 2010;15:253–8.
72. Maizlin ZV, Wiseman SM, Vora P, Kirby JM, Mason AC, Filipenko D, et al. Hürthle cell neoplasms of the thyroid: Sonographic appearance and histologic characteristics. J Ultrasound Med. 2008;27:751–7.
73. Nesland JM, Sobrinho-Simões MA, Holm R, Sambade MC, Johannessen JV. Hürthle-cell lesions of the thyroid: a combined study using transmission electron microscopy, scanning electron microscopy, and immunocytochemistry. Ultrastruct Pathol. 1985;8:269–90.
74. Satoh M, Yagawa K. Electron microscopic study on mitochondria in Hürthle cell adenoma of thyroid. Pathol Int. 1981;31:1079–87.
75. Sobrinho-Simões MA, Nesland JM, Holm R, Sambade MC, Johannessen JV. Hürthle cell and mitochondrion-rich papillary carcinomas of the thyroid gland: an ultrastructural and immunocytochemical study. Ultrastruct Pathol. 1985;8:131–42.
76. Máximo V, Sobrinho-Simões M. Mitochondrial DNA “common” deletion in Hürthle cell lesions of the thyroid. J Pathol. 2000;192:561–2.
77. Máximo V, Soares P, Lima J, Cameselle-Teijeiro J, Sobrinho-Simões M. Mitochondrial DNA somatic mutations (point mutations and large deletions) and mitochondrial DNA variants in human thyroid pathology: a study with emphasis on Hürthle cell tumors. Am J Pathol. 2002;160:1857–65.
78. Gasparre G, Porcelli AM, Bonora E, Pennisi LF, Toller M, Iommarini L, et al. Disruptive mitochondrial DNA mutations in complex I subunits are markers of oncocytic phenotype in thyroid tumors. Proc Natl Acad Sci USA. 2007;104:9001–6.
79. Bonora E, Porcelli AM, Gasparre G, Biondi A, Ghelli A, Carelli V, et al. Defective oxidative phosphorylation in thyroid oncocytic carcinoma is associated with pathogenic mitochondrial DNA mutations affecting complexes I and III. Cancer Res. 2006;66:6087–96.
80. Pathak KA, Klonisch T, Nason RW, Leslie WD. FDG-PET characteristics of Hürthle cell and follicular adenomas. Ann Nucl Med. 2016;30:506–9.

81. Kim JM, Ryu J-S, Kim TY, Kim WB, Kwon GY, Gong G, et al. 18F-fluorodeoxyglucose positron emission tomography does not predict malignancy in thyroid nodules cytologically diagnosed as follicular neoplasm. J Clin Endocrinol Metab. 2007;92:1630–4.
82. Deandreis D, Al Ghuzlan A, Auperin A, Vielh P, Caillou B, Chami L, et al. Is (18) F-fluorodeoxyglucose–PET/CT useful for the presurgical characterization of thyroid nodules with indeterminate fine needle aspiration cytology? Thyroid. 2012;22:165–72.
83. de Koster EJ, de Geus-Oei LF, Brouwers AH, van Dam E, Dijkhorst-Oei LT, van Engen-van Grunsven ACH, et al. [(18)F]FDG-PET/CT to prevent futile surgery in indeterminate thyroid nodules: A blinded, randomised controlled multicentre trial. Eur J Nucl Med Mol Imaging. 2022;49:1970–84.
84. Cooper DS, Doherty GM, Haugen BR, Kloos RT, Lee SL, Mandel SJ, et al. Revised American Thyroid Association management guidelines for patients with thyroid nodules and differentiated thyroid cancer. Thyroid. 2009;11:1167–214.
85. Stojadinovic A, Hoos A, Ghossein RA, Urist MJ, Leung DH, Spiro RH, et al. Hurthle cell carcinoma: a 60-year experience. Ann Surg Oncol. 2002;9(2):197–203.
86. Petric R, Besic H, Besic N. Preoperative serum thyroglobulin concentration as a predictive factor of malignancy in small follicular and Hürthle cell neoplasms of the thyroid gland. World J Surg Oncol. 2014;12(1):1–7.
87. Chindris AM, Casler JD, Bernet VJ, Rivera M, Thomas C, Kachergus JM, et al. Clinical and molecular features of Hurthle cell carcinoma of the thyroid. J Clin Endocrinol Metab. 2015;100(1):55–62.
88. Wong KS, Jo VY, Lowe AC, Faquin WC, Renshaw AA, Shah AA, et al. Malignancy risk for solitary and multiple nodules in Hürthle cell-predominant thyroid fine-needle aspirations: a multi-institutional study. Cancer Cytopathol. 2020;128(1):68–75.
89. Sulaiman S, Chirukandath R, Krishnan SK, Rajesh N, Antony M, Mohan KSS. Unraveling the enigma: a five-year comprehensive analysis of hurthle cell tumors in south India's tertiary care center. Cureus. 2024;16(3):e57166.
90. Hoos A, Stojadinovic A, Singh B, Dudas ME, Leung DH, Shaha AR, et al. Clinical significance of molecular expression profiles of Hurthle cell tumors of the thyroid gland analyzed via tissue microarrays. Am J Pathol. 2002;160(1):175–83.
91. Erickson LA, Jin L, Goellner JR, Lohse C, Pankratz VS, Zukerberg LR, et al. Pathologic features, proliferative activity, and cyclin D1 expression in Hurthle cell neoplasms of the thyroid. Mod Pathol. 2000;13(2):186–92.
92. Tsybrovskyy O, Rößmann-Tsybrovskyy M. Oncocytic versus mitochondrion-rich follicular thyroid tumors: Should we make a difference? Histopathology. 2009;55:665–82.
93. Kitano M, Rahbari R, Patterson EE, Xiong Y, Prasad NB, Wang Y, et al. Expression profiling of difficult-to-diagnose thyroid histologic subtypes shows distinct expression profiles and identify candidate diagnostic microRNAs. Ann Surg Oncol. 2011;18:34–43.
94. Alexander EK, Kennedy GC, Baloch ZW, Cibas ES, Chudova D, Diggans J, et al. Preoperative diagnosis of benign thyroid nodules with indeterminate cytology. N Engl J Med. 2012;367(8):705–15.
95. McIver B, Castro MR, Morris JC, Bernet V, Smallridge R, Henry M, et al. An independent study of a gene expression classifier (Afirma) in the evaluation of cytologically indeterminate thyroid nodules. J Clin Endocrinol Metab. 2014;99(11):4069–77.
96. Brauner E, Holmes BJ, Krane JF, Nishino M, Zurakowski D, Hennessey JV, et al. Performance of the Afirma gene expression classifier in Hurthle cell thyroid nodules differs from other indeterminate thyroid nodules. Thyroid. 2015;25(7):789–96.
97. Lastra RR, Pramick MR, Crammer CJ, LiVolsi VA, Baloch ZW. Implications of a suspicious afirma test result in thyroid fine-needle aspiration cytology: an institutional experience. Cancer Cytopathol. 2014;122(10):737–44.
98. Wu JX, Young S, Hung ML, Li N, Yang SE, Cheung DS, et al. Clinical factors influencing the performance of gene expression classifier testing in indeterminate thyroid nodules. Thyroid. 2016;26(7):916–22.

99. Nikiforov YE, Carty SE, Chiosea SI, Coyne C, Duvvuri U, Ferris RL, et al. Highly accurate diagnosis of cancer in thyroid nodules with follicular neoplasm/suspicious for a follicular neoplasm cytology by ThyroSeq v2 next-generation sequencing assay. Cancer. 2014;120(23):3627–34.
100. Trovisco V, Vieira de Castro I, Soares P, Máximo V, Silva P, Magalhães J, et al. BRAF mutations are associated with some histological types of papillary thyroid carcinoma. J Pathol. 2004;202(2):247–51.
101. Soares P, Trovisco V, Rocha AS, Lima J, Castro P, Preto A, et al. BRAF mutations and RET/PTC rearrangements are alternative events in the etiopathogenesis of PTC. Oncogene. 2003;22(29):4578–80.
102. Chiappetta G, Toti P, Cetta F, Giuliano A, Pentimalli F, Amendola I, et al. The RET/PTC oncogene is frequently activated in oncocytic thyroid tumors (Hurthle cell adenomas and carcinomas), but not in oncocytic hyperplastic lesions. J Clin Endocrinol Metab. 2002;87(1):364–9.
103. Wirtschafter A, Schmidt R, Rosen D, Kundu N, Santoro M, Fusco A, et al. Expression of the RET/PTC fusion gene as a marker for papillary carcinoma in Hashimoto's thyroiditis. Laryngoscope. 1997;107(1):95–100.
104. Cheung CC, Ezzat S, Ramyar L, Freeman JL, Asa SL. Molecular basis off hurthle cell papillary thyroid carcinoma. J Clin Endocrinol Metab. 2000;85(2):878–82.
105. Belchetz G, Cheung CC, Freeman J, Rosen IB, Witterick IJ, Asa SL. Hürthle cell tumors: using molecular techniques to define a novel classification system. Arch Otolaryngol Head Neck Surg. 2002;128(3):237–40.
106. de Vries MM, Celestino R, Castro P, Eloy C, Maximo V, van der Wal JE, et al. RET/PTC rearrangement is prevalent in follicular hurthle cell carcinomas. Histopathology. 2012;61:833–43.
107. Doerfler WR, Nikitski AV, Morariu EM, Ohori NP, Chiosea SI, Landau MS, et al. Molecular alterations in hurthle cell nodules and preoperative cancer risk. Endocr Relat Cancer. 2021;28(5):301–9.
108. Endo M, Nabhan F, Angell TE, Harrell RM, Nasr C, Wei S, et al. Letter to the editor: use of molecular diagnostic tests in thyroid nodules with hurthle cell-dominant cytology. Thyroid. 2020;30:1390–2.
109. Ganly I, Makarov V, Deraje S, Dong Y, Reznik E, Seshan V, et al. Integrated genomic analysis of hurthle cell cancer reveals oncogenic drivers, recurrent mitochondrial mutations, and unique chromosomal landscapes. Cancer Cell. 2018;34:256–70.e5.
110. Ganly I, Ricarte Filho J, Eng S, Ghossein R, Morris LG, Liang Y, et al. Genomic dissection of hurthle cell carcinoma reveals a unique class of thyroid malignancy. J Clin Endocrinol Metab. 2013;98:E962–72.
111. Gopal RK, Kubler K, Calvo SE, Polak P, Livitz D, Rosebrock D, et al. Widespread chromosomal losses and mitochondrial DNA alterations as genetic drivers in hurthle cell carcinoma. Cancer Cell. 2018;34:242–55.e5.
112. Schatz-Siemers N, Brandler TC, Oweity T, Sun W, Hernandez A, Levine P. Hurthle cell lesions on thyroid fine needle aspiration cytology: molecular and histologic correlation. Diagn Cytopathol. 2019;47:977–85.
113. Evangelisti C, de Biase D, Kurelac I, Ceccarelli C, Prokisch H, Meitinger T, et al. A mutation screening of oncogenes, tumor suppressor gene TP53 and nuclear encoded mitochondrial complex I genes in oncocytic thyroid tumors. BMC Cancer. 2015;15:157.
114. Kasaian K, Chindris AM, Wiseman SM, Mungall KL, Zeng T, Tse K, et al. MEN1 mutations in hurthle cell (oncocytic) thyroid carcinoma. J Clin Endocrinol Metab. 2015;100:E611–5.
115. Landa I, Ibrahimpasic T, Boucai L, Sinha R, Knauf JA, Shah RH, et al. Genomic and transcriptomic hallmarks of poorly differentiated and anaplastic thyroid cancers. J Clin Invest. 2016;126:1052–66.
116. Nikiforova MN, Wald AI, Roy S, Durso MB, Nikiforov YE. Targeted next-generation sequencing panel (ThyroSeq) for detection of mutations in thyroid cancer. J Clin Endocrinol Metab. 2013;98:E1852–60.
117. Wei S, LiVolsi VA, Montone KT, Morrissette JJ, Baloch ZW. PTEN and TP53 mutations in oncocytic follicular carcinoma. Endocr Pathol. 2015;26:365–9.

118. Pecce V, Verrienti A, Abballe L, Carletti R, Grani G, Falcone R, et al. Loss of function Setd2 mutations in poorly differentiated metastases from two hurthle cell carcinomas of the thyroid. Cancers (Basel). 1892;2020(12):1–15.
119. Saqcena M, Leandro-Garcia LJ, Maag JLV, Tchekmedyian V, Krishnamoorthy GP, Tamarapu PP, et al. SWI/SNF complex mutations promote thyroid tumor progression and insensitivity to redifferentiation therapies. Cancer Discov. 2020;11:1158–75.
120. Nikiforov YE, Ohori NP, Hodak SP, Carty SE, LeBeau SO, Ferris RL, et al. Impact of mutational testing on the diagnosis and management of patients with cytologically indeterminate thyroid nodules: a prospective analysis of 1056 FNA samples. J Clin Endocrinol Metab. 2011;96(11):3390–7.
121. Ganly I, Ricarte Filho J, Eng S, Eng S, Ghossein R, Morris LG, et al. Genomic dissection of Hurthle cell carcinoma reveals a unique class of thyroid malignancy. J Clin Endocrinol Metab. 2013;98(5):E962–72.
122. Wallace DC, Mitochondrial DNA. Sequence variation in human evolution and disease. Proc Natl Acad Sci USA. 1994;91:8739–46.
123. Wredenberg A, Wibom R, Wilhelmsson H, Graff C, Wiener HH, Burden SJ, et al. Increased mitochondrial mass in mitochondrial myopathy mice. Proc Natl Acad Sci USA. 2002;99:15066–71.
124. Sheu SY, Handke S, Bröcker-Preuss M, Görges R, Frey UH, Ensinger C, et al. The C allele of the GNB3 C825T polymorphism of the G protein beta3-subunit is associated with an increased risk for the development of oncocytic thyroid tumours. J Pathol. 2007;211(1):60–6.
125. Gasparre G, Porcelli AM, Bonora E, Pennisi LF, Toller M, Iommarini Let al. Disruptive mitochondrial DNA mutations in complex I subunits are markers of oncocytic phenotype in thyroid tumors. Proc Natl Acad Sci USA 2007; 104(21): 9001–9006.
126. Yeh JJ, Lunetta KL, van Orsouw NJ, Moore FD Jr, Mutter GL, Vijg J, et al. (mtDNA) mutations in papillary thyroid carcinomas and differential mtDNA sequence variants in cases with thyroid tumours. Oncogene. 2000;19:2060–6.
127. Savagner F, Franc B, Guyetant S, Rodien P, Reynier P, Malthiery Y. Defective mitochondrial ATP synthesis in oxyphilic thyroid tumors. J Clin Endocrinol Metab. 2001;86:4920–5.
128. Zielke A, Tezelman S, Jossart GH, Wong M, Siperstein AE, Duh QY, et al. Establishment of a highly differentiated thyroid cancer cell line of hurthle cell origin. Thyroid. 1998;8:475–83.
129. Gopal RK, Calvo SE, Shih AR, Chaves FL, McGuone D, Mick E, et al. Early loss of mitochondrial complex i and rewiring of glutathione metabolism in renal oncocytoma. Proc Natl Acad Sci USA. 2018;115:E6283–90.
130. Yuan Y, Ju YS, Kim Y, Li J, Wang Y, Yoon CJ, et al. Comprehensive molecular characterization of mitochondrial genomes in human cancers. Nat Genet. 2020;52:342–52.
131. Rainwater LM, Farrow GM, Hay ID, Lieber MM. Oncocytic tumours of the salivary gland, kidney, and thyroid: nuclear DNA patterns studied by flow cytometry. Br J Cancer. 1986;53:799–804.
132. Mazzucchelli L, Burckhardt E, Hirsiger H, Kappeler A, Laissue JA. Interphase cytogenetics in oncocytic adenomas and carcinomas of the thyroid gland. Hum Pathol. 2000;31:854–9.
133. Erickson LA, Jalal SM, Goellner JR, Law ME, Harwood A, Jin L, et al. Analysis of hurthle cell neoplasms of the thyroid by interphase fluorescence in situ hybridization. Am J Surg Pathol. 2001;25:911–7.
134. Corver WE, Ruano D, Weijers K, den Hartog WC, van Nieuwenhuizen MP, de Miranda N, et al. Genome haploidisation with chromosome 7 retention in oncocytic follicular thyroid carcinoma. PLoS One. 2012;7:e38287.
135. Máximo V, Botelho T, Capela J, Soares P, Lima J, Taveira A, et al. Somatic and germline mutation in GRIM-19, a dual function gene involved in mitochondrial metabolism and cell death, is linked to mitochondrion-rich (Hurthle cell) tumours of the thyroid. Br J Cancer. 2005;92(10):1892–8.
136. Canzian F, Amati P, Harach HR, Kraimps JL, Lesueur F, Barbier J, et al. A gene predisposing to familial thyroid tumors with cell oxyphilia maps to chromosome 19p13.2. Am J Hum Genet. 1998;63(6):1743–8.

137. Harach HR, Lesueur F, Amati P, Brown A, Canzian F, Kraimps JL, et al. Histology of familial thyroid tumours linked to a gene mapping to chromosome 19p13.2. J Pathol. 1999;189(3):387–93.
138. Baris O, Mirebeau-Prunier D, Savagner F, Rodien P, Ballester B, Loriod B, Granjeaud S, Guyetant S, Franc B, Houlgatte R, Reynier P, Malthiery Y. Gene profiling reveals specific oncogenic mechanisms and signaling pathways in oncocytic and papillary thyroid carcinoma. Oncogene. 2005;24(25):4155–61.
139. Bonora E, Evangelisti C, Bonichon F, Tallini G, Romeo G. Novel germline variants identified in the inner mitochondrial membrane transporter TIMM44 and their role in predisposition to oncocytic thyroid carcinomas. Br J Cancer. 2006;95(11):1529–36.
140. Addie RD, Kostidis S, Corver WE, Oosting J, Aminzadeh-Gohari S, Feichtinger RG, et al. Metabolic reprogramming related to whole-chromosome instability in models for hurthle cell carcinoma. Sci Rep. 2020;10:9578.
141. Corver WE, Demmers J, Oosting J, Sahraeian S, Boot A, Ruano D, et al. ROS-induced near-homozygous genomes in thyroid cancer. Endocr Relat Cancer. 2018;25:83–97.
142. Arbajian E, Koster J, Vult von Steyern F, Mertens F. Inflammatory leiomyosarcoma is a distinct tumor characterized by near-haploidization, few somatic mutations, and a primitive myogenic gene expression signature. Mod Pathol. 2018;31:93–100.
143. Assie G, Letouze E, Fassnacht M, Jouinot A, Luscap W, Barreau O, et al. Integrated genomic characterization of adrenocortical carcinoma. Nat Genet. 2014;46:607–12.
144. Baker TG, Alden J, Dubuc AM, Welsh CT, Znoyko I, Cooley LD, et al. Near haploidization is a genomic hallmark which defines a molecular subgroup of giant cell glioblastoma. Neurooncol Adv. 2020;2:vdaa155.
145. Bovee JV, van Royen M, Bardoel AF, Rosenberg C, Cornelisse CJ, Cleton-Jansen AM, et al. Near-haploidy and subsequent polyploidization characterize the progression of peripheral chondrosarcoma. Am J Pathol. 2000;157:1587–95.
146. Holmfeldt L, Wei L, Diaz-Flores E, Walsh M, Zhang J, Ding L, et al. The genomic landscape of hypodiploid acute lymphoblastic leukemia. Nat Genet. 2013;45:242–52.
147. Joshi S, Tolkunov D, Aviv H, Hakimi AA, Yao M, Hsieh JJ, et al. The genomic landscape of renal oncocytoma identifies a metabolic barrier to tumorigenesis. Cell Rep. 2015;13:1895–908.
148. Kang HC, Kim HK, Lee S, Mendez P, Kim JW, Woodard G, et al. Whole exome and targeted deep sequencing identify genome-wide allelic loss and frequent SETDB1 mutations in malignant pleural mesotheliomas. Oncotarget. 2016;7:8321–31.
149. Zheng S, Cherniack AD, Dewal N, Moffitt RA, Danilova L, Murray BA, et al. Comprehensive pan-genomic characterization of adrenocortical carcinoma. Cancer Cell. 2016;30:363.
150. Baloch ZW, Asa SL, Barletta JA, Ghossein RA, Juhlin CC, Jung CK, et al. Overview of the 2022 WHO classification of thyroid neoplasms. Endocr Pathol. 2022;33(1):27–63.
151. National Comprehensive Cancer Network. Clinical practice guidelines in oncology (NCCN Guidelines), 2015. (Thyroid Carcinoma, Version 2.2015).

Oncocytic (Hürthle Cell) Neoplasm: Controversy of Clinical Behavior

10

10.1 Demographic Data

Oncocytic adenomas (Hürthle cell adenomas—HCAs) are most likely diagnosed much more frequently than oncocytic carcinomas of the thyroid (Hürthle cell carcinomas—HCCs). The female-to-male ratio is 8:1 for HCAs and 2:1 for HCCs [1]. In 2018, Malith et al. reported that a total of 2641 medical records were reviewed of which 25.6% (676/2641) were for neoplasms. 15.8% (107/676) of the neoplasms were Hürthle cell neoplasms (HCNs) and 25.2% (27/107) of HCNs were HCCs. 77.2% (71/92) of HCAs and 77.8% (21/27) of HCCs were from female patients [2]. However, they added that the patient's gender is not useful for predicting malignancy in HCNs. Hürthle cell cancer tends to occur in older patients than oncocytic adenoma (Hürthle cell adenoma), with a median age at diagnosis of approximately 61 years [1–3]. However, the difference was not statistically significant in the study by Malith et al. [2] who concluded that no demographic parameter was found to be useful in predicting final diagnosis of oncocytic/HCC in their study.

10.2 Clinical Presentation

Typically, a painless thyroid mass is found in patients with oncocytic/Hürthle cell neoplasm [1]. Malith et al. from South Africa (2018) reported that out of 107 cases of oncocytic/Hürthle cell neoplasms in their study, the average *tumor size* for HCCs and HCAs was 4.9 ± 2.7 cm and 3.5 ± 2.0 cm, respectively. The difference was statistically significant ($p = 0.016$). They added that the risk of malignancy increased from 11.1% in HCNs less than 1 cm to 53.8% for tumors, which were greater than 4 cm in diameter [2]. Several other authors have reported that the risk of malignancy rises as the size of oncocytic/HCN increases. Straziser et al. [4] reported that malignancy rate in patients with tumor size between 1 cm and 4 cm and greater than 4 cm were 20% and 40%, respectively. Chen et al. [5] also reported that HCN of the size

M. Sakr, *Oncocytic (Hürthle Cell) Thyroid Lesions*,
https://doi.org/10.1007/978-3-032-03115-0_10

of 1 cm or less had 17% chance of being malignant. Malignancy risk is 23% for tumors 1–4 cm in diameter and 65% for those which are 4 cm or larger [4]. Although, as may be expected, patients with oncocytic/HCC usually present with larger tumors than those with oncocytic adenoma (Hürthle cell adenoma); yet, the size and growth pattern of the tumor cannot, in general, be used to determine malignancy.

Rarely, oncocytic/HCCs can spread to the lymph nodes (LNs) [2, 6] and, on few occasions, have distant metastases in the lungs or surrounding bones [1]. By definition, an indolent course lacking recurrence or metastasis is the clinical hallmark of "benign" tumors. However, for oncocytic/Hürthle cell neoplasms (HCNs), this concept is confused by the occasional reports of recurrence or metastasis in histologically proven oncocytic adenomas (Hürthle cell adenomas—HCAs) [7]. Asa [8] suggested that such lesions may be unrecognized cases of Hürthle cell papillary carcinoma (HCPC). To resolve this confusion, HCA has been suggested to be restricted to oncocytic/HCNs not only lacking capsular invasion (CI) and vascular invasion (VI) but also lacking RET/PTC rearrangement; oncocytic/HCNs showing this molecular event would be considered HCPC [9]. Tumors displaying only capsular invasion tend to behave less aggressively than those with vascular invasion [10].

The clinical course of oncocytic/HCC has been a subject of varying interpretations among researchers. Some have reported a very favorable clinical outcome for this tumor, while others have regarded it as a relatively aggressive malignancy of the thyroid gland. This diversity of perspectives highlights the complexity of understanding and managing oncocytic/Hürthle cell carcinoma, warranting further investigation and consensus-building to improve patient outcomes [11].

Oncocytic/Hürthle cell carcinomas are recognized as being either minimally invasive (miHCC) or less commonly, widely invasive (wiHCC). While the miHCC (or encapsulated carcinoma) is fully surrounded by a fibrous capsule, the wiHCC shows extensive area of both capsular and vascular invasion with the leftover capsule typically difficult to identify [1]. Classification is important since widely invasive tumors can present with local invasion of adjacent structures such as strap muscles, prevertebral fascia, trachea, and esophagus, and can have worse outcomes with a mortality rate reaching up to 55% [1].

Several investigators have reported in the literature that oncocytic/HCC with focal vascular invasion (<4 foci) can be associated with less aggressive behavior similar to that of oncocytic/HCCs with minimal capsular invasion and no vascular invasion. In a retrospective study of 50 patients with encapsulated oncocytic/HCC, Ghossein et al. [12] reported that the pathological finding of >4 foci of vascular invasion is the most powerful predictor of recurrence and compromised recurrence-free survival ($p < 0.001$) among patients with encapsulated oncocytic/HCC. In their study, patients with no vascular invasion or < 4 foci of vascular invasion had 100% recurrence-free survival at 5 years compared to only 20% recurrence-free survival among patients with >4 foci of vascular invasion. More recently, a retrospective study by Xu et al. that included 276 patients with encapsulated differentiated thyroid cancers (DTCs) showed that extensive vascular invasion (≥4 foci of vascular invasion) is an independent predictor of recurrence in patients with encapsulated

DTCs. The risk of recurrence was 42% in patients with extensive vascular invasion compared to only 1% in patients with no vascular invasion or focal vascular invasion (<4 sites) [13].

Recently, in 2021, Jin et al. [14] reported persistent/recurrent disease in only 8.2% of the patients with oncocytic/HCC, and none of their patients died of oncocytic/HCC during a median follow-up of 8.5 years. Similarly, Oluic et al. [15] reported a rate of 12% of persistence/recurrence, with a slightly worse survival rate than that reported by Jin et al.

It is important to note that aggressive clinical behavior is well-established primarily in patients presenting with widely invasive disease (extra-thyroidal extension or extensive vascular invasion). Patients presenting with minimally invasive HCC exhibit excellent prognoses similar to FTC, based on available studies [16–18].

10.3 Clinical Behavior Compared to Follicular Carcinoma

Of note, the American Thyroid Association (ATA) considers HCC a variant of follicular thyroid carcinoma (FTC); therefore, they are stratified using the same guidelines [19]. However, Hürthle cell tumors are now considered a distinct pathological entity of differentiated thyroid carcinoma (DTC) in the most recent (2022) World Health Organization (WHO) classification scheme (fifth edition) given the clinicopathological differences with FTC. Despite this separation of the two entities, the authors acknowledge the controversy and inconsistency in the literature regarding the biological and clinical behavior of FTC in comparison with oncocytic/HCC (likely due in part to ambiguous criteria for defining oncocytic/HCC in previous studies) [20].

There has been a considerable controversy in the literature as to oncocytic/HCC has a similar or more aggressive clinical behavior as compared to FTC. Some authors found that both tumors behave in an identical fashion [21, 22] as there was no statistically significant difference between both in terms of size, extra-thyroidal extension (ETE), nodal or distant metastasis, local recurrence, and patient survival [23–26]. On the other hand, other investigators [27–29] suggested that oncocytic/HCCs are clinically more aggressive than FTCs based on the facts of more frequent nodal [23, 30] and distal metastasis [31, 32], less radioactive iodine (RAI) avidity [24, 30, 33], and greater likelihood of local recurrence [23, 34]. In a study by Shaha et al. [35], the Hürthle variety of FTC categorized it into higher risk groups.

Oncocytic/Hürthle cell neoplasms exhibit high ^{18}fluoro-deoxy glucose (^{18}FDG) uptake compared to other forms of thyroid cancer [36, 37]. Conversely, oncocytic/HCCs are reported to exhibit less avidity for radioactive iodine (RAI), at least compared to FTC [3, 17, 38]. Whether RAI has therapeutic benefit in oncocytic/HCC patients remains muddled.

Several authors reported that both FTC and oncocytic/HCC have relatively high rates of distant metastases, consistent with hematogenous spread [21, 27, 31, 39, 40], but oncocytic/HCCs also have been found to have higher rates of locoregional metastases in some studies [27, 39]. Interestingly, Bishop et al. [41] reported that all cases of locoregional metastases in their cohort of oncocytic/HCC consisted of tumor nodules in soft tissue without associated lymphoid tissue, with approximately 50% of cases demonstrating tumor nodules within veins. True lymph node (LN) metastases were present in a minority of cases and were predominantly microscopic deposits. Their study suggests that soft tissue implants through venous invasion, rather than true LN metastases, appear to be a major source of locoregional recurrence in oncocytic/HCC.

Not surprisingly, the survival data on oncocytic/HCC and FTC are variable as well. In some studies, the oncocytic phenotype has been found to be prognostic [27, 35, 42, 43]. For example, although Hundahl et al. [42] found a similar 5-year overall survival between oncocytic/HCC and FTC, the 10-year overall survival was worse in oncocytic/HCC (76% *versus* 85%, respectively). Similar findings were reported by Shaha and colleagues in 1995 [35] and in 1996 [31] with survival of oncocytic/HCC and FTC similar at 5 years, but diverging with longer follow-up (20-year survival 65% *versus* 81%, respectively). However, in studies accounting for other clinicopathological factors such as tumor size and stage, multivariate analysis did *not* find oncocytic (Hürthle) cell morphology to be prognostic as more recently reported by Haigh et al. [21] and later by Sugino et al. [44].

10.4 Clinical Behavior Compared to Papillary Carcinoma

The clinical behavior of Hürthle cell papillary carcinoma (HCPC) is also controversial; Herrera et al. reported a more aggressive behavior with higher rates of recurrence and cause-specific mortality [45] while few years later, Berho and Suster reported a behavior identical to conventional type papillary thyroid carcinoma (PTC) [46]. Recently (2023), Abdulhaleem and Aldajani reported that oncocytic/HCC tends to present in larger thyroid nodules, unlike papillary thyroid cancer (PTC) [47].

References

1. Schwab M. Encyclopedia of cancer. 2011. https://doi.org/10.1016/B0-12-227555-1/00151-9.
2. Malith V, Bombil I, Harran N, Luvhengo TE. Demographic and histological subtypes of Hurthle cell tumours of the thyroid in a South African setting. S Afr J Surg. 2018;56(3):20–3.
3. Lopez-Penabad L, Chiu AC, Hoff AO, Schultz P, Gaztambide S, Ordonez NG, et al. Prognostic factors in patients with Hurthle cell neoplasms of the thyroid. Cancer. 2003;97:1186–94.
4. Strazisar B, Petric B, Sesek M, Zgajnar J, Hocevar M, Besic N. Predictive factors of carcinoma in 279 patients with Hurthle cell neoplasm of the thyroid gland. J Surg Oncol. 2010;101(7):582–6.
5. Chen H, Nicol TL, Zelger MA, et al. Hurthle cell neoplasms of the thyroid, are there factors predictive of malignancy? Ann Surg. 1998;227(4):542–6.
6. Montone KT, Baloch ZW, LiVolsi VA. The thyroid Hurthle (oncocytic) cell and its associated pathologic conditions: a surgical pathology and cytopathology review. Arch Pathol Lab Med. 2008;132(8):1241–50.
7. Ain K. Unusual types of thyroid cancer. Rev Endocr Metab Disord. 2000;1(3):225–31.

8. Asa S. My approach to oncocytic tumours of the thyroid. J Clin Pathol. 2004;57(3):225–32.
9. Belchetz G, Cheung CC, Freeman J, Rosen IB, Witterick IJ, Asa SL. Hürthle cell tumors: using molecular techniques to define a novel classification system. Arch Otolaryngol Head Neck Surg. 2002;128(3):237–40.
10. Erickson LA. Hurthle cell thyroid neoplasms. In: Atlas of endocrine pathology. New York: Springer; 2014. p. 63–6.
11. Sulaiman S, Chirukandath R, Krishnan SK, Rajesh N, Antony M, Mohan KSS. Unraveling the enigma: a five-year comprehensive analysis of hurthle cell tumors in South India's tertiary care center. Cureus. 2024;16(3):e57166.
12. Ghossein RA, Hiltzik DH, Carlson DL, Patel S, Shaha A, Shah JP, et al. Prognostic factors of recurrence in encapsulated Hurthle cell carcinoma of the thyroid gland: a clinicopathologic study of 50 cases. Cancer. 2006;106(8):1669–76.
13. Xu B, Wang L, Tuttle RM, Ganly I, Ghossein R. Prognostic impact of extent of vascular invasion in low-grade encapsulated follicular cell-derived thyroid carcinomas: a clinicopathologic study of 276 cases. Hum Pathol. 2015;46(12):1789–98.
14. Jin M, Kim ES, Kim BH, Kim HK, Kang YE, Jeon MJ, et al. Clinicopathological characteristics and disease-free survival in patients with Hürthle cell carcinoma: a multicenter cohort study in South Korea. Endocrinol Metab. 2021;36(5):1078–85.
15. Oluic B, Paunovic I, Loncar Z, Djukic V, Diklic A, Jovanovic M, et al. Survival and prognostic factors for survival, cancer specific survival and disease free interval in 239 patients with Hurthle cell carcinoma: a single center experience. BMC Cancer. 2017;17(1):371.
16. Stojadinovic A, Hoos A, Ghossein RA, Urist MJ, Leung DH, Spiro RH, et al. Hurthle cell carcinoma: a 60-year experience. Ann Surg Oncol. 2002;9:197–203.
17. Sanders LE, Silverman M. Follicular and Hurthle cell carcinoma: predicting outcome and directing therapy. Surgery. 1998;124:967–74.
18. van Heerden JA, Hay ID, Goellner JR, Salomao D, Ebersold JR, Bergstralh EJ, et al. Follicular thyroid carcinoma with capsular invasion alone: a nonthreatening malignancy. Surgery. 1992;112:1130–6.
19. Haugen BR, Alexander EK, Bible KC, Oherty GM, Mandel SJ, Nikiforov YE, et al. American Thyroid Association management guidelines for adult patients with thyroid nodules and differentiated thyroid cancer. Thyroid 2016. 2015;26(1):1–133.
20. Lloyd RV, Osamura RY, Klöppel GRJ, Raosai J, editors. World Health Organization classification of tumours of endocrine organs, vol. 10. 4th ed. Lyon: IARC Press; 2017.
21. Haigh PI, Urbach DR. The treatment and prognosis of Hürthle cell follicular thyroid carcinoma compared with its non-Hürthle cell counterpart. Surgery. 2005;138(6):1152–8.
22. Bhattacharyya N. Survival and prognosis in Hürthle cell carcinoma of the thyroid gland. Arch Otolaryngol Head Neck Surg. 2003;129(2):207–10.
23. Evans HL, Vassilopoulou-Sellin R. Follicular and Hurthle cell carcinomas of the thyroid: a comparative study. Am J Surg Pathol. 1998;22(12):1512–20.
24. Sanders LE, Silverman M. Follicular and Hürthle cell carcinoma: predicting outcome and directing therapy. Surgery. 1998;124(6):967–74.
25. Khafif A, Khafif RA, Attie JN. Hürthle cell carcinoma: a malignancy of low-grade potential. Head Neck. 1999;21(6):506–11.
26. Ozlem Kucuk N, Kulak H, Tokmak E, Okmak E, Tar P, Ibiş E, Aras G. Hurthle cell carcinoma: a clinicopathological study of thirteen cases. Nucl Med Commun. 2006;27(4):377–9.
27. Kushchayeva Y, Duh Q-Y, Kebebew E, D'Avanzo A, Clark OH. Comparison of clinical characteristics at diagnosis and during follow-up in 118 patients with Hurthle cell or follicular thyroid cancer. Am J Surg. 2008;195(4):457–62.
28. Carcangiu ML, Bianchi S, Savino D, Voynick IM, Rosai J. Follicular Hurthle cell tumors of the thyroid gland. Cancer. 1991;68(9):1944–53.
29. Grani G, Lamartina L, Durante C, Filetti S, Cooper DS. Follicular thyroid cancer and Hurthle cell carcinoma: challenges in diagnosis, treatment, and clinical management. Lancet Diabetes Endocrinol. 2018;6(6):500–14.
30. Yutan E, Clark O. Hürthle cell carcinoma. Curr Treat Options in Oncol. 2001;2(4):331–5.

31. Shaha AR, Shah JP, Loree TR. Patterns of nodal and distant metastasis based on histologic varieties in differentiated carcinoma of the thyroid. Am J Surg. 1996;172(6):692–4.
32. Ruegemer JJ, Hay ID, Bergstralh EJ, Ryan JJ, Offord KP, Gorman CA. Distant metastases in differentiated thyroid carcinoma: a multivariate analysis of prognostic variables. J Clin Endocrinol Metab. 1988;67(3):501–8.
33. Schneider DF, Chen H. New developments in the diagnosis and treatment of thyroid cancer. CA Cancer J Clin. 2013;63(6):373–94.
34. Mills SC, Haq M, Smellie WJ, Harmer C. Hurthle cell carcinoma of the thyroid: retrospective review of 62 patients treated at the Royal Marsden Hospital between 1946 and 2003. Eur J Surg Oncol. 2009;35(3):230–4.
35. Shaha AR, Loree TR, Shah JP. Prognostic factors and risk group analysis in follicular carcinoma of the thyroid. Surgery. 1995;118(6):1131–8.
36. Pathak KA, Klonisch T, Nason RW, Leslie WD. Fdg-PET characteristics of Hurthle cell and follicular adenomas. Ann Nucl Med. 2016;30:506–9.
37. Pryma DA, Schoder H, Gonen M, Robbins RJ, Larson SM, Yeung HW. Diagnostic accuracy and prognostic value of 18F-FDG PET in Hurthle cell thyroid cancer patients. J Nucl Med. 2006;47:1260–6.
38. Sabra MM, Ghossein R, Tuttle RM. Time course and predictors of structural disease progression in pulmonary metastases arising from follicular cell-derived thyroid cancer. Thyroid. 2016;26:518–24.
39. Goffredo P, Roman SA, Sosa JA. Hurthle cell carcinoma: a population-level analysis of 3311 patients. Cancer. 2013;119:504–11.
40. Chindris AM, Casler JD, Bernet VJ, Rivera M, Thomas C, Kachergus JM, et al. Clinical and molecular features of Hürthle cell carcinoma of the thyroid. J Clin Endocrinol Metab. 2015;100:55–62.
41. Bishop JA, Wu G, Tufano RP, Westra WH. Histological patterns of locoregional recurrence in Hürthle cell carcinoma of the thyroid gland. Thyroid. 2012;22:690–4.
42. Hundahl SA, Fleming ID, Fremgen AM, Menck HR. A national cancer data base report on 53,856 cases of thyroid carcinoma treated in the U.S., 1985-1995. Cancer. 1998;83:2638–48.
43. Samaan NA, Maheshwari YK, Nader S, Hill CS Jr, Schultz PN, Haynie TP, et al. Impact of therapy for differentiated carcinoma of the thyroid: an analysis of 706 cases. J Clin Endocrinol Metab. 1983;56:1131–8.
44. Sugino K, Kameyama K, Ito K, Nagahama M, Kitagawa W, Shibuya H, et al. Does Hürthle cell carcinoma of the thyroid have a poorer prognosis than ordinary follicular thyroid carcinoma? Ann Surg Oncol. 2013;20:2944–50.
45. Herrera M, Hay I, Wu PC, Goellner JR, Ryan JJ, Ebersold JR, et al. Hürthle cell (oxyphilic) papillary thyroid carcinoma: a variant with more aggressive biologic behavior. World J Surg. 1992;16(4):669–74.
46. Berho M, Suster S. The oncocytic variant of papillary carcinoma of the thyroid: a clinicopathologic study of 15 cases. Hum Pathol. 1997;28(1):47–53.
47. Abdulhaleem M, Aldajani A. Thyroid Hurthle cell neoplasms: review article. Am J Otolaryngol Head Neck Surg. 2023;6(5):1243.

Oncocytic (Hürthle Cell) Adenoma: Controversy of Diagnosis and Treatment

11

11.1 Definition

Oncocytic adenoma (Hürthle cell adenoma—HCA) is a rare benign thyroid tumor that can only be confirmed through postoperative histopathological findings. It is characterized by follicular architecture with more than 75% tumor cells configured as "oncocytes" (Hürthle cells) demonstrating intracytoplasmic accumulation of numerous dysfunctional mitochondria, and without any capsular or vascular invasion [1]. Designated as oncocytic adenoma, HCA, oncocytic cell adenoma, Askanazy cell adenoma, eosinophilic adenoma, or oxyphilic cell adenoma, the exogenous factors influencing the emergence of this neoplasm remain undefined [2].

11.2 Risk Factors and Clinical Significance

The Worldwide incidence of oncocytic adenoma (Hürthle cell adenoma—HCA) of the thyroid gland is extremely low, accounting for less than 5% of all thyroid tumors [3]. Oncocytic/Hürthle cell adenoma affects women more than men with a female-to-male ratio of 8:1, and it typically occurs at a young age (> 40 years) than oncocytic carcinoma (Hürthle cell carcinoma—HCC), which occurs at a median age of approximately 60 years**.** HCA of the thyroid lacks typical clinical manifestations. The most common clinical sign is a palpable thyroid mass that can grow slowly for up to 10 years without causing any symptoms. According to its location and size, the tumor may cause pressure and pain to the patient; however, often the tumor goes undetected. Although HCA is "benign," it has, similar to all adenomas, the potential to become malignant, transforming to the malignant counterpart, HCC, and to metastasize to other bodily organs [4, 5].

Oncocytic/Hürthle cell adenomas (and carcinomas) have a higher incidence in people who have other, nonmalignant thyroid problems such a Graves' disease, colloid nodular disease, chronic lymphocytic thyroiditis (Hashimoto's thyroiditis),

M. Sakr, *Oncocytic (Hürthle Cell) Thyroid Lesions*,
https://doi.org/10.1007/978-3-032-03115-0_11

thyroid hyperplasia, and follicular adenomas, in addition to parathyroid adenoma. Patients who have experienced excessive irradiation of the head and neck are also at increased risk, especially for malignancy.

Oncocytic/Hürthle cell adenoma (HCA) is the benign analogue of oncocytic/Hürthle cell carcinoma (HCC). Often oncocytic/HCA is harmless and even large clusters of oncocytic (Hürthle) cells may not be life-threatening, but this tumor should be removed after detection because its future course cannot be trusted and it is not easy to predict whether it will transform into oncocytic/HCC [4, 5].

11.3 Workup

Color Doppler ultrasonography (US), contrast-enhanced computed tomography (CT) scan, positron emission tomography–CT (PET–CT), fine-needle aspiration cytology (FNAC), and postoperative histopathological pathological examination are generally used to diagnose oncocytic/HCA. Due to its extremely low incidence, lack of special clinical manifestations, and lack of typical imaging features, preoperative diagnosis of HCA is very difficult. The mis-diagnosis rate of oncocytic/HCA of the thyroid is high because it is easily confused with nodular goiter and other thyroid tumors. However, oncocytic/HCA of the thyroid can be diagnosed by postoperative pathological findings [3] due to its unique histological features. Thyroid function tests are generally normal or TSH levels can be slightly elevated [6]. Preliminary data about the location and size of the tumor is usually gleaned through imaging such as ultrasound (US) or computed tomography (CT) scans.

After detection, the mass is tested using an invasive fine-needle aspiration biopsy (FNAB) in an attempt at determining whether the tumor is malignant or benign. Fine-needle aspiration biopsy (FNAB) of oncocytic/Hürthle cell neoplasms (HCNs) are usually "indeterminate" for malignancy, challenging the preoperative diagnosis of oncocytic/Hürthle cell carcinomas (HCCs). Even current molecular preoperative tests are unable to distinguish oncocytic/HCAs from oncocytic/HCCs correctly [7]. Therefore, surgery is still required to distinguish benign from malignant oncocytic neoplasms [8–10].

11.4 Imaging Studies

11.4.1 Ultrasonography (US)

In oncocytic/HCAs, ultrasonographic features usually include a hypo-echoic, solid mass with a smooth margin, an oval shape, a characteristic halo sign, and no microcalcification (Fig. 11.1) [6, 11–14]. It may also show multiple nodules, with a small number of cystic echoes. During ultrasonography (US), the following nine US characteristics and Korean-Thyroid Imaging Reporting and Data System (K-TIRADS) categories of the lesions are better evaluated: tumor size, internal content,

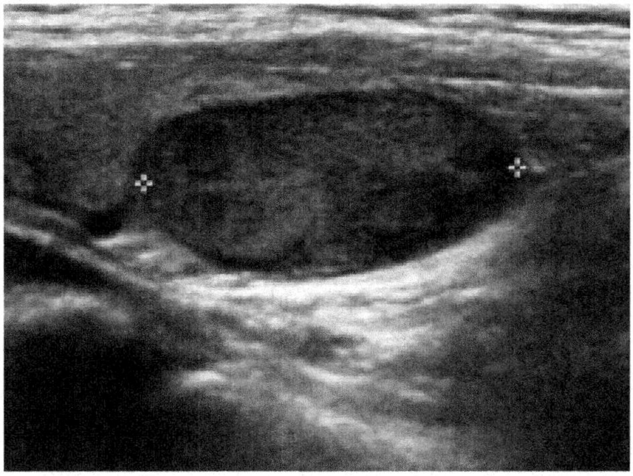

Fig. 11.1 Ultrasonographic image of the thyroid gland showing a hypo-echoic solid mass with a smooth margin, an oval shape, a halo sign, and no microcalcification; features consistent with a benign lesion that proved by histopathology to be an oncocytic adenoma (Hürthle cell adenoma)

echogenicity, margin, orientation, shape, internal calcification, presence of a halo sign, and vascularity [15].

Kim et al. [16] studied the preoperative sonographic characteristics of 139 oncocytic/Hürthle cell neoplasms and correlated them with their postoperative histopathological results (99 lesions were oncocytic adenomas). Univariate analysis showed that three features were significantly associated with oncocytic/HCA versus oncocytic/HCC: internal content, US tumor size, and pathological tumor size. The oncocytic/HCC masses more frequently showed cystic changes than oncocytic/HCAs (38% versus 17%, respectively; $P < 0.001$). Other factors such as echogenicity, margin, orientation, calcification, halo sign, vascularity, K-TIRADS category, and Bethesda category did *not* show statistical significance for differentiating carcinoma from adenoma. Multiple logistic regression analysis revealed that the US tumor size was an independent significant predictor of malignancy ($P = 0.001$). The best cutoff value of US tumor size for predicting malignancy was 3.35 cm (sensitivity, 53.1%; specificity, 87.9%) [16].

11.4.2 Computed Tomography (CT) Scan

In oncocytic/HCA, contrast-enhanced CT scan usually shows a heterogeneously enhancing mass in the thyroid. The enhancement degree of the mass may be lower than thyroid gland and adjacent blood vessels [17]. There is no enhanced necrotic area in the center of the lesion. Radiation-like, low-density scarring are sometimes seen in the lesion with intact capsule enhancement around the lesion [17].

Dayong et al. [17] reported that contrast-enhanced CT imaging of their patient with oncocytic/HCA showed an expansive growth and clear boundary, intact lesion capsule, radiation-like low-density scarring in the center of the lesion, enhanced surrounding area, and no abnormal enlargement of lymph nodes (LNs) in the bilateral neck, which indicated the lesion is a benign tumor. In addition, it was consistent with the growth characteristics of a benign tumor for her history of more than 10 years. Finally, left thyroidectomy was performed and postoperative histopathology confirmed the diagnosis of oncocytic/HCA, which was in line with the diagnosis revealed by contrast-enhanced CT examination. The authors concluded that the typical imaging features of oncocytic/HCA on contrast-enhanced CT are helpful for the early diagnosis of this benign neoplasm. This will provide an important basis for the preoperative diagnosis and treatment strategy of oncocytic/HCA of the thyroid in the future [17].

It is noteworthy that oncocytic/HCC of the thyroid has the same imaging features in contrast-enhanced CT as oncocytic/HCA except the incomplete lesion capsule. However, thyroid cancer usually has blurred boundary, irregular shape, discontinuous capsule, inhomogeneous enhancement in contrast-enhanced CT scan, accompanied by abnormal enlargement of cervical LNs [18]. Radiation-like low-density scarring in the center of the lesion helps to differentiate oncocytic/HCA from other benign tumors of the thyroid.

11.4.3 Positron Emission Tomography–Computed Tomography (PET–CT)

Although positron emission tomography–computed tomography (PET–CT) images can detect the area of abnormal radiopharmaceutical uptake corresponding to oncocytic/HCAs [19] and improve its diagnostic rate, it is an unpopular modality because of its high price and radiation damage.

11.5 Cytology/Histopathology

11.5.1 Cytology

Fine-needle aspiration cytology (FNAC) is a simple, safe, and reliable procedure with a high diagnostic accuracy, but it is impossible to judge whether capsular or vascular invasion is present [20]. In addition, oncocytic/HCNs tend to undergo spontaneous necrosis or show extensive degenerative necrosis following fine-needle aspiration biopsy (FNAB). In these situations, viable lesional cells are often not present, and it is difficult to fully evaluate the lesion pathologically [21]. In general, FNAB cannot reliably diagnose neoplasia versus hyperplasia and carcinoma versus adenoma [22].

Oncocytic (Hürthle) cells arise from the follicular epithelium. They tend to be polygonal cells with distinct cell borders, larger in size than follicular cells. The principal features of these oncocytic cells include an abundant, eosinophilic, granular cytoplasm and a spherical nucleus with intracytoplasmic lumina or vacant vacuoles and a large nucleolus [23]. Predominantly cellular cytological aspirate is composed of $\geq 75\%$ enlarged, pleomorphic, discohesive oncocytic (Hürthle) cells. Upon staining with Diff-Quik, the aforesaid vacuoles appear magenta or represent as green vacuoles with Papanicolaou stain. Transgressing vascular articulations or capillaries appear to circumscribe clusters of oncocytic (Hürthle) cells [2].

Morphological features as tumor magnitude, nuclear atypia, multinucleated cells, cellular or nuclear pleomorphism, enhanced mitotic activity, or definitive histological configurations appear non-indicative of malignant metamorphosis [2]. The hallmark of malignant transformation or the presence of oncocytic/HCC is vascular invasion and/or capsular invasion. Generally, the aspirate is devoid of colloid, inflammatory cells such as lymphocytes, histiocytes or plasma cells, or normal follicular epithelial cells. On the other hand, "malignant cells" appear discohesive, miniature, or enlarged and exhibit significant dysplasia with nuclear crowding [2, 24].

11.5.2 Histopathology

The tumor cells of oncocytic/Hürthle cell neoplasms (HCNs) can be trabecular or small follicles and they can form glial calcification, containing thick colloid, a focal nipple structure. Numerous methods have been tried to identify benign and malignant disease of oncocytic/HCNs [25–27] such as cytological morphometry, immunohistochemical features, and gene rearrangements. However, preoperative clinical, cytological, and genetic studies have *not* reliably discriminated between benign and malignant lesions of oncocytic/HCNs. Therefore, histopathology remains the gold standard for diagnosis of oncocytic/HCA.

Upon microscopy, tumefaction is comprised of ≥75% oncocytic cells or enlarged cells with distinct cellular outline, granular intensely eosinophilic cytoplasm, enlarged nucleus with prominent nucleolus, and an absence of cellular polarity. Nuclear grooves or nuclear pseudo-inclusions are occasional. Nuclear atypia is common and random, although nonrepresentative of malignant transformation. Tumor configurations as follicular, trabecular, solid, or papillary patterns may be observed [2]. Follicular lumen is impacted with calcific concretions as nonlaminated, psammoma body-like aggregates, as opposed to laminated, psammoma bodies confined to stroma of papillary thyroid carcinoma [1].

The histopathological diagnostic criteria of thyroid oncocytic/HCA are thyroid tumor cells consisting entirely or predominantly (>75%) of follicular cells, characterized by eosinophils [20], and thyroid tumor tissue with an intact capsule, and no vascular invasion [28].

11.6 Differential Diagnosis

Oncocytic/Hürthle cell adenoma (HCA) should be differentiated from oncocytic/HCC. Upon imaging with radioactive iodine (RAI), oncocytic/HCA usually manifests as a "cold" nodule. "Warm" or "hot" nodules are exceptional [29, 30]. Oncocytic/HCC represents with characteristic histological features and decimated uptake of RAI upon imaging. While oncocytic/HCA is immune reactive to thyroglobulin (Tg), TTF1 or CK7, poorly differentiated oncocytic carcinoma is immune nonreactive to TTF1 or Tg [29, 30].

Oncocytic/Hürthle cell adenoma requires also segregation from other thyroid disorders such as chronic lymphocytic thyroiditis (Hashimoto's thyroiditis), medullary thyroid carcinoma (MTC), nodular colloid goiter with prominent oncocytic cells, follicular thyroid carcinoma (FTC), or papillary thyroid carcinoma (PTC) with subtypes such as oncocytic variant, Warthin-like variant, or tall-cell variant [29, 30].

11.7 Treatment

Regardless of whether or not the oncocytic/Hürthle cell tumor is malignant, oncocytic/Hürthle cell adenomas and carcinomas should be both excised promptly to prevent the disease from progressing further. A total thyroidectomy (TT) is often performed, but some patients may only undergo hemithyroidectomy or lobectomy without the need for any adjuvant therapy due to its good prognosis [29, 30].

Oncocytic (Hürthle) cells are generally resistant to radiation treatment, so it is difficult to treat recurrences, although several authors have reported some success with using radioactive iodine (RAI) treatment to slow the progress of the disease and reduce the recurrence rate [31].

11.8 Hürthle Cell Adenoma in Hashimoto's Thyroiditis

Oncocytic/Hürthle cell neoplasms (HCNs) represent less than 5% of all thyroid tumors [32]. These are composed predominantly of oncocytic (Hürthle) cells, which are thyroglobulin-producing, mitochondria-rich thyroid epithelial cells [33]. They are often an associated finding in various benign thyroid conditions such as Hashimoto's thyroiditis, nonspecific chronic thyroiditis, long-standing hyperthyroidism, nodular goiter, and thyroid neoplasms where they represent oncocytic metaplasia [34]. Diagnosis of an oncocytic/Hürthle cell neoplasm can be made only if 75% or more of the tumor cells are oncocytic (Hürthle) cells [35].

The association of autoimmune thyroiditis especially chronic lymphocytic thyroiditis (Hashimoto's thyroiditis) with thyroid neoplasms has often been reported and detailed research has been carried out in this area. Oncocytic/Hürthle cell neoplasms are also known to arise in a background of thyroiditis, though the frequency is much less in comparison to the occurrence of follicular/papillary carcinomas. As with follicular neoplasms, it is often difficult to differentiate a benign oncocytic/HCA from an oncocytic/HCC based on cytology, hence surgery is advisable whenever there is a suspicion.

Hashimoto's thyroiditis is a well-known cause of hypothyroidism and is characterized by autoimmune destruction of the thyroid gland. Antibodies against various thyroid antigens are present, especially anti-TSH (thyroid-stimulating hormone) receptor antibody, anti-thyroglobulin (Tg) and antithyroid peroxidase (TPO) antibody [36]. It is commonly seen in the fifth andsixth decade and is ten times more prevalent in females than in males [4]. Various synonyms for Hashimoto's thyroiditis include chronic lymphocytic thyroiditis (CLT), diffuse lymphocytic thyroiditis, goitrous autoimmune thyroiditis, and struma lymphomatosa [33].

Clinically, most of the patients are either euthyroid or present with features of mild hypothyroidism with a mild to moderately enlarged, painless thyroid gland [33]. It is associated with various thyroid neoplasms; follicular adenoma, follicular thyroid carcinoma (FTC), papillary thyroid carcinoma (PTC), medullary thyroid carcinoma (MTC), lymphomas, Hürthle cell adenoma (HCA), and Hürthle cell carcinoma (HCC) [37].

The majority of these tumors are benign and are labeled as oncocytic/Hürthle cell adenomas (HCAs), but up to 40% are malignant oncocytic/(Hürthle cell carcinoma—HCC) [38]. As mentioned before, documentation of the presence of capsular and/or vascular invasion or lymphatic spread is necessary for the diagnosis of oncocytic/HCC [35]. However, some of these adenomas exhibit few features of invasion, but lack unequivocal signs of malignancy and patients have remained well on follow-up. Such tumors are considered "atypical HCAs" or Hürthle cell tumors of uncertain malignant potential [35]. Persistent autoimmune cell response may lead to oxyphil cell hyperplasia in autoimmune thyroiditis [39]. In addition, the mitochondrial DNA common deletion (mtDNA CD), which encodes for oxidative phosphorylation (OXPHOS) proteins, has been identified in cases of Hashimoto's thyroiditis with oxyphil cells, resulting in deficient energy production and compensatory mitochondrial proliferation, and pointing to the possible role of genetic defects in the respiratory chain in the development of oxyphil cell change in these cases [2, 39].

The 4977 base pair deletion (mtDNA CD) has been detected in oncocytic/Hürthle cell tumors as well. In one series, up to 16% deletion frequency was detected in every oncocytic/Hürthle cell tumor [40]. This is again suggestive of a possible association between oncocytic/Hürthle cell tumors and germline polymorphisms of ATPase-6 (Adenosine triphosphatase-6) [40]. It is thought that the decreased efficiency of mtDNA replication could have a pathogenetic role in the development of oncocytic/Hürthle cell tumors. The increased mitochondrial content may be a compensatory process arising from defective energy productions of the cell [40].

In 1998, Katoh et al. [41] stated that oxyphilia in thyroid tumors may be a "primary" development, due to somatic mutations, or a "secondary phenomenon" linked to oxidative damage or environmental aggression such as associated thyroiditis. More recently (2000), a specific gene, GRIM-19 (a 552 base pair gene and it encodes a 16 kDa protein), which is a dual function gene, associated with both interferon β/retinoic acid-induced cell death and mitochondrial metabolism [42] has been linked to oncocytic/Hürthle cell tumors through somatic and germline mutations [43]. In fact, the GRIM-19 mutation is the first nuclear mutation specifically linked to oncocytic/Hürthle cell tumors [43].

It is often difficult to differentiate a benign from a malignant oncocytic/Hürthle cell neoplasm on fine-needle aspiration cytology (FNAC). Moreover, a diagnosis of malignancy can be confirmed only on histopathology through detection of capsular/

vascular invasion or lymphatic spread. Statistically significant features on cytology that indicate a neoplastic process include a high proportion (>75–90%) of oncocytic (Hürthle) cells, cellular discohesiveness, nuclear pleomorphism, large nucleoli, and the lack of accompanying inflammatory cells [44].

Diagnosis of oncocytic/HCA in association with Hashimoto's disease is therefore achieved by subjecting the postoperative (thyroidectomy) specimen to histopathological examination. The gross pathology usually reveals an encapsulated nodular mass, firm-to-hard in consistency and tan-brown cut-section. Microscopic examination shows a diffuse lymphocytic infiltrate with formation of many lymphoid follicles, and reduced or atrophic thyroid follicles. A large focal encapsulated area is composed of clusters and sheets of oxyphil cells, which are round to oval in shape with abundant granular cytoplasm and enlarged hyper-chromatic nuclei. Some cells may have prominent nucleoli. In oncocytic/HCA, there is no evidence of vascular or capsular invasion. The final histopathological diagnosis in such a case is "Hashimoto's thyroiditis with oncocytic/HCA."

References

1. Bajaj A. Fuchsia and roseate – hürthle cell adenoma. Acta Scient Clin Case Rep. 2023;4(2):1–3.
2. Mulita F, Anjum F. Thyroid adenoma. Treasure Island: Stat Pearls International; 2022.
3. Cannon J. The significance of Hurthle cells in thyroid disease. Oncologist. 2011;16:1380–7.
4. Ristevska N, Stojanoski S, Gjorceva DP. Appearance of Hürthle cell carcinoma soon after surgical extirpation of Hürthle cell adenoma and follicular adenoma of the thyroid gland. Radiol Oncol. 2015;49(1):26–31.
5. Wasvary H, Czako P, Poulik J, Lucas R. Unilateral lobectomy for Hürthle cell adenoma. Am Surg. 1998;64(8):729–32.
6. Li P, Liu P, Zhang H. Ultrasonic diagnosis for thyroid Hurthle cell tumor. Cancer Biomark. 2017;20:235–40.
7. Harrell R, Bimston D. Surgical utility of Afirma: effects of high cancer prevalence and Oncocytic cell types in patients with indeterminate thyroid cytology. Endocr Pract. 2014;20(4):364–9.
8. Pu RT, Yang J, Wasserman PG, Bhuiya T, Griffith KA, Michael CW. Does Hurthle cell lesion/neoplasm predict malignancy more than follicular lesion/neoplasm on thyroid fine-needle aspiration? Diagn Cytopathol. 2006;34(5):330–4.
9. Roh MH, Jo VY, Stelow EB, Faquin WC, Zou KH, Alexander EK, et al. The predictive value of the fine-needle aspiration diagnosis "suspicious for a follicular neoplasm, Hürthle cell type" in patients with Hashimoto thyroiditis. Am J Clin Pathol. 2011;135(1):139–45.
10. Giorgadze T, Rossi ED, Fadda G, Gupta PK, Livolsi VA, Baloch Z. Does the fine-needle aspiration diagnosis of "Hürthle-cell neoplasm/follicular neoplasm with oncocytic features" denote increased risk of malignancy? Diagn Cytopathol. 2004;31(5):307–12.
11. Lee KH, Shin JH, Ko ES, Hahn SY, Kim JS, Kim JH, et al. Predictive factors of malignancy in patients with cytologically suspicious for Hurthle cell neoplasm of thyroid nodules. Int J Surg. 2013;11:898–902.
12. Maizlin ZV, Wiseman SM, Vora P, Kirby JM, Mason AC, Filipenko D, et al. Hurthle cell neoplasms of the thyroid: sonographic appearance and histologic characteristics. J Ultrasound Med. 2008;27:751–7.
13. Santana NO, Freitas RM, Marcos VN, Chammas MC, Camargo RY, Schmerling CK, et al. Diagnostic performance of thyroid ultrasound in Hurthle cell carcinomas. Arch Endocrinol Metab. 2019;63:300–5.

14. Lee SK, Rho BH, Woo SK. Hurthle cell neoplasm: correlation of gray-scale and power Doppler sonographic findings with gross pathology. J Clin Ultrasound. 2010;38:169–76.
15. Shin JH, Baek JH, Chung J, Ha EJ, Kim JH, Lee YH, et al. Ultrasonography diagnosis and imaging-based management of thyroid nodules: revised Korean Society of Thyroid Radiology consensus statement and recommendations. Korean J Radiol. 2016;17:370–95.
16. Kim MJ, Shin JH, Hahn SY, Oh YL, Kim SW, Kim TH, Lim Y, Lee S. Ultrasonographic characteristics of Hürthle cell neoplasms: prediction of malignancy. Ultrasonography. 2022;41(4):689–97.
17. Dayong D, Xi C, Hongru W, Haidi W. Typical manifestations of Hürthle cell adenoma of the thyroid on contrast-enhanced CT: a case report. Medicine. 2019;98(22):e15866.
18. Ben HY. Diagnosis and differential diagnosis of thyroid carcinoma by multi-slice spiral CT. Chin J Med Imaging. 2011;19:749–52.
19. Paone G, Treglia G, Bongiovanni M, Ruberto T, Ceriani L, Giovanella L. Incidental detection of Hurthle cell adenoma by 18F-choline PET/CT scan in a patient with prostate cancer. Rev Esp Med Nucl Imagen Mol. 2013;32:340–1.
20. Kochummen E, Tong S, Umpaichitra V, Chin VL. A unique case of bilateral Hurthle cell adenoma in an adolescent. Horm Res Paediatr. 2017;87:136–42.
21. Montone KT, Baloch ZW, LiVolsi VA. The thyroid Hurthle (oncocytic) cell and its associated pathologic conditions: a surgical pathology and cytopathology review. Arch Pathol Lab Med. 2008;132:1241–50.
22. Shawky M, Sakr M. Hurthle cell lesion: controversies, challenges, and debates. Indian J Surg. 2016;78:41–8.
23. Schwab M. Encyclopedia of cancer; 2011. https://doi.org/10.1016/B0-12-227555-1/00151-9.
24. Zhou X, Zheng Z, Chen C, Zhao B, Cao H, Li T, et al. Clinical characteristics and prognostic factors of Hurthle cell carcinoma: a population based study. BMC Cancer. 2020;20(1):407.
25. Tai P, Korzeniowski M, Sadikov E, Joseph K, Kirby A, Tonita J, et al. Issues in managing Hurthle cell carcinoma of thyroid: a case report. Cureus. 2017;9:e1167.
26. Gonzalez JL, Wang HH, Ducatman BS. Fine-needle aspiration of Hurthle cell lesions. A cytomorphologic approach to diagnosis. Am J Clin Pathol. 1993;100:231–5.
27. Cheung CC, Ezzat S, Ramyar L, Freeman JL, Asa SL. Molecular basis off Hurthle cell papillary thyroid carcinoma. J Clin Endocrinol Metab. 2000;85:878–82.
28. Baloch ZW, LiVolsi VA, Asa SL, Rosai J, Merino MJ, Randolph G, et al. Diagnostic terminology and morphologic criteria for cytologic diagnosis of thyroid lesions: a synopsis of the National Cancer Institute thyroid fine-needle aspiration state of the science conference. Diagn Cytopathol. 2008;36:425–37.
29. Chiapponi C, Hartmann MJM, Schmidt M, Faust M, Burns CJ, Schulteis AM, et al. Hürthle cell carcinoma: single center analysis and considerations for surgical management based on the recent literature. Front Endocrinol (Lausanne). 2022;13:904986.
30. Yeap ZH, Arman S, Stenhouse G, Isa A. Synchronous Hürthle cell and medullary thyroid carcinomas. BMJ Case Rep. 2022;15(5):e248879.
31. Aydemirli MD, Corver W, Beuk R, Roepman P, Solleveld-Westerink N, van Wezel T, et al. Targeted treatment options of recurrent radioactive iodine refractory Hürthle cell cancer. Cancers (Basel). 2019;11(8):1185.
32. Stojadinovic A, Hoos A, Ghossein RA, Urist MJ, Leung DHY, Spiro RH, et al. Hurthle cell carcinoma: a 60 year experience. Ann Surg Oncol. 2002;9:197–203.
33. Franssila KO. Thyroid gland. In: Kisane JM, Anderson WAD, editors. Anderson's pathology. 8th ed. St. Louis: CV Mosby Company; 1985. p. 1399–419.
34. Baloch ZW, Livolsi VA. Pathology of thyroid and parathyroid disease. In: Mills SE, Carter D, Reuter VE, Greenson JK, Oberman HA, Stoler MH, editors. Sternberg's diagnostic surgical pathology. 4th ed. Philadelphia: Lippincott Williams and Wilkins; 2004. p. 578–9.
35. Rosai J. Rosai and Ackermann's surgical pathology. 9th ed. New Delhi: Elsevier; 2004. p. 544–7.
36. Maitra A, Abbas AK. The endocrine system. In: Kumar V, Abbas AK, Fausto N, editors. Robbins and Cotran-pathologic basis of disease. 7th ed. New Delhi: Elsevier; 2004. p. 1169–70.

37. Sah SP, Agarwal CS, Mishra A, Rani S. Latent Paillary carcinoma of thyroid with Hashimoto's thyroiditis: diagnosis by fine needle aspiration cytology. J Nep Med Assoc. 2000;39:222–5.
38. LiVolsi VA. Surgical pathology of the thyroid. In: Bennington JL, editor. Major problems in pathology, vol. 22. Philadelphia: WB Saunders; 1990. p. 357–63.
39. Muller-Hocker J, Jacob U, Seibel P. Hashimoto's thyroiditis is associated with defects of cytochrome c oxidase in oxyphil Ashkanazy cells and with the common deletion (4,977) of mitochondrial DNA. Ultrastruct Pathol. 1998;22:91–100.
40. Maximo V, Soares P, Lima J, Cameslle-Teijeiro J, Sobrinho-Simoes M. Mitochondrial DNA somatic mutations (point mutatioms and large deletions) and mitochondrial DNA variants in human thyroid pathology-a study with emphasis on Hurthle cell tumours. Am J Pathol. 2002;160:1857–65.
41. Katoh R, Harach HR, Williams ED. Solitary, multiple and familial oxyphil tumours of the thyroid gland. J Pathol. 1998;186:292–9.
42. Angell JE, Lindner DJ, Shapiro PS, Hoffman ER, Kalvakolanu DU. Identification of GRIM-19, a novel cell death-regulatory gene induced by the interferon P and retinoic acid combination, using a genetic approach. J Biol Chem. 2000;275:33416–26.
43. Maximo V, Botelho T, Capela J, Soares P, Lima J, Taveira A, et al. Somatic and germline mutations in GRIM-19, a dual function gene involved in mitochondrial metabolism and cell death is linked to mitochondrion rich (Hurthle cell) tumour of the thyroid. Br J Cancer. 2005;92:1892–8.
44. Gonzalez JL, Wang HH, Ducatman BS. Fine needle aspiration of Hurthle cell lesions. A cytomorphologic approach to diagnosis. Am J Clin Pathol. 1993;100:231–5.

Oncocytic (Hürthle Cell) Carcinoma: Controversy of Pathophysiology, Diagnosis, and Treatment

12

12.1 Background

Oncocytic tumors are found in various organs, including salivary glands, lacrimal glands, pancreas, liver, kidney, thyroid, parathyroid, and pituitary glands. Oncocytic carcinoma (Hürthle cell carcinoma—HCC) of the thyroid gland is an unusual and relatively rare tumor accounting for approximately 3–10% of all differentiated thyroid cancers (DTCs). Thus, few institutions only have extensive experience with these neoplasms [1]. Oncocytic/Hürthle cell tumors are identified by the World Health Organization (WHO) classification as a special type of tumor derived from thyroid follicles, and distinguished from thyroid follicular tumor [2].

Oncocytic/Hürthle cell neoplasms (HCNs) can be benign (oncocytic adenoma, also known as Hürthle cell adenoma—HCA) or malignant (oncocytic carcinoma, also known as Hürthle cell carcinoma—HCC). Both tumors cannot be distinguished from each other on the basis of cytological analysis of fine-needle aspiration biopsy (FNAB). Features such as pleomorphism, anaplasia, hyperchromatism, and atypia are also observed in benign follicular adenomas. Definitive differentiation of oncocytic/HCC from oncocytic/HCA is based on vascular invasion (VI) and/or capsular invasion (CI), as well as on permanent histological sections or extra-thyroidal extension (ETE), tumor spread to lymph nodes (LNs), and systemic metastases [1].

Oncocytic/HCC represents 3–4% of all thyroid carcinoma cases [3, 4]. In the literature, the incidence of oncocytic/HCC in Hürthle-cell neoplasms (HCNs) is widely variable, ranging from 13% to 67%. Overall, only about one-third (approximately 33%) of oncocytic/Hürthle cell tumors show signs of that invasive growth that indicates malignancy and the possibility of metastasizing. Oncocytic/HCC has been considered as a more aggressive form of carcinoma compared to non-oncocytic thyroid carcinomas. In comparison, oncocytic/HCC may be considered to be more likely to metastasize than follicular thyroid carcinoma (FTC). The likelihood of nodal metastases is greater in oncocytic/HCC than in FTC; but is not as great as with papillary thyroid carcinoma (PTC) [1].

M. Sakr, *Oncocytic (Hürthle Cell) Thyroid Lesions*,
https://doi.org/10.1007/978-3-032-03115-0_12

There is still no consensus on the optimal treatment method for oncocytic/HCC, and the postoperative effect of radioactive iodine treatment is unclear. Histological interpretation may result in the designation of some nonneoplastic Hürthle cell lesions (HCLs) as malignant tumors. Obviously, this factor has a major impact in interpreting the natural history of this disease and adds to the controversy about the aggressiveness of HCC. This leads to reported high overall mortality rates ranging from 9% to 28%.

12.2 Epidemiology

12.2.1 General Incidence

12.2.1.1 USA

Thyroid cancer is uncommon, and among all cancers, it accounts for 0.74% in men and 2.3% in women in the USA. The average age-adjusted annual incidence for thyroid cancer is less than 40 cases per 1 million people. Oncocytic/Hürthle cell carcinomas account for about 3–10% of these cases. However, thyroid cancer is reported to be the most rapidly increasing malignancy in the USA, with rates rising by 5.1% per year from 2003 to 2012 [5]. For thyroid cancer as a whole, 64,300 new cases (49,350 in females and 14,950 in males) were projected in the USA during the year 2016. The estimated deaths were 1980 (1070 in females and 910 in males) [5]. It is conceivable that oncocytic/HCC cases will be about 3–10% of these. A recent (2022) retrospective analysis of oncocytic/HCC primarily treated with surgery at Memorial Sloan Kettering Cancer Center between 1986 and 2015 identified a total of 111 patients only [6].

12.2.1.2 International (Worldwide)

Worldwide, thyroid cancer rates have been increasing over the past few decades [5]. International frequency likely approximates that of the USA. In general, the annual incidence of thyroid cancer in various parts of the world is 0.5–10 cases per 100,000 individuals. Approximately 3–10% of these cases are oncocytic/HCCs. Jin et al. from South Korea (2021) reported that oncocytic/Hürthle cell carcinoma (HCC) of the thyroid is rare, accounting for only 3–4% of all thyroid tumors [7].

12.2.1.3 Race- and Age-Related Demographics

All races appear to be affected with oncocytic/HCC equally. The tumor is more often observed in females, and the reported female to male ratio of oncocytic/HCC is 1.6–4.8:1 [8–11]. The typical age range of patients presenting with this condition is 20–85 years. The mean age is usually 54–62 years, approximately 10 years older than the age associated with other types of differentiated thyroid cancers (DTCs) [8, 10, 12–15].

12.3 Pathophysiology

The cellular origin of oncocytic/HCC, as well as other thyroid cancer types, is still *not* completely understood. Thyroid cancer stem cell (CSC) model is one hypothesis to explain thyroid carcinogenesis. To identify thyroid CSCs, various research with CD133 [16, 17], CD44 [17, 18], multidrug resistance (MDR1) [19], ATP-binding cassette subfamily G member 2 (ABCG2) [19, 20], multidrug-associated protein 1 (MRP1) [20], aldehyde dehydrogenase (ALDH) [21], as well as sphere formation assay [22] and side population assay [21] have been carried out. These studies focused on differentiated and undifferentiated thyroid carcinomas, not on oncocytic/HCC, and no common CSC markers have been reported to date. Further studies on the isolation and characterization of CSCs in oncocytic/HCC will improve knowledge regarding oncocytic/HCC initiation.

There is no accepted paradigm for the pathogenesis of FTC and oncocytic/HCC. It is conceivable that a multistep adenoma-to-carcinoma pathway is involved; however, this concept is not universally accepted. Many of the cells probably develop from preexisting adenomas, but a FTC in situ is *not* recognized pathologically. Progressive transformations through somatic mutations of genes that are important in growth control are involved in FTC formation. Low iodide intake is a key environmental factor determining the relative incidence of follicular and papillary cancers. Most follicular adenomas and all follicular carcinomas are thought to have monoclonal origin.

Oncogene activation, particularly by mutation or translocation of the *RAS* oncogene, is common in both follicular adenomas and FTC (approximately 40%), supporting a role in early tumorigenesis. Such *ras* oncogene mutations are not specific for follicular tumors and also occur in papillary thyroid cancer (PTC). The *RAS* oncogene is frequently involved in the pathogenesis of oncocytic/Hürthle cell neoplasms (HCNs). In PTC and in many oncocytic/HCNs, *RET* rearrangements are found; these are not found in follicular tumors. Local spread may be found in *RET*-positive cases; *RET*- negative cases, as in follicular cancer cases, are more likely to spread hematogenously to distant metastatic sites.

Unlike FTC, oncocytic/HCC genetic analysis shows a low rate of RAS mutations and PAX8-PPARG fusions. Until the last decade, the genetic mechanism of developing oncocytic/HCC was not entirely clear. It was believed that chromosomal disturbances, in terms of chromosomal gains or losses, played a role in oncocytic (Hürthle) cell tumorigenesis. In 2012, Corver et al. reported that Copy Number Alterations (CNAs) leading to genome haploidization are the genetic mechanism of oncocytic/HCC [23]. CNAs are considered driver alterations in thyroid carcinogenesis, defined as a "section of DNA that presents variable copy numbers in comparison with a reference genome." Several genetic studies have supported that CNA is a hallmark of the oncocytic/HCC process. Recently, Doerfler et al. (2021) investigated whether CNAs are a hallmark of oncocytic/HCC specifically or oncocytic/

HCA as well [24]. They concluded that CNAs could present in both conditions. Moreover, the presence of CNAs with other aggressive mutations, such as TERT mutation, suggests an aggressive malignant histology rather than a benign process. In addition to CNAs, Doerfler et al. identified RAS and EIF1AX mutations as common in both oncocytic/HCC and oncocytic/HCA in similar frequency [24].

An association was also found between overexpression of the *p53* gene product and a subset of oncocytic/HCCs. Several authors reported a high prevalence of TP53 among widely invasive HCC (wiHCC) compared to minimally invasive HCC (miHCC) [25]. Additionally, gene expression analysis can reveal differences between miHCC and wiHCC. One of the significant differences observed was an enriched gene set related to beta-catenin (CTNNB1). In wiHCC, beta-catenin plays a crucial role in the regulation of processes that govern vascular invasion [26].

Reduced immuno-expression of E-cadherin exists, with a trend to a diffuse cytoplasmic pattern, both in benign and malignant oncocytic/HCNs and in papillary, poorly differentiated, and undifferentiated thyroid carcinomas. Isolated studies indicate overexpression of the *N-myc* oncogene, (*TGF-α*), tumor growth factor-beta (*TGF-β*), insulin-like growth factor-1 (*IGF-1*), and somatostatin receptor in oncocytic/HCCs.

Cytogenetic abnormalities and evidence of genetic loss are more common in FTC than in PTC. These abnormalities occur in follicular adenomas, suggesting that cell cycle control, mitotic spindle formation, DNA repair, or more than one of these mechanisms may be impaired in these neoplasms, possibly at an earlier stage.

Activating mutations of genes encoding the thyrotropin receptor and the α- subunit of the stimulatory G-protein are also reported in some follicular carcinomas. These losses are associated particularly with chromosomes *3, 10, 11,* and *17*. The deletions and/or rearrangements involving the p (short) arm of chromosome *3* are the most common. Loss of a tumor suppressor on chromosome arm 3p has been postulated to be specific for FTC and may be involved in adenoma-to-carcinoma progression.

Restriction fragment length polymorphism (RFLP) analysis demonstrates that unbalanced losses of genetic material are relatively common in oncocytic/Hürthle cell neoplasms. Loss of heterozygosity from the q (long) arm of chromosome *10* is also detected in oncocytic tumors. Evidence suggests that some Hürthle cell adenomas and carcinomas can express an *RET/PTC* gene arrangement, which is more unique to PTC. Because of this gene arrangement, another subclassification of Hürthle cell neoplasms has been proposed, namely, the papillary variant of HCC (i.e., Hürthle cell papillary thyroid carcinoma), in addition to oncocytic/HCC and oncocytic adenoma. Clinically, tumors in this group tend to behave like PTC; however, they are more indolent, with a propensity for lymph node (LN) metastasis rather than hematogenous spread. In 2006, Maxwell et al. [27] reported that the Hürthle cell tumors with *RET/PTC*—positive gene arrangement have higher incidence of regional metastatic disease and more aggressive treatment has been recommended.

As reported by Asa [28], many oncocytic/HCNs, whether benign or malignant, show papillary change. This is a pseudo-papillary phenomenon because oncocytic/

HCNs have only scant stroma and may fall apart during manipulation, fixation, and processing. True oxyphilic or oncocytic (Hürthle) cell papillary carcinoma has been reported to comprise 1–11% of all PTCs. These tumors have a papillary architecture, but are composed predominantly, or entirely, of oncocytic (Hürthle) cells.

Mitochondrion-related alterations, such as mutations in mitochondrial DNA (mtDNA), are also described in Hürthle cell tumors. Defects of cytochrome c oxidase and deletion of mitochondrial DNA occur frequently in oncocytic/HCCs and in oncocytic (Hürthle) cells of Hashimoto's thyroiditis. In one study, almost all oncocytic (Hürthle) cells displayed a common deletion, somatic mitochondrial point mutations, or both. Activating gene mutations encoding the thyrotropin receptor and the α-subunit of the stimulatory G-protein are also reported in some follicular carcinomas.

DNA content profiles after flow cytometry are commonly abnormal. Hürthle cell neoplasms, including histologically benign tumors, are often aneuploid. This finding parallels with nuclear atypia and anisocytosis. The demonstration of aneuploidy may indicate aggressive clinical behavior compared with euploid tumors. In a recent Italian study, p27 and cyclin D3 proteins were found to be overexpressed in oncocytic/HCC cell lines and clinical samples of thyroid cancer [29]. Accumulation of p27 was found to be associated with the overexpression of cyclin D3 in oncocytic/HCC of the thyroid.

In a study analyzing genomic dissection of oncocytic/HCC reported that unsupervised hierarchical clustering of gene expression showed three groups of Hürthle cell tumors: Hürthle cell adenomas, minimally invasive Hürthle cell carcinoma (miHCC), and widely invasive Hürthle cell carcinoma (wiHCC). These are clustered separately, with a marked difference between wiHCC and Hürthle cell adenoma. Molecular pathways that differentiate Hürthle cell adenomas from wiHCC included the PIK3CA-Akt-mTOR and Wnt/β -catenin pathways, potentially providing a rationale for new targets for the treatment of this type of thyroid carcinoma [26].

12.4 Etiology/Risk Factors

12.4.1 Etiological Factors

Etiological factors of oncocytic/HCC may be summarized as follows:

- Radiation to the neck.
- Iodide deficiency.
- Overexpression of the *p53* oncogene.
- Oncogene activation, particularly by mutation or translocation of the *ras* oncogene.
- Activating mutations of genes encoding the thyrotropin receptor and the α-subunit of the stimulatory of G-protein (reported in some follicular carcinomas).
- Somatic mutations of genes important in growth control.

- Mitochondrion-related alterations (e.g., mutations in mitochondrial DNA). A study by Maximo et al. [30] (2005) linked somatic and germline mutation in *GRIM-19* (a dual-function gene involved in mitochondrial metabolism and cell death) to Hürthle cell tumors of the thyroid. This is the first nuclear gene mutation described for a subgroup of oncocytic/HCCs.

12.4.2 Clinical Indicators of Malignancy

Indicators of malignancy among oncocytic/Hürthle cell neoplasms (HCNs) include male gender [31], older age (mean age for oncocytic/HCC 51.8 years versus 43.1 years for oncocytic/HCA) [32], tumor size more than 4 cm [11, 31–33], and ultrasound class (USC) ≥ 3 [33]. Subsequently, surgical indications of oncocytic/HCNs are reported as USC ≥ 3, tumor size >4 cm, and thyroglobulin >500 ng/dL (with negative anti-thyroglobulin-antibody) [33].

12.5 Clinical Presentation

12.5.1 History-Taking

The history in patients with a thyroid nodule or a known follicular or oncocytic/Hürthle cell neoplasm is neither sensitive nor specific for a diagnosis of malignancy. However, the following clinical features are more suggestive of malignancy: (1) a palpable mass in the thyroid (most common clinical sign), (2) pressure symptoms (e.g., dysphagia, dyspnea, coughing, choking spells, and hoarseness of voice), (3) rapid growth or significant compressive symptoms, and (4) pain.

Other features of oncocytic/HCC include the following: (1) multifocality and bilaterality, (2) LN metastasis and symptoms confined to metastatic sites can be the first clinical presentation in a subgroup of cases, (3) a history of head and neck external beam irradiation should alert the clinician to a possible malignancy (multifocal and bilateral disease is more common in such cases), and (4) a family history of thyroid cancer and endocrinopathies can also be present, and patients are usually euthyroid, but hyperthyroidism or hypothyroidism occurs in a small percentage of patients.

Other benign thyroid and parathyroid disorders can be observed, such as Graves' disease, colloid nodular disease, chronic lymphocytic thyroiditis (Hashimoto's thyroiditis), thyroid hyperplasia, parathyroid adenoma, and follicular adenomas.

12.5.2 Physical Examination

The most common physical examination finding is a palpable single neck mass; however, the contralateral lobe may harbor impalpable malignancy in such cases.

Less often, patients may have multiple palpable masses. The main findings on physical examination may include the following:

- Regional lymph nodes (LNs) may sometimes be felt in the neck and locoregionally, though less common than in PTC. In 2022, Chiapponi et al. [34] reported that the rate of LN involvement in oncocytic/HCC in their study was 4.3%, which is similar to that of Goffredo et al. (2013) [12], who documented node-positive disease in 5.3% of patients. In their meta-analysis, Coca Pelaz et al. (2021) included 9638 patients and found LN metastasis in only 9% of patients [35]. However, Lopez-Penabad et al. [32] and Chindris et al. [8] reported a high nodal involvement of approximately 20%. It needs to be mentioned that in the study by Chindris et al., LNs were not examined in the majority of cases (57.8%), therefore the rate of LN involvement is probably not representative. The study of Lopez-Penabad et al. [32] included 127 patients with oncocytic/Hürthle cell neoplasms (89 oncocytic/HCC and 38 oncocytic/HCA). Seven tumors had anaplastic foci, which may have influenced the nodal involvement rate.
- The trachea can be compressed and/or deviated from the midline secondary to the mass effect of the tumor.
- Hoarseness of voice may occur if vocal cords were involved.
- A hard, fixed thyroid nodule, cervical lymphadenopathy, and vocal cord paralysis are features that may indicate carcinoma.
- Horner's syndrome may be present in patients with involvement of the cervical sympathetic ganglia.
- If the tumor extends into the upper mediastinum, superior mediastinal syndrome may ensue, with facial swelling and dilated veins.
- Most patients with oncocytic/HCC (and oncocytic/HCA) are euthyroid, but in rare cases, signs of thyrotoxicosis may be present caused by either massive tumor burden or functioning metastatic disease.

Complications of oncocytic/HCCs are similar to those of thyroid cancer in general. They can cause complications in the neck by local invasion into the larynx, vocal cords, esophagus, trachea, or mediastinum and by compression of major nerves and vessels in the neck from bulky adenopathy. Metastases tend to occur in LNs, lungs, bone, and infrequently the brain. Physical findings of metastases and pathological bone fractures may be found in long and flat bones.

12.6 Differential Diagnosis

Oncocytic/Hürthle cell carcinoma (HCC) shares many clinical and histological features with other types of thyroid cancers, in particular with follicular thyroid carcinoma (FTC). Oncocytic adenoma (Hürthle cell adenoma—HCA) is the principal consideration in the differential diagnosis of oncocytic/HCC. Other pathologies to consider include follicular adenoma, thyroid cysts, thyrotoxicosis, and metastatic tumors to the thyroid (usually result from renal cell carcinoma, but may also originate from Hürthle cell tumors in other organs that harbor oncocytic (Hürthle) cells, such as salivary glands, pharynx, larynx, trachea, parathyroid gland, esophagus, pituitary gland, and liver.

In general, the list of thyroid diseases from which oncocytic/HCC should be differentiated from is long and variable. It includes anaplastic thyroid carcinoma (ATC), differentiated thyroid cancer (DTC) (FTC and PTC), medullary thyroid carcinoma (MTC), thyroid lymphoma, diffuse toxic goiter (Graves' disease), Hashimoto's thyroiditis, simple (nontoxic) goiter, thyroid nodule, and toxic nodular goiter.

Compared to follicular thyroid carcinoma, oncocytic/HCCs tend to be larger, multifocal, have a higher rate of local thyroid invasion, lymph node metastases, and distant metastases [36, 37]. In addition, oncocytic/HCCs have characteristic histological features and also have a low tendency to take up radioactive iodine (RAI) on imaging.

Rapidly growing thyroid carcinomas should always be evaluated for anaplastic thyroid carcinoma (ATC) as these tumors carry a significantly worse prognosis and need immediate treatment with systemic chemotherapy and sometimes combined with radiation of the neck.

12.7 Investigations (Workup)

12.7.1 Laboratory Studies

A full set of thyroid function tests should be ordered, including thyroid-stimulating hormone (TSH), thyroxine (T4), triiodothyronine (T3), and free T4. In addition, the following antibody studies should be ordered: anti-peroxidase antibodies and anti-thyroglobulin antibodies. If TSH is low, indicating a functional nodule, this can be confirmed by a radioiodine imaging scan. These functionally hyperthyroid or "hot" nodules are rarely cancerous and require management of hyperthyroidism or thyrotoxicosis.

Thyroglobulin (Tg) production varies by case. Both high Tg production (>500 ng/dL) [33, 38, 39] and limited production [40], which reflects less active follicular cells, have been reported in patients with oncocytic/HCC. An increased Tg level is a biomarker for recurrence after thyroidectomy; however, some recurrent oncocytic/HCC cases have undetectable Tg levels. Clinical follow-up by Tg levels should be decided depending on the case [41].

Petric et al. (2014) reported that while oncocytic/HCC may not always have a high Tg value, a level > 80 ng/mL in a oncocytic/Hürthle cell neoplasm (HCN) predicts malignancy [42]. In their study, the median preoperative Tg concentration in benign tumors, PTCs, FTCs, and oncocytic/HCC was 41, 87, 72, and 106 ng/ml ($P = 0.05$), respectively [42].

12.7.2 Imaging Studies

Imaging studies for the evaluation of oncocytic/HCC include the following:

12.7.2.1 Radioiodine Thyroid Uptake and Scan

The typical finding of oncocytic/HCC in thyroid scan is an area of decreased uptake, which corresponds to the tumor. However, oncocytic/HCC may not be iodine avid.

12.7.2.2 Octreotide Scintigraphy

A significant proportion of thyroid cancers may be non-iodine avid. Thyroid tumors are known to express somatostatin receptors. Octreotide, a synthetic analogue of somatostatin with a considerably longer half-life, can be combined with a radioactive isotope, such as 111 Indium-diethylenetriaminepentaacetic acid-d-phenylalanine-octreotide (^{111}In-DTPA$^{0)}$ to visualize tumors with high concentrations of somatostatin receptors. Octreotide scintigraphy can be considered for patients with recurrent or metastatic oncocytic/HCC because evidence suggests the higher expression of "somatostatin" receptors by oncocytic/Hürthle cell neoplasms than the surrounding normal thyroid tissue [43].

Imaging with octreotide does *not* provide an alternative to conventional radiology in the staging of non-iodine avid thyroid cancer, but may provide additional useful information, particularly in the case of widespread bone metastases [44]. A major advantage of scintigraphy using octreotide compared to radioiodine is that patients do not have to withdraw thyroid hormone. This was emphasized by Haslinghuis et al. (2001) in a series of 25 patients with differentiated thyroid cancer, who also showed that 75% patients with lesions that did not concentrate radioiodine did show uptake of octreotide [45]. In addition, the major interest in imaging with octreotide lies in its potential for peptide receptor targeted therapy.

Gulect et al. (1998) described three patients with oncocytic/HCC and found all to have positive octreotide scintigraphy [46]. In a study by Gorges et al. (1999), eight of nine patients with metastatic HCC showed ^{111}In-pentetreotide accumulation of various intensity, while ^{131}I scans were negative except for one patient. The octreotide scans were compared to FDG-PET scans and found to be slightly inferior [47]. Tisell et al. (1999) reported that two patients with HCC, previously thyroidectomized, had their metastases visualized by octreotide scintigraphy. The tissue/blood ^{111}In concentration ratios for tumor samples showed clearly higher values than observed for normal connective tissue, muscle, or lymph nodes [48].

Kostoglou-Athanassiou et al. (2003) described a locally recurrent lesion in the tumor bed by [^{111}In] Octreotide in a patient with known thyroid oncocytic/HCC, increased thyroglobulin levels, and a negative radio-iodine total-body scan. The recurrent lesion was then successfully excised by surgery. On histology, the tumor proved to be an oncocytic/HCC, and within the tumor somatostatin receptors were detected by reverse transcription polymerase chain reaction (RT-PCR) [49].

Christian et al. (2003) assessed 18 patients with histologically proven metastatic or locally recurrent non-iodine avid thyroid carcinoma to determine the usefulness of ^{111}In-DTPA octreotide scintigraphy compared to conventional radiology in diagnosing sites of metastasis. Of the 18 patients, 14 had octreotide-positive scans. In one patient with widespread bone metastases, octreotide gave a more detailed assessment of metastatic disease than conventional radiology. In addition, one patient with oncotic/HCC metastatic to bone and a positive octreotide scan has been treated with ^{90}yttrium-labeled octreotide. They concluded that ^{111}In-DTPA octreotide imaging for patients with non-iodine avid carcinoma of the thyroid may be a useful diagnostic and staging tool, and monitoring of patients with non-iodine avid carcinoma. They added that for unresectable disease, diagnostic scan-positive patients may progress to somatostatin receptor-targeted therapy [44].

More recently, in 2020, Jahanpanah et al. reported that a 75-year-old male patient with non-avid radioiodine HCC was evaluated by ^{99m} Tc-octreotide scintigraphy in order to find possible metastatic lesions. A bony metastatic lesion was detected by this procedure, which was confirmed by histopathology. They concluded that ^{99m}Tc-octreotide scintigraphy is a precise and cost-effective imaging modality for detection of non-iodine avid lesions in metastatic oncocytic/HCCs [50].

12.7.2.3 Thyroid Ultrasound (US)

Ultrasound (US) is typically the first imaging method used for any thyroid condition, but preoperative diagnosis of oncocytic/HCC by US is challenging and almost impossible. However, certain features may suggest a malignant or aggressive condition. On ultrasound, oncocytic/HCC shows a range of sonographic appearances from predominantly hypoechoic to hyper-echoic lesions [11, 51]. Ultrasound usually demonstrates a solid mass (Fig. 12.1), can characterize the solid/cystic nature of the lesion (Fig. 12.2), and is also helpful in diagnosing enlarged LNs in the

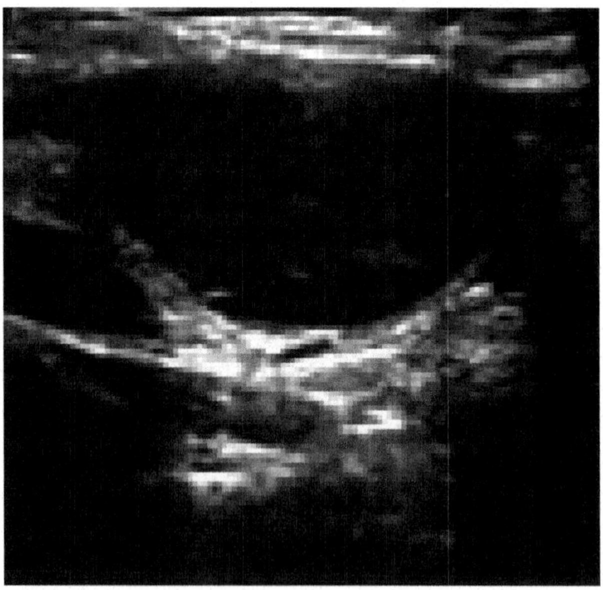

Fig. 12.1 Ultrasound of the thyroid gland demonstrating an oncocytic/Hürthle cell carcinoma as a solid hypoechoic nodule

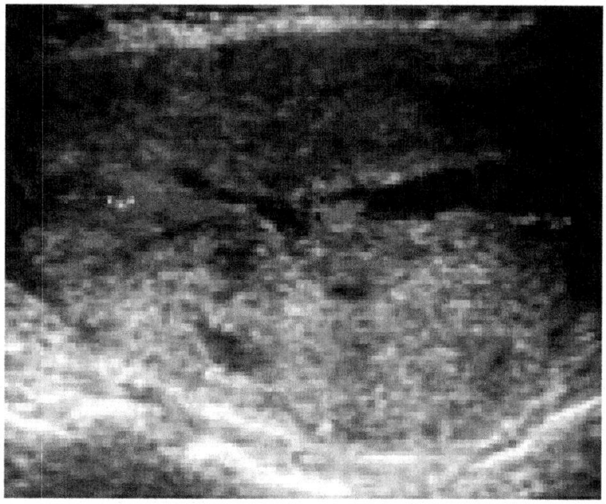

Fig. 12.2 Ultrasound of the thyroid gland demonstrating an oncocytic/Hürthle cell carcinoma as a partially cystic isoechoic nodule

neck. However, no preoperative features can differentiate oncocytic/HCC from oncocytic/HCA [11, 51].

Several attempts have been made by many researchers to predict oncocytic/HCC before the operation. Ito et al. (2007) classified thyroid nodules into classes 1–5 with intermediate steps of 0.5 for classes 2–5, called ultrasound classes (USC) [52]. USC2 is defined as having a round and cystic nodule/isoechoic solid nodule—an adenomatous nodule or follicular adenoma. USC3 is defined as a round, hypoechoic solid nodule—a follicular adenoma, adenomatous nodule, or possibly carcinoma. USC4 is a solid nodule with an irregular border or the presence of psammoma calcifications—a carcinoma. Although USC is not related to the incidence of oncocytic/HCC, among patients diagnosed with oncocytic cell tumors by fine-needle aspiration cytology (FNAC), such patients are more likely to show malignancy when USC is 3 or greater.

In 2008, Maizlin et al. attempted to distinguish oncocytic/HCNs in US. They reviewed 15 proven cases of oncocytic/HCNs and reported that the lesions varied from hypo- to hyper-echoic and from low- to high-vascularity, and no feature suggested oncocytic/HCNs by US at that time [51]. With advances in US technology, a review of 139 cases of oncocytic/HCNs found that size was the only suggestive feature of oncocytic/HCC, particularly when the size was above 3.35 cm [53]. In another study, it was found that malignant tumors displayed a higher probability of hypoechoic and hyper-echoic nodules as opposed to benign tumors. Conversely, iso-echogenicity was a more dependable indicator of benignity [54].

More recently, Ito and colleagues [33] reported that they observed round and hypoechoic solid nodules and solid nodules with irregular borders or with psammoma calcifications represented 83% of oncocytic/HCCs and 78% of oncocytic/HCAs. However, the authors concluded that such sonographic presentations were independent predictors of malignancy in patients with oncocytic (Hürthle) cells in FNAC. In contrast, lesions with a flat, isoechoic, or hyper-echoic pattern with a peripheral halo were frequent among the oncocytic/HCCs in the present study at rates of 83.3%, 62.5%, and 79.2%, respectively.

Oncocytic/HCC typically presents as TIRADS 3, 4, or 5 in thyroid US. Few studies have assessed the ability of preoperative sonographic characteristics in differentiating oncocytic/HCCs from oncocytic/HCAs due to the low prevalence of both lesions. Santana et al. [11] conducted a retrospective study to compare the preoperative features of oncocytic/HCCs and oncocytic/HCAs and evaluate the diagnostic performance of ultrasound (US) in distinguishing between both conditions. The study included 101 patients (52 oncocytic/HCCs and 49 oncocytic/HCAs) who underwent thyroid surgery (total thyroidectomy or lobectomy) from 2000 to 2016. Diagnostic performance of suspicious sonographic features was analyzed in 51 cases (24 oncocytic/HCCs and 27 oncocytic/HCAs). Among the oncocytic/HCCs, the lesions were purely solid in 54.2% of cases, hypoechoic in 37.5%, and had coarse calcifications (Fig. 12.3) in 12.5%, microcalcifications (Fig. 12.4) in 8.3%, irregular contours in 4.2%, and a taller-than-wide shape in 16.7%. Predominantly/exclusive intra-nodular vascularization (Fig. 12.4) was observed in 52.6%. Overall, 58% of the oncocytic/HCCs were classified as TI-RADS 4 (moderately suspicious) or 5 (highly suspicious) compared with 48% of the HCAs. TI-RADS 4 or 5 had a specificity of only 51.8% and a positive likelihood ratio of only 1.21.

In general, several sonographic features are usually associated with a higher risk of malignancy in a thyroid nodule. According to the American Thyroid Association (ATA), a highly suspicious sonographic pattern is represented by a solid hypoechoic nodule or solid hypoechoic component of a partially cystic nodule associated with at least one of the following findings: irregular margins, microcalcifications, taller-than-wide shape, rim calcifications with a small protruding soft tissue component, or evidence of extra-thyroidal extension (ETE). The absence of a peripheral halo and increased intra-nodular vascularization are also considered suspicious for malignancy [55]. These suspicious characteristics are mainly observed in papillary thyroid carcinomas (PTCs) [55, 56]. From their study, Santana and colleagues

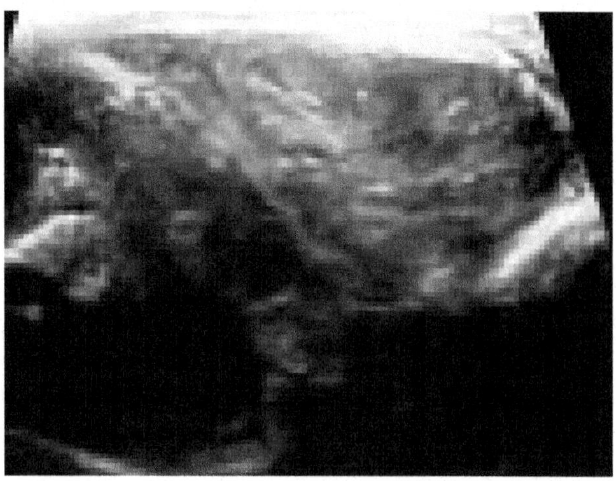

Fig. 12.3 Ultrasound of the thyroid gland demonstrating an oncocytic/Hürthle cell carcinoma as a solid hypoechoic nodule with microcalcifications and coarse calcifications

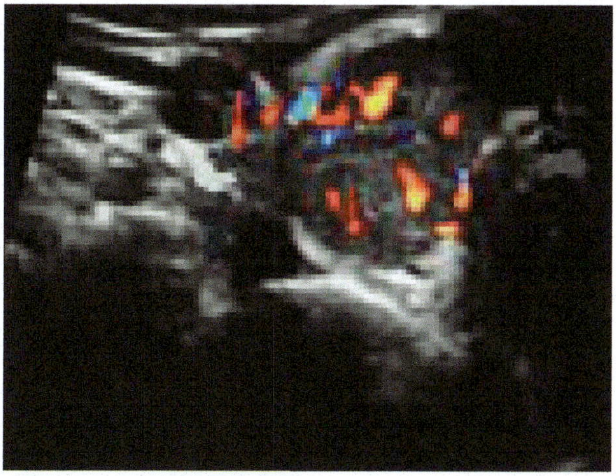

Fig. 12.4 Ultrasound of the thyroid gland demonstrating an oncocytic/Hürthle cell carcinoma as a solid hypoechoic nodule with intra-nodular vascularization

(2019) [11] concluded that sonographic characteristics raising suspicion for malignancy, which are mostly present in PTCs, were "infrequent" in oncocytic/HCCs, and that new tools must be developed in order to improve preoperative diagnosis and deferral of surgery in cases of benign oncocytic/Hürthle cell neoplasms (HCAs).

More recently, Kim et al. [53] studied the preoperative sonographic characteristics of 139 oncocytic/Hürthle cell neoplasms (HCNs) and correlated them with their postoperative histopathological results, which showed that 99 lesions were adenomas, 32 were carcinomas, and 8 were HCNs with UMB (uncertain malignant behavior). Univariate analysis, showed that the significant features associated with oncocytic/HCA versus oncocytic/HCC were internal content, US tumor size, and pathological tumor size. The oncocytic/HCC masses more frequently showed cystic changes than oncocytic/HCAs (38% versus 17%, respectively; $P < 0.001$). Other factors such as echogenicity, margin, orientation, calcification, halo sign, vascularity, K-TIRADS category, and Bethesda category did not show statistical significance between oncocytic/HCC and oncocytic/HCA. Their multiple logistic regression analysis, revealed that the US tumor size was an independent significant predictor of malignancy ($P = 0.001$) with the best cutoff value of 3.35 cm (sensitivity, 53.1%; specificity, 87.9%) [53].

12.7.2.4 Computed Tomography (CT) Scan

Computed tomography (CT) scan of the neck provides more detailed information about the thyroid tumor (Fig. 12.5) and its relation to the other neck structures. Moreover, it is helpful in assessment of calcifications. Thus, it can help determine the location and size of tumor, whether it has invaded into any nearby structures, and whether it has spread to lymph nodes (LNs) in nearby areas. The CT scan can also be used to look for spread into distant organs such as the lungs. Ultimately, all of these studies will determine the extent of the required surgery. The more aggressive the oncocytic/HCC, the larger it will appear in the CT scan, with a necrotic center and invasion of adjacent structures. In some advanced cases, it may mimic

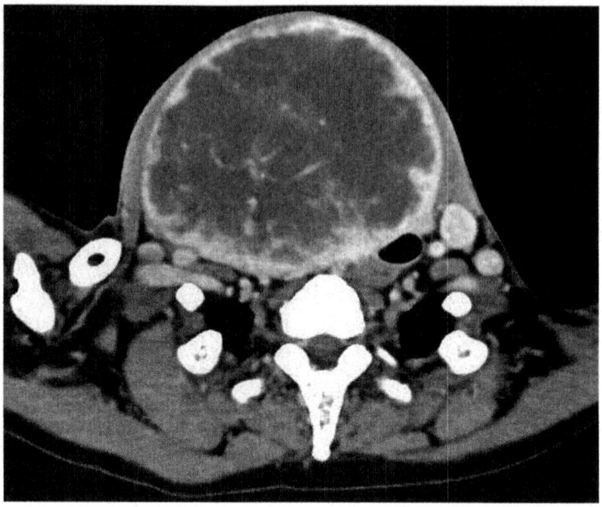

Fig. 12.5 Computed tomography (CT) scan of the thyroid showing a heterogeneously enhancing huge mass with areas of central necrosis that was proven by histopathology to be an oncocytic/Hürthle cell carcinoma

poorly differentiated or undifferentiated thyroid cancer. In general, a CT scan of the neck is *not* needed or required for the more common FNA diagnosis of "Hürthle cell neoplasm" (HCN) of the thyroid. However if the oncocytic/HCN is clinically suggested to be a high-risk lesion for a diagnosis of oncocytic/HCC, then a CT scan of the neck is frequently considered.

Potential indications for obtaining a CT scan of the neck for lesions high risk for a diagnosis of oncocytic/HCC include (1) a large oncocytic/HCN more than 4 cm, (2) a fixed or minimally mobile mass, (3) an ultrasound suggesting soft tissue extension or invasion, and (4) a patient presenting with symptoms of vocal cord paralysis (hoarseness of voice) and/or difficulty in swallowing.

In patients with a diagnosis of oncocytic/HCC, a CT scan of the chest should be obtained. The CT scan of the chest provides an excellent baseline examination of the lungs, the highest risk site for distant spread in patients with oncocytic/HCC.

12.7.2.5 Magnetic Resonance Imaging (MRI)

Magnetic resonance imaging (MRI) of the neck will also provide more detailed information about the tumor and its relation to the other neck structures. Like CT scans, MRI scans can be used to look at a presumed diagnosis of oncocytic/HCC, or cancer that has spread to nearby or distant parts of the body. However, US is usually the first choice for looking at the thyroid and neck structures.

12.7.2.6 Positron Emission Tomography (PET) Scan

Oncocytic/Hürthle cell carcinoma (HCC) is an aggressive thyroid cancer that may require more aggressive locoregional therapy than differentiated thyroid cancer (DTC). This tumor is more commonly metastatic, and a thorough evaluation for distant metastasis is thus highly recommended.

Positron emission tomography (PET) with 18F-2-fluoro-2-deoxy-D-glucose (18F-FDG PET) can identify high-grade cancer because of the high glucose uptake in aggressive, poorly differentiated malignancy. It has been shown to be helpful in diagnosing recurrent and metastatic disease in oncocytic/HCC, particularly with tumors that have low iodine avidity and tumors that have a high blood marker of thyroglobulin [57–60]. Metastatic disease usually involves lymph nodes (Fig. 12.6), lungs, and bones (Fig. 12.7).

Lowe et al. [61] reported that 14 18F-FDG PET scans of 12 patients documented HCC showed intense 18F-FDG uptake in all known HCC lesions except in one. PET showed disease not identified by other imaging methods in 7 of the 14 PET scans. It identified distant metastatic disease ($n = 5$) and local disease ($n = 2$) that was more extensive than otherwise demonstrated. This information provided by PET was used to guide or change therapy due to better characterization of indeterminate abnormalities on CT scan or US in three scans, and to detection of unsuspected disease in four other scans [61].

The results reported by Lowe et al. [61] support those reported previously by Plotkin et al. [62] who described accurate identification of oncocytic/HCC by 18F-FDG PET in a group of 17 patients with indications of recurrent disease. In a more recent study by Pryma et al. [63], 18F-FDG PET was shown to increase diagnostic accuracy over CT scan and radioactive iodine (RAI) scan. In addition, in this study, intense 18F-FDG uptake in lesions was an indicator of poor prognosis.

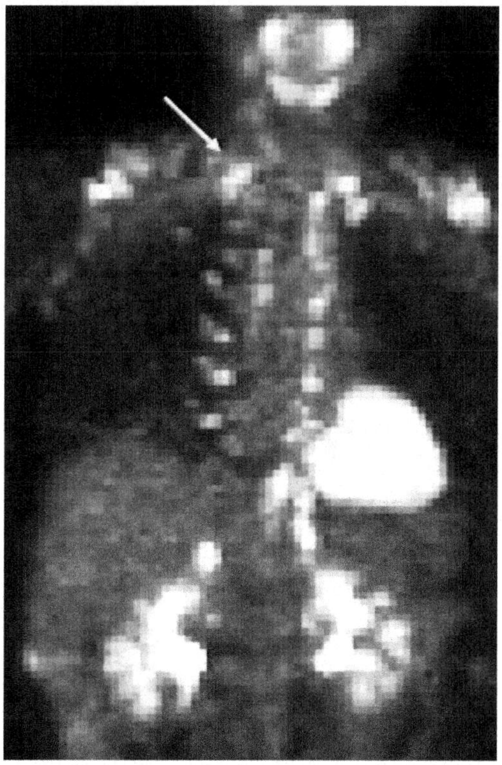

Fig. 12.6 Positron emission tomography (PET) image of a patient treated for documented oncocytic/Hürthle cell carcinoma. Follow-up cervical ultrasonography showed a 1-cm right cervical lymph node. PET scan confirmed metastatic disease (arrow)

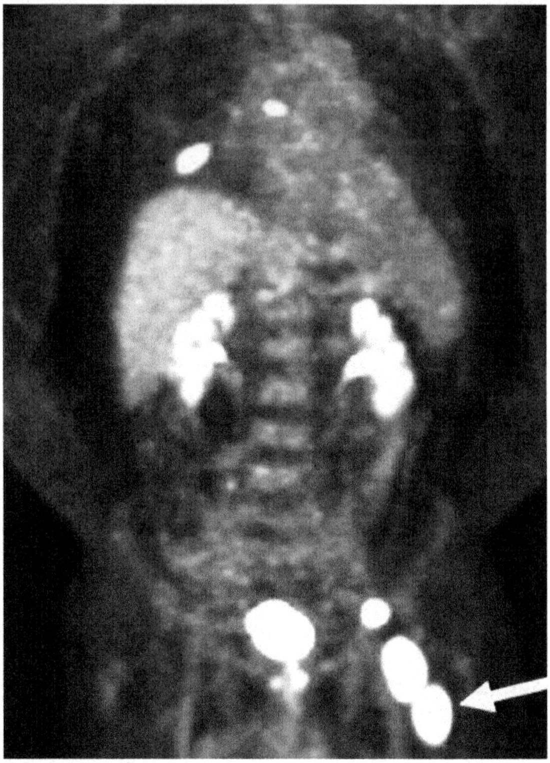

Fig. 12.7 Positron emission tomography (PET) image of a patient treated for documented oncocytic/Hürthle cell carcinoma. Follow-up cervical ultrasonography and ^{131}I scan had negative findings. PET image showed lung, vertebral body, and pelvis/femur (arrow) metastases. Pelvic biopsy confirmed metastatic disease

On the other hand, Pathak et al. (2014) reported that PET scan is not useful in predicting malignancy, as all oncocytic/HCAs and oncocytic/HCCs are 18fludeoxyglucose (18FDG)-PET-positive [64]. Researchers at the University of Vienna reported that the average maximum standardized uptake values (SUv) of oncocytic/HCN was 5.8 (range: 2.6–16) [65]. To increase the sensitivity of PET scan, thyroxine withdrawal or recombinant thyroid-stimulating hormone (rTSH) can be used especially in the setting of suspected non-radioiodine avid recurrence with elevated Tg [66]. Palaniswamy and Subramanyam P (2013) stated that newer PET radiotracers are needed, such as Iodine-124, Fluorine-18 DOPA (3,4-dihydroxy-L-phenylalanine), and Gallium-68 DOTA [67].

PET/CT scanning is commonly positive in patients with oncocytic/HCC. Indications for obtaining a PET/CT scan for a patient with a diagnosis of oncocytic/HCC include (1) de-differentiated or poorly differentiated oncocytic/HCC, (2) a diagnosis of oncocytic/HCC with no/low avidity to RAI, (3) recurrent tumor, (4) metastatic oncocytic/HCC, and (5) a diagnosis of oncocytic/HCC where the previously treated patient has a blood thyroglobulin level higher than anticipated for the disease that has been found.

12.7.3 Fine-Needle Aspiration (FNA)

12.7.3.1 The Bethesda System for Reporting Thyroid Cytopathology (BSRTC) Criteria

Fine-needle aspiration (FNA) is a widely accepted technique and is commonly utilized for the preoperative evaluation of thyroid nodules [68, 69]. Results of FNA are usually reported in a standardized manner using the Bethesda System for Reporting Thyroid Cytopathology (BSRTC) criteria, which have recently been updated, and provide rate of malignancy information that is crucial to guide subsequent treatment [70].

The presence of Hürthle cell/oncocytic change in BSRTC categories further poses a diagnostic challenge for cytopathologists, endocrinologists, and surgeons dealing with thyroid disorders [71]. Hürthle cell/oncocytic change has been shown to be associated with both benign and malignant thyroid lesions, including benign conditions such as Hashimoto's thyroiditis, adenomatous or multi-nodular goiter (MNG) with Hürthle cell metaplasia, as well as neoplasms including oncocytic/Hürthle cell adenoma (HCA) and oncocytic/Hürthle cell carcinoma (HCC) [72]. The 2017 BSRTC classification denotes Hürthle cells as a subcategory in the follicular neoplasm or suspicious for a follicular neoplasm (FN/SFN) category, but does *not* provide specific information to the clinician as to its implication with respect to the rate of malignancy. Moreover, the degree of Hürthle cell presence in FNAC can vary greatly, but little information is provided about the correlation of the degree of Hürthle cell features with the rate of malignancy on final histopathological examination [73].

Given that Hürthle cells may be interpreted by clinicians as "atypical cells" and are frequently reported on FNAC reports, clinicians may be uncertain as to how to interpret the presence of Hürthle cells as it relates to the BSRTC classification and the implied rates of malignancy. Many clinicians assume that the presence of Hürthle cells increases the risk of malignancy beyond the risk predicted by a given BSRTC category [74].

Ren et al. (2020) retrospectively reviewed the records of 300 patients with Hürthle cell/oncocytic change on FNA and final surgical pathology and compared the results with a multi-institutional FNA cohort. The degree of oncocytic (Hürthle) cell presence was correlated with histopathological diagnoses. The aim of this study was to delineate the association between oncocytic (Hürthle) cells in preoperative FNA cytology (FNAC) and subsequent pathology of the indexed thyroid nodule and to report the rates of malignancy [74]. In the oncocytic (Hürthle) cell FNA group, the BSRTC categories were as follows: I (nondiagnostic) ($n = 14$–4.7%); II (benign) ($n = 113$–37.7%); III (atypia of undetermined significance/follicular lesion of undetermined significance—AUS/FLUS) ($n = 33$–11%); IV (follicular neoplasm/suspicious for a follicular neoplasm—FN/SFN) ($n = 125$–41.6%); V (suspicious for malignancy— SM) ($n = 12$–4%); and VI (malignant) ($n = 3$–1%). When categorized based on the degree of Hürthle cell change, 59 cases (29%) were classified as "mild" (Hürthle cells <25% of cellular content), 13 (6%) as "moderate" (Hürthle cells 25–75%), and 131 (65%) as "predominant" (Hürthle cells >75%). The reported risk of malignancy for BSRTC categories were as follows: I (7%), II (7%), III (15%), IV (21%), V (50%), and VI (100%).When comparing the results with a multi-institutional FNA cohort (all with surgical confirmation), the presence of Hürthle cells was found to be associated with a lower risk of malignancy in all BSRTC categories, with a statistically significant difference in the BSRTC IV and V groups. The only exception was when Hürthle cell presence was classified as predominant; the rate of malignancy was significantly elevated in FNAs interpreted as benign/Bethesda II. The authors concluded that, although Hürthle cells have been considered by clinicians as "atypical cells," their presence does not seem to increase the risk of malignancy within BSRTC categories overall. However, when predominant Hürthle cell change is present, the risk of malignancy is increased in the benign cytology/BSRTC category II [74].

Although FNAC can diagnose oncocytic/Hürthle cell neoplasms (HCNs) in most patients, it cannot differentiate oncocytic/HCA from oncocytic/HCC, because it does not permit assessment of vascular invasion (VI) and capsular invasion (CI), which are the two main histological features that differentiate carcinoma from adenoma. There is little information in the literature that discusses how the presence of Hürthle cells affects rates of malignancy within the BSRTC diagnostic categories.

In the 2017 BSRTC update, "Hürthle cell atypia" is described as an additional important criterion in raising concern of malignancy in the setting of Hürthle cell changes. Hürthle cell atypia may be "large cell" or "small cell dysplasia," which involves specific cytoplasmic and nuclear features [73]. FNA specimens that are suspicious of oncocytic/Hürthle cell neoplasm are distinguished from those suspicious for non-Hürthle cell follicular neoplasm because of the striking morphological differences between the two cytological patterns, as well as the divergent genetic underpinnings of follicular carcinoma and HCC [73]. According to the 2017 BSRTC, the terms used are "follicular neoplasm, Hürthle cell type" or the equally acceptable "suspicious for follicular neoplasm, Hürthle cell type." The interpretation of follicular neoplasm Hürthle cell type or suspicious for a follicular neoplasm Hürthle cell type refers to cellular aspirates that consist exclusively or almost exclusively of oncocytic (Hürthle) cells. The World Health Organization guidelines suggest only follicular neoplasms comprised of >75% oncocytic (Hürthle) cell change be termed Hürthle cell neoplasm (HCN) [75, 76]. It is noted that the specificity of FNA for detection of oncocytic/HCC is low with most nodules diagnosed as suspicious of follicular neoplasm Hürthle cell type (also known as follicular neoplasm Hürthle cell type) with a risk of malignancy ranging between 10% and 40%.

In general, the rate of malignancy is most accurately predicted based on the BSRTC diagnostic categories. As reported by Ren et al. [74], there is only one exception to the oncocytic (Hürthle) cell lower risk of malignancy effect. The malignancy risk in benign FNAs (BSRTC II) with a predominance of oncocytic (Hürthle) cells was 27.3%, which was significantly higher than the overall risk of 9.3% for all benign FNAs derived from the multi-institutional control cohort ($p = 0.048$).

In several reported series, the risk of malignancy varied widely from 10% to 45% in patients with cytology consisting of oncocytic (Hürthle) cells and available corresponding final pathology [77, 78]. In a smaller series of 128 FNAs with Hürthle cells compared with 582 FNAs without oncocytic (Hürthle) cells, the presence of oncocytic (Hürthle) cells altered the expected distribution of Bethesda cytological diagnoses, with a higher number of cases in the AUS/FLUS and FN/SFN categories, and an increased risk of malignancy on final pathology in FNAs that were either benign (6.0–15.1%) or FN/SFN (21.9–63.6%) [17]. As mentioned before, in the recent study by Ren et al. (2020), oncocytic (Hürthle) cell presence was not found to increase the risk of malignancy overall.

At the John Hopkins University, specimens diagnosed as containing Hürthle cells have a 19% (9/47) chance of being malignant if they are classified as AUS with Hürthle cells [79, 80]. At Indiana University, the corresponding figure of malignancy is 24% [81]. FNAC can be enhanced by a rapid on-site evaluation, correlating with clinical and US data to classify subtypes of DTC, according to the Bethesda system [82, 83]. Screening by cytotechnologists is another way to improve the efficiency of cytopathologists and to avoid oversights. The American Thyroid Association (ATA) recommends pathologists to be acquainted with the local prevalence of malignancy within each indeterminate cytological category [55, 84]. Despite all the above strategies, it is still very difficult to differentiate oncocytic/HCAs from oncocytic/HCCs. It should be noted that oncocytic/HCC can occur in conjunction with other pathology entities such as follicular adenoma or parathyroid carcinoma [85]. A follicular oncocytic/HCC harboring the BRAF v600e mutation was reported to occur in collision with multifocal PTC [86]. To complicate matters further, FNAC of parathyroid carcinoma can mimic oncocytic/HCC [87].

It is worth mentioning that other factors can influence the rate of malignancy. For example, Silva de Morais et al. (2019) have reported that the association of Hashimoto's thyroiditis resulted in an increased risk of malignancy [88]. However, some researchers believe that this is a result of selection bias resulting from inclusion of only surgical cases [89]. In 2019, Radetti et al. emphasized that the relation between Hashimoto's thyroiditis and thyroid cancer remains unclear [90]. In their study in children and adolescents, the authors reported the association of Hashimoto's thyroiditis with an increased risk of developing thyroid nodules, but not with thyroid malignancy [90]. Prospective studies with longer follow-up may further elucidate this association.

12.7.3.2 Cytological Features/Differential Diagnosis

Fine needle aspiration cytology (FNAC) of oncocytic/HCC lesions characteristically shows clusters of the monotonous follicular cells with large eosinophilic, granular cytoplasm and usually, hypercellularity. The cells often show irregular nuclear outlines, prominent nucleoli, and bland chromatin. The tumor cells appear scarcely accompanied by colloid, and/or inflammation (Fig. 12.8).

Oncocytic (Hürthle) cells are also observed in nodular goiter, chronic lymphocytic thyroiditis (Hashimoto's thyroiditis), and oncocytic variants of papillary thyroid carcinoma (OV-PTCs) and oncocytic variant of medullary thyroid carcinoma (OV-MTC). Therefore, the presence of these cells should not engender a diagnosis of an oncocytic/Hürthle cell lesion [40]. In Hashimoto's thyroiditis and nodular goiter, isolated or small cohesive clusters of oncocytic cells are common,

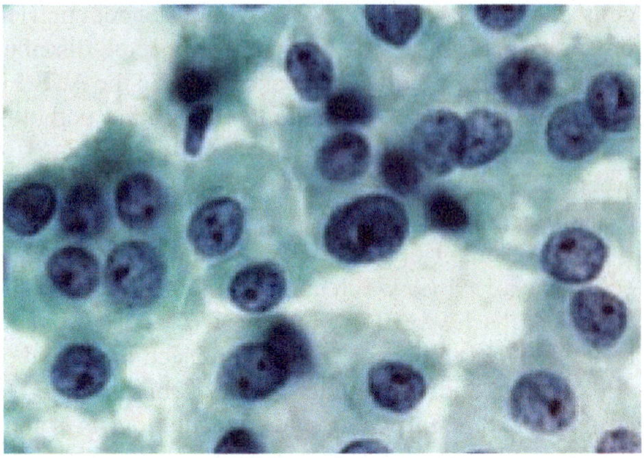

Fig. 12.8 Cytological image of the oncocytic/Hürthle cell carcinoma showing monotonous oncocytic (Hürthle) cells with prominent nucleoli arranged in loosely cohesive clusters. The cells have prominent nucleoli, bland chromatin, and granular cytoplasm. Papanicolaou stain ×600

representing follicular cells with oncocytic metaplasia. In addition, in nodular goiter, follicular cells with abundant colloids are observed, and the follicles are not uniform. In Hashimoto's thyroiditis, lymphoplasmacytic infiltrations are frequently observed. However, when a large irregular sheet of oncocytic cells dominantly appear, differentiating between chronic thyroiditis and Hürthle cell tumor may be difficult. In a study of 139 Hürthle cell lesions by Elliott et al. (2006), they reported that the presence of all of the following cytological features correctly identified Hürthle cell neoplasia in 86% of cases: (1) non-macrofollicular architecture, (2) absence of colloid, (3) absence of inflammation, and (4) presence of transgressing blood vessels [91].

The tumor cells of OV-PTCs show fine granular cytoplasm and elongated nuclei, and a nuclear groove. Intra-cytoplasmic inclusion can be sparse in some cases. The cytological features of papillary fronds and monolayered sheets suggest an OV-PTC rather than oncocytic/Hürthle cell neoplasia (HCN) [92, 93]. In the FNAC sample of the OV-MTC, amyloid deposit supports the diagnosis, but is not always observed [94]. Oncocytic cells in OV-MTC show polygonal, plasmacytoid characteristics with eccentrically placed round nuclei with "salt and pepper" chromatin [95]. In addition, multi-vacuolization resembling histiocytes and loose granularity are observed in OV-MTC. In contrast, granularity in HCC is dense and firm [96]. For accurate diagnosis, immunohistochemistry (IHC) using calcitonin and thyroglobulin in combination [97] in addition to consideration of family history of the patient and laboratory data are needed.

Cytological features such as small cell dysplasia (bland nuclei, cell diameter < twice the nuclear diameter), large cell dysplasia (cell diameter at least twice the nuclear diameter, with prominent nucleoli and irregular nuclear outlines), nuclear crowding, and dyshesion have been proposed by Renshaw et al. (2002) as a diagnostic clue of oncocytic/HCC [98]. These criteria were later shown by Wu et al. (2008) to be significant features in favor of HCC over HCA and other benign lesions [99]. However, distinction of oncocytic/HCC from oncocytic/HCA by FNAC still remains to be challenging due to the lack of other supporting data [100]. In the daily practice using TBSRTC [101], a Hürthle cell neoplasm is typically classified as atypia of undetermined significance or follicular lesion of undetermined significance (AUS/FLUS, Bethesda III) or benign (Bethesda II). The presence of Hürthle cells itself does not increase the risk of malignancy [102], but >75% Hürthle cells in a benign/Bethesda II aspirate may pose an increased risk of malignancy [74].

12.7.3.3 Diagnostic Markers in FNA Samples

MicroRNA expression array has recently identified novel diagnostic markers in FNA samples for conventional and oncocytic cell carcinoma. In a study by Jacques and colleagues [103] in 2013, novel miR-885-5p was strongly upregulated (>40 fold) in oncocytic follicular carcinomas compared with conventional follicular carcinomas, follicular adenomas, and hyperplastic nodules.

A test that measures the expression of 167 genes may help determine whether a cytologically "indeterminate" thyroid nodule is "benign" and thus may be considered for more conservative treatment. In their study of 265 indeterminate nodules 1 cm or larger, Alexander et al. [104] reported that gene-expression classifier testing correctly identified 78 of 85 nodules as suspicious (92% sensitivity; 52% specificity). The negative predictive value (NPV) of follicular neoplasm or lesion was 94%. Analysis of the aspirates with false-negative results showed that six of the seven had a paucity of thyroid follicular cells, suggesting insufficient sampling of the nodule. In this study, 10 malignant Hürthle cell nodules were present, and 9 were correctly identified as malignant (90%); 21 nodules were benign (HCAs), and 17 of them were correctly identified (81%) [104].

Another recent study (2016) by Donatini et al. [105] concluded that the cellular proliferation index (Ki67) and GRIM-19 (a protein involved in cell proliferation and apoptosis) are potential cytological markers of malignancy in HCC. Compared with oncocytic/HCAs, carcinomas showed a significantly elevated Ki67 ($p = 0.0004$) and reduced expression of GRIM-19 ($p = 0.005$).

Nevertheless, until more accurate methods to differentiate benign nodules from malignant ones are available, all patients with the cytological diagnosis of an oncocytic/Hürthle cell neoplasm (HCN) should proceed to surgery to ensure that the carcinomas are identified and managed appropriately. In addition, as with any other thyroid tumor, other factors should be taken into consideration such as tumor size, microcalcification, echogenicity, and vascularity when considering whether to perform hemithyroidectomy or total thyroidectomy, or to choose observation.

12.7.4 Macroscopic Features

Macroscopically, oncocytic/HCC shows a mahogany brown appearance (Fig. 12.9), which is due to air contact [39]. Areas of necrosis and hemorrhage may be observed due to the degenerative nature of the tumor. Calcification, resulting from a physiochemical reaction to altered thyroglobulin within the colloid of the tumor follicles, may be observed in some cases and is more often found in oncocytic/HCC than in oncocytic/HCA.

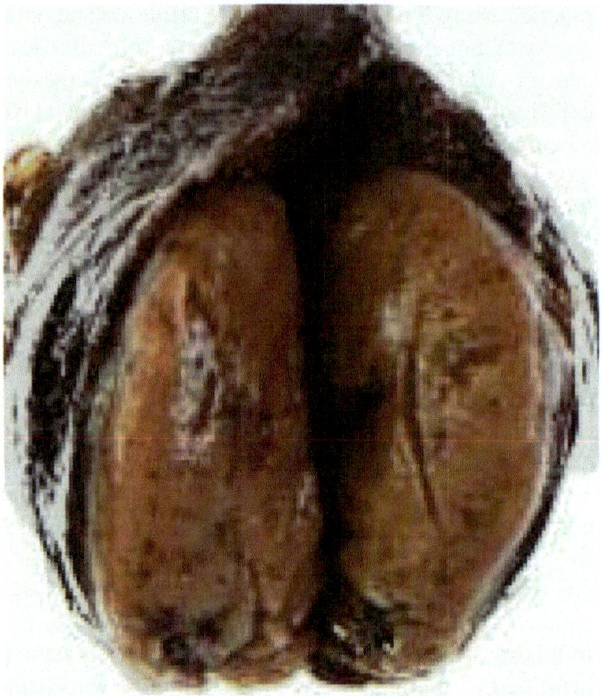

Fig. 12.9 Gross appearance of oncocytic/Hürthle cell carcinoma. The tumor is mahogany brown in color with several foci of hemorrhage and capsular invasion

12.7.5 Histological Features/Differential Diagnosis

Common histological malignancy criteria, such as architectural distortion, cellular atypia, or pleomorphism, are encountered in both benign and malignant follicular adenomas; these histological criteria are therefore *not* helpful while evaluating a thyroid mass. The cytological features of oncocytic/Hürthle cell neoplasms are hypercellularity, with a predominance of oncocytic (Hürthle) cells usually above 75%, few or no lymphocytes, and scanty or absent colloid. Oncocytic (Hürthle) cells are large and polygonal in shape, with indistinct cell borders. They have a large pleomorphic hyperchromatic nucleus, a prominent nucleolus, and intensely pink fine granular cytoplasm with hematoxylin-eosin staining (Fig. 12.10).

Papillary structures and intranuclear inclusions, features that are not ordinarily associated with oncocytic/Hürthle cell lesions, are occasionally noted [106].

Cytoplasmic granularity in oncocytic (Hürthle) cells is due to the presence of numerous mitochondria (Fig. 12.11). The amount and morphological characteristics of the mitochondria vary greatly from case to case [107]. However, according to the diagnostic criteria, more than 75% of oxyphilic cells must be observed for diagnosis. The high prevalence of oncocytic (Hürthle) cell changing into thyroid lesions may reflect high oxidative stress and reactive oxygen species production in thyroid cells during normal iodine and thyroid hormone metabolism [108, 109]. These high

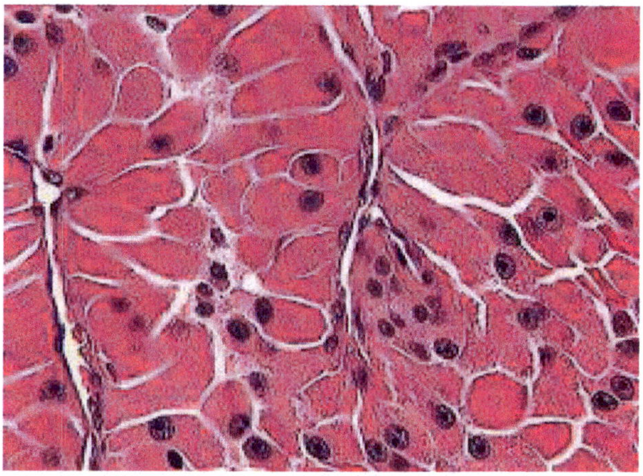

Fig. 12.10 Histology showing oncocytic (Hürthle) cells as large polygonal cells with well-defined borders and eosinophilic granular cytoplasm. The nuclei are enlarged and have a central prominent macro-nucleolus

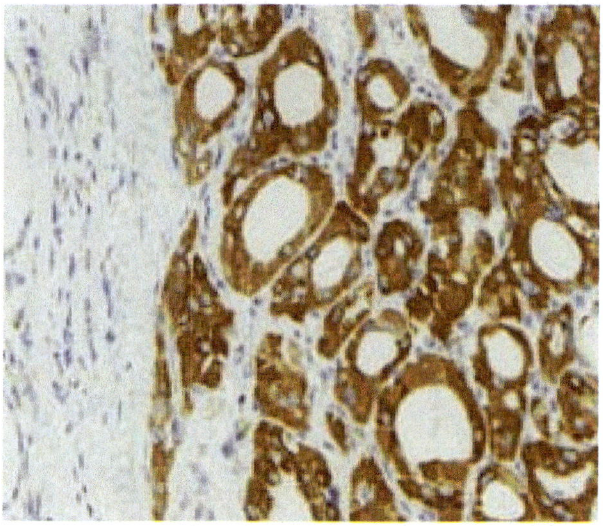

Fig. 12.11 Immunohistochemistry of oncocytic/Hürthle cell carcinoma showing tumor cells that are diffuse and strongly positive for anti-mitochondria antibodies (×100)

reactive oxygen species levels can result in mutagenic genetic events in mitochondrial DNA, leading to mitochondrial dysfunction [110, 111]. Abnormality of mitochondria leads to defects in the energy production process, and consequently a compensatory mechanism [111]. This results in increased proliferation of numerous mitochondria, which is observed as oncocytic cytoplasm [106]. Over time, as the number of the mitochondria increases, a continuous process of Hürthle cell appearance is expressed [111]. In cases of oncocytic/HCC, necrosis frequently appears either spontaneously or after fine-needle aspiration (FNA). This observation is reported to be a consequence of mitochondrial abnormalities [112].

Histopathological differentiation of oncocytic/HCC from oncocytic/HCA is based mainly on vascular invasion (VI) and capsular invasion (CI). Vascular invasion is defined by the presence of tumor penetration of blood vessels within or outside of the capsule of the oncocytic/Hürthle cell lesion (Fig. 12.12). Capsular invasion refers to tumor cell penetration of the capsule of the neoplasm (Fig. 12.13). Capsular invasion, vascular invasion, or both diagnose oncocytic/HCC. Based on its histology, the tumor is subcategorized as either minimally invasive or widely invasive. Minimally invasive HCC (miHCC) refers to encapsulated tumors with microscopically identifiable foci with capsular or vascular invasion <4 foci. Widely invasive HCC (wiHCC) shows extensive capsular invasion and/or vascular invasion of 4 foci or greater [41].

Infarction following FNAC is often seen in oncocytic/HCC, making it difficult to observe capsular invasions. The exact mechanism leading to infarction is still

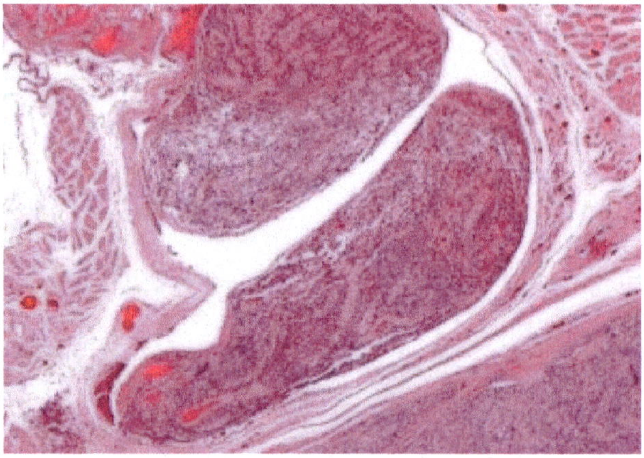

Fig. 12.12 Histological image of Hürthle cell carcinoma (HCC) showing an adjacent focus of overt vascular invasion in a large vessel located within the adjacent muscle. H&E stain × 40

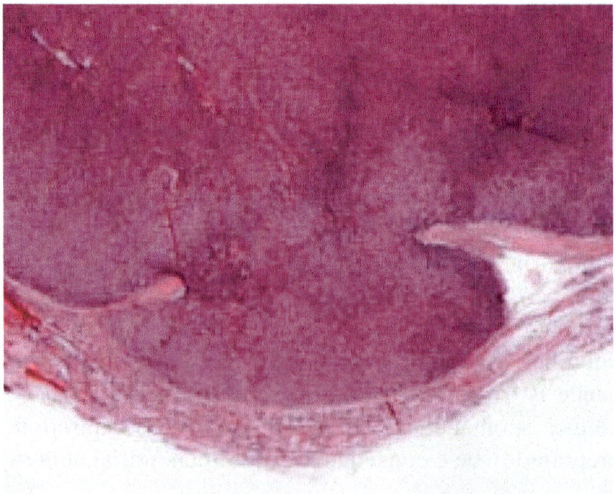

Fig. 12.13 Histological image of oncocytic/Hürthle cell carcinoma showing the diagnostic capsular invasion of the tumor

unknown [113]. Mitochondrial DNA deletion is reported to be less frequent in infarcted oncocytic/Hürthle cell tumors than in non-infarcted ones. For clear identification of capsular invasion, clinical information such as where the tumor cells were aspirated by FNAC is considered important. Widely invasive HCC often shows capsular invasion in the form of compacted nodules, lacking stromal desmoplastic reaction. In some cases, determining whether there is a capsule is quite difficult [113]. Benign diseases such as chronic lymphocytic thyroiditis (Hashimoto's thyroiditis), nodular goiter, or toxic goiter usually have no encapsulation. Hürthle cell changes are part of an inflammatory process.

Oncocytic/Hürthle cell carcinoma (HCC) often shows follicular, trabecular, and/or solid architecture, and rarely shows a predominantly papillary pattern [39]. A pure follicular pattern is rather uncommon in oncocytic/HCC [2], but when such a follicular pattern is seen, the tumor accompanies fibrous bands between nests.

In a study by Volante et al. [114], the role of galectin-3 and HBME-1 tumor markers (an anti-mesothelial monoclonal antibody that recognizes an unknown antigen on microvilli of mesothelial cells), as well as the peroxisome proliferator-activated receptor (PPAR) gamma protein expression, were assessed in oncocytic Hürthle cell tumors, including HCAs, HCCs, and an oncocytic variant of papillary thyroid carcinoma (PTC). In this study of 152 oncocytic/Hürthle cell tumors (70 HCCs, 50 HCAs, and 32 oncocytic variant of PTC), the sensitivity of galectin-3 was 95.1%, the sensitivity of HBME-1 was 53%, and a combination of both, galectin-3 and HBME-1, was as high as 99%. However, the specificity for both markers was 88%, lower than for non-oncocytic follicular tumors. Interestingly, PPAR gamma protein overexpression was absent in all adenomas tested and present in only 10% of carcinomas, similar to other reports that confirm the low prevalence of PAX8-PPAR gamma translocations in oncocytic/HCCs.

It is believed by some authors that transformation of poorly differentiated and anaplastic forms may occur in some oncocytic/HCCs [115–117]. This is supported by the rare finding of Hürthle cell tumors in association with anaplastic thyroid carcinomas [117]. This association has led to the speculation that HCNs can behave in a manner similar to low-grade PTC and FTC, that is, they can undergo transformation to high-grade malignancies. The exact frequency of this occurrence is unknown and the transformation is more commonly seen in recurrences and metastases than in primary tumors.

Thyroid lesions containing oncocytic cells are nodular goiter, oncocytic variants of PTC and MTC, both of which are rare, showing extensive mitochondrial hyperplasia, prominent nucleoli, well-defined cytoplasm, and polygonal cells, which is in contrast with the spindle-shaped cells of conventional MTC. Although MTC is derived from C-cells (parafollicular cells), not follicular cells, oncocytic variant MTC may be difficult to histologically differentiate. The presence of amyloid deposits in MTC aids in diagnosis. However, amyloid deposits sometimes occur as a result of systemic or secondary amyloidosis [118]. Oncocytic/HCC with neuroendocrine differentiation [119] or thyroid tumors in patients with basal high calcitonin levels should be diagnosed with caution. For the appropriate diagnosis, consideration of molecular testing, as well as family history and serum calcitonin levels, is essential [120].

Oncocytic parathyroid adenoma and adenocarcinoma are also included in the differential diagnosis of oncocytic/HCC. Neoplastic lesions showing extensive invasion without hormone production are especially difficult to differentiate. Immunohistochemically, parathyroid tissue tests positive for chromogranin A, GATA3, while thyroid tissue tests positive for TTF-1, PAX8. However, in the hormone nonproducing tumors, neither calcitonin nor PTH is clearly expressed. Tumor location with images and invasive patterns can be diagnostic clues in these cases. Immunohistochemistry is *not* mandatory for the diagnosis of oncocytic/HCC, except in cases to distinguish MTC or parathyroid tumors, and a specific diagnostic marker for oncocytic/HCC has not yet been obtained. Oncocytic/HCC cells test positive for thyroid transcription factor-1 (TTF-1) and thyroglobulin (Tg), and negative for calcitonin and parathyroid hormone (PTH). Thyroglobulin may show peri-nuclear positivity. According to the literature, genes associated with Retinoid-interferon-induced Mortality-19 (GRIM-19) [121], p53 [112], and Cyclin D [122, 123] can be immunohistochemically detected.

12.7.6 Electron Microscopy

The electron microscopic examination of oncocytic (Hürthle) cells in tumor formation is unique, revealing an irregular surface and a large cytoplasm that is almost completely filled with mitochondria (Fig. 12.14). A full-brown oncocytic cell is estimated to contain 4000–5000 mitochondria [124]. These mitochondria display two types of morphology. One is larger mitochondria with stacking "shelf-like" cristae) [125, 126]. The other is smaller and oval, and short cristae are peripherally arranged [125]. The amount and morphological characteristics of the mitochondria vary greatly from case to case [106, 107].

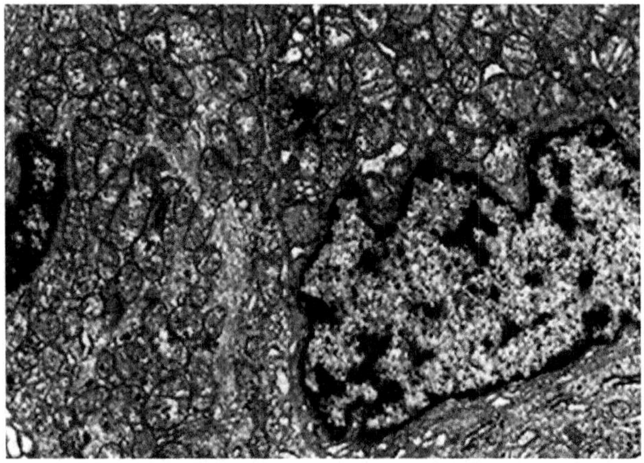

Fig. 12.14 Electron microscopy of oncocytic/Hürthle cell carcinoma of the thyroid gland showing an oncocytic (Hürthle) cell with a large cytoplasm that is almost completely filled with mitochondria

Other structural abnormalities seen under electron microscopy are large lysosome-like dense bodies and dilated Golgi zones confined to the apical portion of the cytoplasm. Unusual richness of chromatin is clumped against the inner nuclear membrane [40, 106, 127].

The oncocytic (Hürthle) cell contains an irregular nucleus with a deep notch containing one to several nucleoli. Nuclei are observed as round and dense bodies, with separation of fibrillar and granular substances [125].

12.7.7 Molecular Changes in Hürthle Cell Carcinoma (HCC)

Hürthle cell neoplasms typically manifest as Bethesda category III or IV on fine needle aspiration biopsy (FNAB), and until recently, were managed with diagnostic hemi- or subtotal thyroidectomy. With molecular genetic advances, active surveillance is now used more frequently, avoiding unnecessary surgery. However, no definitive point mutation has been associated with the incidence of oncocytic/HCC.

The genetic profile of oncocytic/HCC differs from PTC and FTC. Molecular pathways that differentiate oncocytic/HCA from widely invasive HCC (wiHCC) include the PIK3CA-Akt-mTOR and Wnt, providing rationale toward new targets of this type of malignancy [128]. Despite having a common origin in the follicular cell, FTC and oncocytic/HCC should be considered as two separate entities due to the significant difference in oncogene expression between both [129]. Changes in both nuclear DNA and mitochondrial DNA (mtDNA) suggest the diagnosis of HCC. Molecular changes in nuclear DNA involve several signaling pathways and mitochondrial functions. Mitochondrial genetic changes involve interaction between mutations in the mitochondrial and nuclear genomes [110].

12.8 Staging of Hürthle Cell Carcinoma

Different prognostic criteria and staging systems are used in differentiated thyroid cancer (DTC) and oncocytic/HCC. However, there is no uniformly accepted staging system and prognostic classification for oncocytic/HCC.

Thyroid cancer staging is done using American Joint Committee on Cancer (AJCC)'s TNM system presently in the eighth edition as of 2017, which is the most widely used staging system. It uses tumor size and extra-thyroidal extension (T), regional cervical, mediastinal and retropharyngeal lymph node involvement status (N), and distant metastases (M) into account as depicted in Table 12.1. All different types of thyroid cancers are classified using the same system with a few noteworthy characteristics.

All patients with differentiated thyroid carcinomas under 45 years are considered to have a good prognosis, and even the most widely metastatic tumors get a maximum stage II. All anaplastic thyroid tumors are considered to have a poor prognosis and start at a minimum stage of IV-A. Medullary carcinoma of the thyroid has some

Table 12.1 TNM staging system for papillary thyroid carcinoma

Stage	Age (<45 years)	Age (>45 years)
I	Any T, any N, M0	T1, N0, M0
II	Any T, any N, M1	T2 or T3, N0, M0
II		T4 or N1, M0
IV		Any T, any N, M1

T1 < 1 cm, T2 2–4 cm, T3 > 4 cm, T4E extending beyond the capsule

differences in tumor (T) definitions for its staging compared to Hürthle cell and follicular carcinomas.

Most classification systems used in the evaluation of patients with oncocytic/HCC consider such factors as tumor size, patient age, presence of metastases, and major capsular invasion (extensive CI in multiple sites).

The other classification systems used for assessing oncocytic/HCC are conducted with scoring systems, using the generally accepted prognostic factors, such as age, metastasis, extent of disease at operation, and size *(AMES)* and age, grade, extent, and size *(AGES)*.

12.9 Treatment of Oncocytic (Hürthle Cell) Carcinoma

At presentation, treatment decision should be made by a multidisciplinary team (MDT). It is important for clinicians and pathologists to correlate the entire information collected from clinical history, physical examination, laboratory tests (thyroid function, calcium, thyroglobulin, etc.), fine needle aspiration biopsy (FNAB), immunohistochemistry (IHC), imaging (ultrasonography, CT scan, RAI scans, etc.), and histopathology.

Surgical excision is the main treatment of patients with oncocytic/HCC. Postoperative iodine-131 (^{131}I) scanning is usually performed 4–6 weeks after surgery. No thyroid hormone treatment is administered to the patient in the interim. If uptake occurs in the thyroid bed or other sites, a treatment dose of ^{131}I is administered, and another total body scan is obtained 4–7 days later.

12.9.1 Surgical Treatment

Surgery is the mainstay of treatment for patients with oncocytic/HCC. It aims at removing the entire cancer, thereby minimizing the risk of locally persistent or recurrent disease, providing adequate staging information, minimizing risk without compromise to optimal cancer management, improving efforts for postoperative adjunctive treatment (e.g., RAI), and facilitating follow-up care.

Total thyroidectomy (TT) is usually recommended for patients with oncocytic/HCC, whereas those with oncocytic/HCAs are generally treated with a thyroid lobectomy. Although total thyroidectomy is generally considered the treatment of choice for oncocytic/HCC, a "lobectomy" is usually performed first; if histological sections show oncocytic/HCC, as evidenced by vascular and/or capsular invasion, then a "completion" thyroidectomy is performed in a second surgery [130, 131]. In clinically high-risk patients and in some institutions, a total thyroidectomy is performed as the first surgery based on frozen-section results. Unfortunately, the majority of series have insufficient numbers of patients to allow statistically valid conclusions regarding which of those approaches should become the standard.

In general, thyroid surgery is approached with preference for diagnostic thyroid lobectomy unless clinical features prompt considering removal of the entire thyroid gland at the primary surgery. A personal history of cranio-cervical radiation does *not* increase the risk of oncocytic/HCC; however, it is an independent risk factor for developing papillary thyroid cancer (PTC), and significant exposure (particularly in childhood or adolescence) warrants upfront total thyroidectomy [55]. Other clinical considerations that would prompt initial total thyroidectomy include presence of dominant contralateral nodules or preexisting diminished hormone production necessitating thyroxine replacement [55].

As previously mentioned, the predominant clinical feature associated with an increased risk of oncocytic/HCC in those patients with indeterminate oncocytic (Hürthle) cell findings on FNA is the "size" of the nodule. A nodule ≥4 cm is associated with an increased risk of oncocytic/HCC, and the ATA guidelines accordingly prescribe upfront total thyroidectomy.

A thorough history taking and physical examination are critical in the initial evaluation of patients with the potential diagnosis of oncocytic/HCC, since dysphagia, dyspnea, and voice change as well as the clinical finding of a palpable hard, immobile mass are concerning for an invasive process. Preoperatively, these patients require laryngoscopy to evaluate vocal cord function and the integrity of the recurrent laryngeal nerves (RLNs). Cross-sectional imaging such as computed tomography (CT) scan and magnetic resonance imaging (MRI) is essential in patients with a suspicion of a locally advanced disease, including concern for invasion of the aero-digestive tract and/or major vessels of the neck, as it can visualize deeper anatomical compartments not readily imaged by ultrasound. In the past, clinicians were advised against CT scan performed with intravenous contrast, as the iodine load was felt to delay treatment with RAI; however, more recent studies have clarified adequate clearance of this iodine, with return of urinary iodine levels to baseline within 1 month for most patients with normal renal function [132].

Since oncocytic/HCC has been classified as a variant of follicular thyroid carcinoma (FTC), many believe that it spreads hematogenously, with rare lymph node (LN) metastasis as is the case for FTC [13]. However, several studies have documented LN metastasis in 5.3–13% of patients with HCC [8, 12, 133]. Therefore, the finding of an oncocytic/HCN should prompt thorough ultrasound evaluation of all compartments of the neck prior to surgery. In a study of 39 cases of oncocytic/HCC, 3 (8%) were found to have LN metastasis at presentation (1 ipsilateral central compartment, 2 ipsilateral central and lateral neck compartments) and warranted neck dissections [134]. All three cases of node-positive disease were associated with a primary tumor >5 cm in size. Another study examining 173 oncocytic/HCCs treated from 2001 to 2012 found a 9.2% incidence of node-positive disease; all cases were associated with a widely invasive or poorly differentiated phenotype [8]. Seven of 173 cases (4.0%) were limited to the central compartment, while nine (5.2%) involved the lateral compartments. The largest study to date examined 3311 cases of oncocytic/HCC, with documentation of node-positive disease in 5.3% [12]. Implications of this study are limited, since only 73.9% of patients had any LNs pathologically examined.

Once an oncocytic/HCC is histologically confirmed following diagnostic thyroid lobectomy, consideration should be given to performing a completion thyroidectomy. Minimally invasive HCC (miHCC) is considered to be at a low risk of recurrence by both the American Thyroid Association (ATA) and National Comprehensive Cancer Network (NCCN) guidelines, and is very often treated with lobectomy alone. In one of the large clinical studies examining outcome for miHCC, all 39 cases (100%) were found to be without evidence of recurrence or disease-specific mortality, with a median follow-up of 69.8 months [8]. However, most patients were indeed treated with either total thyroidectomy or lobectomy followed by completion thyroidectomy. Of 23 patients with miHCC treated over 60 years, none experienced a recurrence or succumbed to their disease [133]. The majority (88%) of patients with miHCC were managed conservatively with thyroid lobectomy alone.

Thyroid cancers less than 1 cm usually do not prompt aggressive surgical treatment or completion thyroidectomy. However, it is important to note that not all sub-centimeter thyroid cancers have the same excellent prognosis. Oncocytic (Hürthle) cell histology is reported to be an independent risk factor for reduced survival even among tumors that are less than 1 cm. Studying 564 cases of FTCs ($N = 371$) and oncocytic/HCCs ($N = 193$) <1 cm compared to 22,174 cases of papillary thyroid micro-carcinomas from the SEER database between 1988 and 2009, Kuo et al. (2013) reported that follicular and oncocytic (Hürthle) cell histologies remain independent risk factors for reduced 10-year disease-specific survival even after adjustment for patient age, type of surgery, RAI treatment, extra-thyroidal extension, and nodal and distant metastases (hazard ratio 5.3, 95% CI 2.78–10.10) [130].

In cases of widely invasive HCC (wiHCC), the risk of recurrence is 73%, and therefore, they should be placed in the ATA intermediate- or high-risk categories, prompting adjuvant treatment with RAI [133]. For these patients, completion thyroidectomy is mandated.

Intraoperative frozen-section examination of the thyroid gland has variable diagnostic value, based on institutional experience. This procedure requires processing of an average of 6–15 slides per patient, which is impractical in many institutions. Other limitations include sampling error, variable thickness, irregularity of the capsule, freezing artifact, difficulty in distinguishing capsular entrapment from invasion, and freezing-induced distortion and collapse of the blood vessels. Frozen-section provides no additional value in most studies. However, in one study (1997), the diagnosis of FTC or oncocytic/HCC was established correctly in 78% of cases, thereby permitting immediate definitive surgical management and eliminating the need for two-stage operations [135]. In general, routine frozen-section analysis in patients with follicular lesions is not necessary secondary to the poor sensitivity and significant cost.

Standard surgical wound care is usually appropriate. Postoperative care includes careful monitoring for infection, hematoma, signs of recurrent laryngeal nerve injury (e.g., hoarseness of voice), airway compromise, signs of hypoparathyroidism and hypocalcemia (e.g., circumoral numbness, carpopedal spasm).

According to the German Guidelines [136], a routine prophylactic central lymph node (LN) dissection is recommended in case of preoperative or intraoperative oncocytic/HCC diagnosis. This recommendation is explained by high rates of LN involvement and impaired iodine avidity of oncocytic/HCC. In case of postoperative diagnosis, prophylactic central lymphadenectomy is recommended for biochemical residual disease, consisting in elevated thyroglobulin (Tg) level. These recommendations are based on seven studies [32, 40, 137–141]: two reviews [40, 137], and four retrospective analyses [32, 139, 141, 142]. They included Lopez-Penabad et al. [32] reporting a 25% LN involvement and a 40% mortality rate in 89 patients, Kushchayeva et al. [138] with 3% LN metastasis at presentation and 13% in follow-up in 33 patients, and Guerrero et al. (2010) [141] with LN involvement in only 3 (8%) of their 39 patients and in no tumor <5 cm. The fourth study quoted in the guidelines is Besic et al. [140]. It describes 30.9% of LN involvement and 45% of extra-thyroidal extension (ETE) in 42 patients. However, these patients were diagnosed with papillary Hürthle cell carcinoma, which is a variant of papillary thyroid cancer (PTC).

12.9.2 Adjuvant Therapy

12.9.2.1 Levothyroxine (L-T4) Treatment

The goals of pharmacotherapy are to reduce morbidity, induce remission, and prevent complications. Thyroid hormone therapy is used to replace endogenous production after thyroidectomy and radioactive iodine (RAI) therapy. Differentiated thyroid cancer (DTC) cells express the thyroid-stimulating hormone (TSH) receptor and respond to TSH by promoting cell division and tumor growth. Employing supraphysiological doses of levothyroxine can suppress TSH levels, potentially decreasing the risk of recurrence and improving survival [55]. Thus, L-T4 should be administered to all patients with thyroid carcinoma, regardless of the extent of thyroid surgery and other treatments. The aim for the degree of TSH suppression following surgery is determined by the patient's overall risk of recurrence, incorporating the patient's response to therapy as well as any comorbid conditions that could be associated with an increased risk of complications with prolonged TSH suppression.

Levothyroxine treatment is started after the treatment dose of ^{131}I is administered. The effective dose of L-T4 in adults is 2.2–2.8 μg/kg; however, children require higher doses. The adequacy of therapy is monitored by measuring serum TSH about 8–12 weeks after the beginning of treatment. The initial goal is a serum TSH concentration of 0.1 μU/mL or less and a serum triiodothyronine concentration within the reference range. When these guidelines are followed, L-T4 therapy does not have deleterious effects on the heart or bone.

Completely resected minimally invasive HCC is categorized by both the ATA and NCCN as being at low risk of recurrence, and it does not require TSH-suppressive therapy; serum TSH may be kept within the low-normal reference range (0.5–2 mU/L). In patients with structurally incomplete response to therapy, serum TSH should be kept at <0.1 mU/L indefinitely, unless there is a contraindication. In patients with an incomplete biochemical response to therapy and those with high-risk HCC and an excellent or indeterminate response to therapy, TSH should be maintained at between 0.1 and 0.5 mU/L, taking into account thyroglobulin levels, trends in those levels over time, and the risks of TSH suppression [55].

12.9.2.2 Radioactive Iodine (RAI) Treatment

Radioactive iodine (RAI) is commonly used in the adjuvant setting for high-risk features such as tumor size >2 cm, cervical LN metastases, positive margins, microvascular invasion, or when postoperative thyroglobulin (Tg) levels are >1 ng/mL. It is estimated that only around 10% of patients with oncocytic/HCCs take up radioiodine; hence responses to treatment with RAI are much lower in these patients when compared to other types of thyroid carcinomas [142, 143]. Since the majority of oncocytic/HCCs are non-iodine avid, a negative postoperative RAI scan may not necessarily rule out distant disease, and it is recommended in patients with high-risk features to undergo fluorodeoxyglucose-positron emission tomography (FDG-PET).

Treatment with radioactive ^{131}I (RAI) is usually administered if postoperative iodine scanning shows uptake in the thyroid bed or elsewhere. This ^{131}I therapy is used after surgery for three reasons. First, RAI destroys any remaining normal thyroid tissue, thereby enhancing the sensitivity of subsequent ^{131}I total-body scanning and increasing the specificity of measurements of serum thyroglobulin (Tg) for the detection of persistent or recurrent disease. Second, ^{131}I therapy may destroy occult microscopic carcinoma. Third, the use of a large amount of ^{131}I allows for total-body scanning, which is a more sensitive test for detecting persistent carcinoma.

There is a controversy with regard to RAI avidity of oncocytic/HCC and the effect of RAI treatment on survival of these patients. Most studies that have evaluated the efficacy of RAI for oncocytic/HCC are small, retrospective, single-institutional series, likely due to the rarity of oncocytic/HCC. Compared with other thyroid carcinomas, HCC has a lower avidity for ^{131}I; therefore, treatment with RAI has a limited efficacy.

There is limited evidence in the literature that redifferentiation therapy with "retinoic acid" may restore ^{131}I uptake in some thyroid carcinomas that have lost their capability of radioiodine concentration. The benefits of this approach remain uncertain to date [144, 145]. Retinoic acid therapy may also be considered in patients with oncocytic/HCC that does not take up RAI, although this is not yet a standard form of therapy.

In an old study (2003), Lopez-Penabad et al. [32] reviewed 127 patients with oncocytic/HCN (89 patients with oncocytic/HCC and 38 patients with oncocytic/

HCA) who were treated from 1944 to 1955 and reported a 38% RAI avidity in patients with oncocytic/HCC. This study showed that RAI therapy is associated with survival benefit in patients with oncocytic/HCC when it is used primarily for ablation rather than when residual disease is believed to be present. In a retrospective single-institution study, Besic et al. [146] reviewed 16 patients with oncocytic/HCC and distant metastases; all these patients underwent thyroid hormone withdrawal. Scanning demonstrated uptake (range 0.1%–12%) in 11 of 16 patients (69%) [146]. In another recent study (2016), Besic et al. [147] evaluated 30 oncocytic/HCC patients with distant metastases and reported RAI uptake in metastases in 16 of 30 patients (53%), with uptake of ≥0.5% in 9 of 30 patients (30%).

At a nationwide level, Jillard et al. [148] identified 1909 patients with oncocytic/HCC who underwent total thyroidectomy in the National Cancer Database (NCDB) between 1998 and 2006. Patients were included if they had AJCC-TNM pT1 tumors with N1or M1 disease, and pT2–4 tumors with any N or M disease status. They reported that post-thyroidectomy ^{131}I therapy improves survival in patients with oncocytic/HCC. In their review of 1909 patients, those who received ^{131}I ($n = 1162$) had superior 5-year and 10-year survival rates compared with patients who did not (88.9% versus 83.1% and 74.4% versus 65.0%, respectively, $p < 0.001$). From their study, they suggested that RAI therapy should be advocated for patients with tumors >2 cm, and those with nodal and distant metastatic disease.

Present guidelines are inconsistent with regard to indications for using RAI for oncocytic/HCC. Administration of RAI is advocated for tumors >2 cm or nodal/distant metastatic disease as reported by Ahmadi et al. [134]. The NCCN guideline recommends RAI ablation for (1) gross extra-thyroidal extension (ETE), (2) primary tumor size >4 cm, (3) extensive vascular invasion, and (4) postoperative unstimulated Tg >5–10 ng/L [36]. RAI ablation can be "selectively" recommended for (1) primary tumor 2–4 cm, and (2) minor vascular invasion/cervical LN metastases. On the other hand, RAI ablation is *not* indicated for intrathyroidal tumor <2 cm without vascular invasion, or for node involvement/detectable anti-Tg antibodies/postoperative unstimulated Tg <1 ng/mL.

12.9.2.3 External Radiotherapy

Oncocytic/Hürthle cell carcinoma is considered a "radio-sensitive" tumor. Radiation therapy may provide palliative relief from symptomatic metastases, control recurrent tumors, and prevent recurrence of advanced resected tumors [149–152].

External beam radiation therapy (EBRT) to the neck and mediastinum is indicated in patients in whom surgical excision is incomplete or impossible. This therapy can also be considered for tumors that do *not* take up ^{131}I. However, it is important to balance the potential benefit of radiation with potential complications, which include dental decay, tracheal stenosis, esophageal stricture, osteonecrosis, fibrosis, and xerostomia [153].

Intensity-modulated radiation therapy *(IMRT)* uses three-dimensional (3D) CT to map the tumor and also computerizes dose calculations. It allows higher radiation doses to be delivered to the tumor and minimizes the dose received by surrounding tissues. In a study using the NCDB, 106,374 patients with differentiated thyroid cancer (DTC) were evaluated; they included patients over 18 years of age, without distant metastases, who underwent cervical radiation therapy to assess the impact of IMRT versus 3D-conformal radiotherapy (3D-CT). Although not statistically significant, comparison of overall survival between patients undergoing IMRT versus 3D-CT demonstrated a hazard ratio of 0.67 (95% CI 0.4–1.1; $P = 0.115$) and trend toward improved overall survival with IMRT [154].

The role of radiation as an adjuvant therapy in patients who have had complete resection of all locally invasive disease is controversial [155–159]. In the absence of persistent gross residual disease, radiation is usually reserved for older patients (>50 years) with tumors that are more likely to be iodine-refractory (including oncocytic/HCC) and who are at high risk of early cervical recurrence not amenable to surgical resection. Radiation is seldom recommended as an adjuvant therapy in young patients, and especially those with iodine-avid tumors.

12.9.2.4 Directed Therapy for Distant Metastases

Targeted therapies in patients with advanced thyroid cancer are valuable tools to address malignant foci that arise in critical locations and that are at high risk of causing significant morbidity or mortality secondary to tumor infiltration or compression of vital structures if they are not treated expeditiously [55]. Such critical locations include the brain, spine, and bone (at risk of pathological fracture). Cervical and mediastinal disease places key airway structures (e.g., trachea, larynx, major bronchi), as well as the digestive tract and great vessels, at risk. These lesions may require treatment prior to RAI therapy to prevent morbidity related to swelling that can occur in some of these metastatic foci. The choice of specific targeted therapy is dependent on tumor size and location, patient preference, and discussion between all members of the multidisciplinary team (MDT).

12.9.2.5 Bone Metastases

The risk of bone metastases is likely increased in oncocytic/HCC patients. Bone metastases in patients with differentiated thyroid cancer including oncocytic/HCC are associated with significant morbidity, including pain and pathologic fracture [160]. Surgery is the preferred treatment option for bone metastases that are associated with structural instability or that are in critical locations. A retrospective study of 109 patients with bone metastases from thyroid cancer (71% with FTC) reported that complete resection of bone metastases in young patients is associated with a significant improvement in survival [161]. Radiotherapy plays an important role in treatment of bone lesions, since it can be used in isolation or to complement surgery in cases of incomplete resection [55]. In a retrospective study of 32 patients with metastatic oncocytic/HCC, Besic et al. [147] reported that the effect of EBRT on bone metastases lasted from 13 to 165 months (median, 93 months). Another treatment option is embolization of tumor vasculature; this can be used for pain control, and it can also be used in a neoadjuvant fashion prior to surgical resection, as these bony metastases tend to be vascular and prone to intraoperative bleeding. Radiofrequency ablation has also been reported to reduce pain from thyroid cancer skeletal metastases [161–164].

12.9.2.6 Lung Metastases

Localized therapies can also be effective treatment options for oncocytic/HCC that involves the respiratory tract and airways (Fig. 12.15). Options include bronchoscopy with laser therapy for intraluminal disease, endobronchial stenting to maintain patency of airways that are compressed or the subject of local invasion, surgical resection of the metastatic lesion, and focused EBRT.

12.9.2.7 Brain Metastases

Overall, brain metastases are uncommon; they are usually found in the setting of widespread metastatic disease and are associated with a very poor overall prognosis. High-dose glucocorticoids are usually recommended to decrease the surrounding edema once brain metastases are identified. Surgical resection is the preferred treatment option, unless the lesions are very small and/or multifocal. Stereotactic radiation can be effective if <3–5 small lesions are present, and whole-brain radiation is required when there are numerous lesions [165–169].

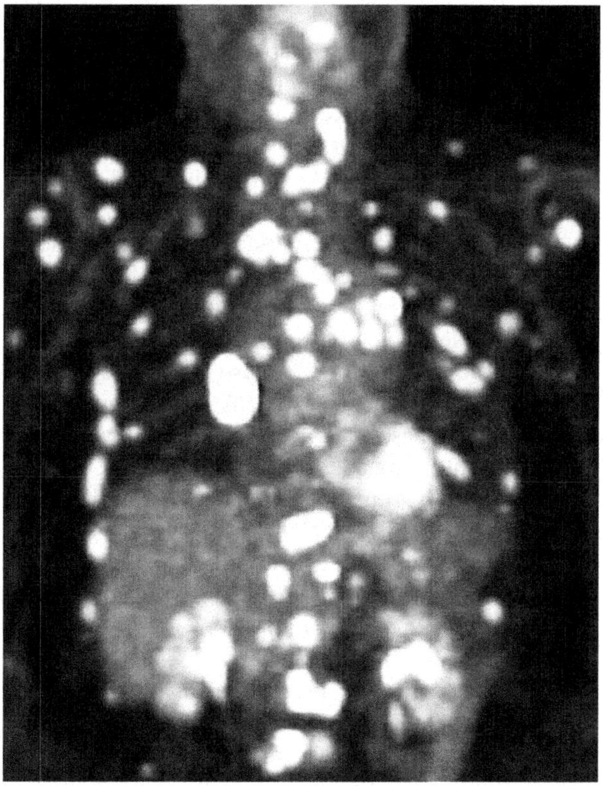

Fig. 12.15 Positron emission tomography (PET) image of a patient who had a history of oncocytic/Hürthle cell carcinoma. Single indeterminate lung nodule with some mediastinal adenopathy was seen on computed tomography scan. Sonography and ^{131}I scans had negative findings. The PET image showed widespread bone and lung metastases, which were confirmed with right hilar biopsy

12.9.3 Systemic Therapy (Chemotherapy)

A particular challenge for systemic therapy is the general lack of actionable somatic alterations in oncocytic/HCC [170]. Alterations amenable to targeted therapy seem to be rare [171, 172]. Some patients with widely metastatic oncocytic/HCC can survive for many years with only minimal disease progression, and they can remain relatively asymptomatic; thus, it is important to identify which patients will likely benefit from a wait-and-watch approach versus systemic therapy. Patients who are asymptomatic with well-differentiated tumors and indolent disease, "observation" is an acceptable option as long as they do not have brain metastases. Factors related to the tumor, patient comorbidities, patients' tolerance of treatment-related morbidity and its impact on quality of life, and patient preference, all should be incorporated into these complex management decisions.

It is unusual to initiate systemic therapy for lesions that are <1 cm; however, not all metastatic lesions >1 cm require systemic therapy. For patients with symptoms or rapidly growing metastatic with iodine avid tumor, RAI is a preferable option. If the patient's tumor is not amenable to RAI, systemic therapy is considered and should be initiated sooner if metastatic lesions are in locations where continued growth would result in compromise of critical surrounding structures. Systemic therapy should be likely considered in the following cases: when patients have symptoms of weight loss, muscle wasting, or fatigue, or other constitutional symptoms attributable to their significant disease burden; when the rate of progression of structural disease is rapid enough that the disease is likely to cause morbidity; or when additional metastatic foci are identified [134].

Chemotherapy for metastatic DTC is usually ineffective. However, some experimental trials have yielded promising results. Over the past decade, good progress has been made in understanding molecular mechanisms of thyroid cancer; accordingly, multiple medications are being developed to target various molecules involved in the development of DTC. These targets are present both in the tumor cell as well as at the vascular endothelial cells providing blood supply to the tumor. The drugs include multikinase inhibitors, selective kinase inhibitors, and combination therapies. Examples include sorafenib, gefitinib, axitinib, motesanib, sunitinib, and pazopanib [173]. Younes et al., in their experimental studies in 2005 [174] and 2006 [175], assessed anti-vascular therapy in mouse models with bone metastasis from FTC [174, 175]. In these studies, a novel dual tyrosine kinase inhibitor of epidermal growth factor receptor (EGFR) and vascular endothelial growth factor (VEGFR) was used alone and in combination with paclitaxel. They showed suppression of tumor growth, with promising outcomes.

Currently, sorafenib and lenvatinib are the only United States Food and Drug Administration-(FDA) approved multi-kinase inhibitors available for RAI-refractory differentiated thyroid cancer. Given the adverse effect profile, lenvatinib is preferred over sorafenib [176, 177]. Due to the relatively small number of such cases, there are no published studies examining outcomes of systemic therapy specifically for HCC. However, most published studies do report the response rate of oncocytic/HCC to treatment. A prospective randomized trial of lenvatinib versus placebo in the treatment of RAI-refractory thyroid cancer included 70 oncocytic/HCC cases (lenvatinib $N = 48$, placebo $N = 22$). Lenvatinib demonstrated a progression-free survival hazard ratio of 0.22 (95% CI 0.10–0.51) in favor of treatment when compared to placebo [176]. The DECISION trial was a multicenter, randomized, double-blind, placebo-controlled Phase III trial of sorafenib in 417 RAI-refractory thyroid cancers; it included 74 oncocytic/HCC cases. The precise hazard ratio and CI for oncocytic/HCC were not published as part of the DECISION trial; however, sorafenib was reported to be associated with overall progression-free survival advantage among the subset of patients with oncocytic/HCC [177].

Vandetanib has also been studied in a European Phase II trial in RAI-refractory DTC. Unfortunately, the study included only two patients categorized as having follicular carcinoma with oncocytic features, and both were randomized to the placebo control group [178]. A multicenter, open-label, single-arm, Phase II study of axitinib in 52 advanced thyroid cancers included 8 oncocytic/HCCs, of which 2 demonstrated a partial response to treatment [179]. There are currently several studies with active recruitment exploring the role of small-molecule inhibitors for iodine-refractory DTC, including oncocytic/HCC. Based on Category 2A evidence, the NCCN guidelines recommend that axitinib, everolimus, pazopanib, and sunitinib be considered in patients with advanced oncocytic/HCC if clinical trials are not available or appropriate [180]. In general, these small-molecule inhibitors can sometimes provide progression-free survival advantages with a side-effect profile that is tolerable in properly selected patients. However, they have not been shown to improve either disease-specific or overall survival, and specific drug activity in oncocytic/HCC is unlikely to be known due to the very small number of oncocytic/HCC cases included in most trials.

Molecular analysis of thyroid cancers can be helpful as there is data for nonspecific use of larotrectinib or entrectinib in cancers with NTRK fusion and pembrolizumab in patients with high tumor mutation burden regardless of the type of cancer [181, 182]. Selpercatinib and pralsetinib have been shown to be beneficial in patients with non-small cell lung cancers and thyroid carcinomas, which have a RET fusion and can be used as a first-line agent in patients with this mutation [183–185]. Most of the patients with RET fusions in the study were medullary carcinoma of the thyroid, but the data can be extrapolated to HCCs with RET fusion. Cytotoxic chemotherapy has been used in small studies but has not been reported to significantly benefit patients with oncocytic/HCC and is usually used as a last option [186].

12.9.4 Management of Locoregional Recurrence/Relapse

Salvage treatment of recurrent oncocytic/HCC includes surgery, RAI or radiofrequency ablation, ethanol ablation, external beam radiotherapy (EBRT), and systemic treatment.

12.9.4.1 Salvage Surgery

Salvage surgery for locoregional relapse can deliver information on the nature of recurrence. In the study by Chiapponi et al. [34], surgery was performed in seven (13.7%) patients and revealed soft tissue metastases instead of LN metastases. Since most of the patients in their study underwent a central lymphadenectomy (in addition to total thyroidectomy), one might speculate that this may have contributed to the absence of lymph nodes in the locoregional recurrences. Bishop et al. (2012) [187] who analyzed 24 metastases also reported that there were no true lymphatic metastases in the majority of their cases, but rather tumor emboli in veins that reimplant along the venous outflow tract. These metastatic nodules were not surrounded by any peripheral cuff of lymphoid tissue or capsule in most cases [187]. This important aspect is probably not given enough clinical attention. These data, together with those recently reported by Coca Pelaz et al. [35], suggest that prophylactic central lymphadenectomy might not be of benefit in patient with oncocytic/HCC. In their meta-analysis Coca Pelaz et al. included 9638 patients and found LN metastasis in only 9% of patients [35].

Soft tissue metastatic nodules can generally be identified in preoperative ^{18}F-FDG PET scan. However, surgeons should be aware of the presence of additional sub-centimeter foci, which might sometimes be found only by accurate palpation and intraoperative sonography, and sometimes are even missed. In fact, only two (28.6%) of the patients undergoing cervical salvage surgery in the Chiapponi et al. analysis could be cured [34]. All others had at least biochemical residual disease.

In patients not eligible for surgery, less invasive approaches such as thermal ablation or extracorporeal radiation and even multiple kinase inhibitors such as lenvatinib or sorafenib are effective alternatives [188–190].

12.9.4.2 Radioactive Iodine (RAI) Therapy

Approximately, 10% of metastases from oncocytic/HCC take up radioiodine, compared with 75% of metastases from follicular thyroid carcinoma (FTC); thus, RAI treatment, which is the most useful nonsurgical therapy for recurrent differentiated thyroid carcinoma (DTC), is *not* always useful in patients with oncocytic/HCC. This causes difficulty in the treatment of recurrences. Nevertheless, RAI is used for most patients with oncocytic/HCC after total and near-total thyroidectomy and in the treatment of patients with recurrent and metastatic disease [191].

Recently, Wenter et al. (2021) systematically evaluated the clinical outcome in a large patient cohort of patients diagnosed with oncocytic/HCC ($n = 126$) and classical FTC ($n = 252$). Patients received thyroidectomy and initial adjuvant RAI therapy, and the mean follow-up was 6.9 years (range 3.7–11.7 years). The authors reported that recurrence was significantly more frequently diagnosed in oncocytic/HCC patients during follow-up than FTC patients (17% versus 8%, respectively; $p = 0.037$). Likewise, oncocytic/HCC patients presented with a reduced mean disease-free survival of 17.9 years versus 20.1 years in FTC patients ($p = 0.027$). Only 19% ($n = 3/16$) of recurrent oncocytic/HCC patients and 17% ($n = 2/12$) of recurrent FTC patients were treated curatively with RAI at the end of follow-up. The difference was not statistically significant ($p = 0.887$) [192].

12.9.4.3 Thermal Ablation

The types of thermal ablation available are hyperthermic [radiofrequency ablation (RFA), microwave ablation (MWA), and laser ablation] and hypothermic (cryoablation).

Combe et al. (2016) reported an 82-year-old man, diagnosed in 2002 with thyroid oncocytic/HCC, which was initially treated by local surgery and was refractory to RAI therapy. The patient had successive secondary recurrences from 2006 onward. Metastases were suspected due to an elevation of serum Tg. Hypermetabolic nodules were targeted using FDG-PET and CT-guided radiofrequency ablations. Tg levels decreased following each procedure. Ten years later, tolerance and efficacy were excellent; 23 lung metastases have been treated during 11 sessions without current relapse. Respiratory function and quality of life were not altered. This report illustrates how radiofrequency ablation can be efficiently integrated into the long-term management of poorly aggressive oligo-metastatic cancer from oncocytic/HCC, in combination with other local and/or systemic therapies [193].

Segkos et al. (2017) stated that oncocytic/HCC rarely metastasizes to the liver, and when it does, the metastasis is almost never isolated. They reported a 62-year-old male with widely invasive Hürthle cell carcinoma (wiHCC) who underwent total thyroidectomy and received adjuvant treatment with RAI with posttreatment scan showing no evidence of metastatic disease. However, his thyroglobulin (Tg) level continued to rise after that and eventually an isolated liver metastasis was identified. He underwent laparoscopic microwave ablation of the liver metastasis, with dramatic decline in Tg and no evidence of disease recurrence. This case highlights the rare occurrence of isolated liver metastasis from oncocytic/HCC and also illustrates the utility of thermo-ablation as an alternative to surgical resection in the treatment of small isolated liver metastases from oncocytic/HCC [189].

12.9.4.4 Ethanol Ablation (EA)

Differentiated thyroid cancer (DTC), including oncocytic/HCC, often metastasizes to cervical lymph nodes (LNs), characteristically with slow growth rate and low-level aggressiveness. Cervical LN resection is the treatment of choice, but ethanol ablation (EA) offers a therapeutic option for patients with few nodes unresponsive to RAI therapy and who are poor surgical candidates. The EA procedure is minimally invasive, guided sonographically, easily and safely repeated, and easily implemented with minimal technology and cost. Transient nerve injury is infrequent and virtually the only important complication [194].

Historically, EA of cervical nodules was developed in response to the need for therapy in poor surgical candidates, initially for parathyroid adenomas [195, 196]. It was later applied to metastatic lymphadenopathy from differentiated thyroid carcinoma (DTC) by the early 2000s but not widely adopted [197]. As recently as 2009, guidelines from the American Thyroid Association (ATA) underscored the need for techniques capable of substituting for surgery, but did not acknowledge that EA fulfilled the desired capabilities, despite being available for two decades since the early reports [4]. The understanding of EA evolved, and by 2016 the ATA-updated guidelines stated that locoregional therapies, such as EA, "may be beneficial in patients with a single or a few metastases and in those with metastases at high risk of local complications" [55]. Eventually, the 2019 National Comprehensive Cancer Network (NCCN) guidelines for thyroid carcinoma stated the preferred therapy for locoregional recurrence is surgery, but EA could be considered in selected patients with unresectable, non-radioiodine-avid, and progressive papillary, follicular, and oncocytic/Hürthle cell carcinoma [198].

According to the criteria outlined in 2013 by Mayo Clinic, appropriate candidates for EA of neck recurrences are those with biopsy-confirmed oligo-metastatic disease (four or fewer nodes), patients unresponsive to RAI therapy, and are deemed poor surgical candidates (or refused surgery) [199]. The typical candidate for EA presents with history of total thyroidectomy and one or more subsequent surgeries for local recurrence of DTC, which could be central compartment dissection, lateral neck dissection, or limited resections of disease found clinically or sonographically, and previous RAI therapy. When recurrences are found in previously operated compartments or the recurrence is single and isolated, EA is a very attractive option.

Treatment with EA is efficacious if the Doppler color flow disappears, the volume reduces, and the node becomes echogenic. On long-term follow-up, nearly 50% of treated nodes become undetectable sonographically and 78–87% volume reduction can be expected. Serum Tg is decreased in 80% of patients [199]. More EA treatments are necessary when previously treated sites show growth, abnormal Doppler color flow persists, or if new abnormalities are found sonographically (especially if accompanied by a rise in Tg). If the recurrence is bulky and multiple, the cancer is aggressive, EA is unlikely to control it, and surgery should be considered. Surgery should also be considered if there is suspicion of invasion near the airway or esophagus [194].

12.9.4.5 External Beam Radiation Therapy (EBRT)

Whether adjuvant external beam radiation therapy (EBRT) might be useful in those patients with oncocytic/HCC is not fully clear to date [200]. There is a lack of evidence on EBRT for thyroid cancer recurrence.

12.9.5 Follow-Up

12.9.6 Further Outpatient Care

Outpatient care of patient with oncocytic/HCC includes the following:

- Monitoring of signs of hypothyroidism after surgical treatment.
- Starting levothyroxine therapy, usually after the treatment dose of ^{131}I is administered.
- Monitoring the patient for signs of hypocalcemia and measure calcium levels.

- Before scanning, the patient is instructed to avoid iodine-containing medications and iodine-rich foods to avoid interference with scanning. Urinary iodine is measured in doubtful cases.
- Pregnancy must be ruled out in women of the child-bearing age.
- Patients should be instructed carefully about radiation precautions prior to ^{131}I treatment and should follow the instructions meticulously when sent home.

12.9.6.1 Levothyroxine Treatment

The adequacy of levothyroxine (L-T4) therapy is monitored by measuring serum TSH approximately 8–12 weeks after treatment begins, with the initial goal being a serum TSH concentration of 0.1 μU/mL or less and a serum T3 concentration within the reference range. In patients who are at low risk and considered cured, the dose of L-T4 is decreased to maintain a low, but detectable, serum TSH concentration (0.1–0.5 μU/mL). In higher-risk patients, higher doses are continued, targeting a serum TSH concentration of 0.1 μU/mL or less.

12.9.6.2 Clinical and Ultrasonographic Examinations

Cervical ultrasound to evaluate the thyroid bed, central, and lateral cervical nodal compartments should be performed every 6–12 months in patients with HCC initially following surgery, and then periodically depending on each patient's risk of recurrence and unique response to therapy [55].

Ultrasonography is recommended in patients at high risk of recurrent disease and in any patient with suspicious clinical findings. Palpable LNs that are small, thin, or reduced in size after an interval of 3 months are considered *benign*.

12.9.6.3 Measurement of Thyroglobulin (Tg) and Anti-Thyroglobulin Antibodies

In the follow-up care of patients, thyroglobulin (Tg) is used as a marker of residual or recurrent disease, and as a prognostic factor. Thyroglobulin is produced only by normal or neoplastic thyroid follicular cells and should be undetectable in patients who have been treated with surgery and radio-ablation. Low Tg concentration (1 ng/mL or lower) can be detected with current assays.

Anti-thyroglobulin antibodies, which are found in approximately 15% of patients with thyroid carcinoma, can produce artifactual alteration in Tg assay results. These antibodies should always be checked when serum Tg is measured.

Serum Tg concentrations are undetectable in a group of patients receiving L-T4 treatment who have isolated LN metastases; therefore, undetectable values do not rule out metastatic LN disease. If the patient is thought to have metastases, a LN biopsy may be performed.

During initial follow-up of patients with HCC, serum thyroglobulin/thyroglobulin antibody (Tg/Tg Ab) levels on levothyroxine therapy should be measured every 6–12 months. In the ATA high-risk patients, more frequent measurements may be appropriate. Time intervals between serum Tg/Tg Ab measurements in the ATA low- to intermediate-risk HCC patients can be lengthened to 12–24 months. The

ATA high-risk HCC patients and all patients with biochemically or structurally incomplete or indeterminate response to therapy should have Tg/Tg Ab levels measured every 6–12 months for several years [55].

12.9.6.4 Chest X-Ray

Most patients with abnormal chest X-ray findings have detectable serum Tg concentrations; therefore, this study might not have an additional value in diagnosing metastatic disease. However, it still can have a limited diagnostic value in a subgroup of patients.

12.9.6.5 Computed Tomography (CT) Scan and Magnetic Resonance Imaging (MRI)

Cross-sectional imaging including CT scan and MRI of the neck and chest should be considered in the setting of bulky recurrent cervical disease, when potential aerodigestive tract invasion requires complete assessment, and in high-risk oncocytic/HCC patients with concern for lung metastases. Cross-sectional imaging of other organs including the brain, skeleton, and abdomen should be considered in high-risk oncocytic/HCC patients with elevated serum Tg and negative neck and chest imaging, and patients who have symptoms referable to those organs [55].

12.9.6.6 ^{131}Iodine Total Body Scanning

If serum Tg concentration becomes detectable in patients receiving L-T4 therapy, recombinant human thyrotropin (thyrotropin-alfa; Thyrogen) should be administered or L-T4 should be withdrawn, an ^{131}I total-body scan should be obtained, and serum Tg should be measured. The uptake of ^{131}I and the level of TSH concentration determine the accuracy of total body scanning. In patients whose L-T4 is withheld, serum TSH concentration should usually be higher than 30 μU/mL when the total-body scan is performed.

Intramuscular injection of thyrotropin-alfa is a promising alternative because L-T4 treatment does not need to be discontinued and the adverse effects are minimal. Thyroglobulin measurement and total body scanning after thyrotropin-alfa administration is currently the standard of care in many institutions. For routine diagnostic scans, 2–5 mCi (74–185 mBq [millibecquerel]) of ^{131}I is administered; higher doses may reduce the uptake of a subsequent therapeutic dose of ^{131}I.

Scanning is performed to measure uptake, if any, 3 days after the thyrotropin-alfa dose has been administered. In certain situations, uptake cannot be detected with diagnostic scans when 2–5 mCi of ^{131}I is administered but may be detectable after the administration of 100 mCi. This is the rationale for administering 100 mCi (or more) of ^{131}I in patients with elevated serum Tg concentrations (usually levels >10 ng/mL after T4 has been withdrawn). If this approach is taken, total-body scanning should be performed 4–7 days later.

If any uptake is detected on ^{131}I total-body scan or serum Tg concentration rises above the previous level, ^{131}I therapy should be administered or a positron emission tomography (PET) scan should be considered to localize the metastasis/recurrence. In the absence of ^{131}I uptake, a CT scan of the neck and lungs, bone scintigraphy, and scintigraphy using a less-specific tracer (e.g., thallium, tetrofosmin, fluorodeoxyglucose) and particularly PET scan should be considered strongly in patients with oncocytic/HCC who are known to have no or low uptake.

Radioactive iodine (RAI) scanning has a high false-negative rate in patients with oncocytic/HCC due to the lack of iodine avidity in a majority of patients; therefore, it is not recommended by many authors as the principle imaging modality for surveillance [8].

12.9.6.7 Fluorine-18-Fluorodeoxyglucose Positron Emission Tomography (FDG-PET)

The ATA guidelines recommend that fluorine-18-fluorodeoxyglucose positron emission tomography (FDG-PET) be considered in patients with high-risk differentiated thyroid cancers, and those cancers with elevated Tg levels and negative RAI scans. FDG-PET may be considered as part of initial staging in patients with invasive HCC [55]. Several studies have shown a high sensitivity of FDG-PET for oncocytic/HCC. In a retrospective single-institution study of 44 patients with oncocytic/HCC, Pryma et al. [63] reported in 2006 a sensitivity of 95.8% and specificity of 95% for FDG PET scans in patients with oncocytic/HCC. In a study of 12 patients with HCC, Lowe et al. [61] found that FDG PET had a sensitivity of 92%; they also noticed that half of the PET scans detected tumors not seen on conventional imaging, which resulted in a change in disease staging and management. In a retrospective study of 17 oncocytic/HCC patients, Plotkin et al. (2002) [62] reported a sensitivity of 92%, specificity of 80%, PPV of 92%, and NPV of 80% for FDG PET/CT for identification of oncocytic/HCC.

12.9.7 Complications

12.9.7.1 Surgical Complications

Surgical complications include laryngeal nerve injury and transient or permanent hypo-parathyroidism. Other surgical complications are infection and hematoma. Surgical scars in the neck can be cosmetically disturbing in certain individuals.

12.9.7.2 Nonsurgical Complications

- Hypothyroidism can occur if replacement therapy is inadequate. On the other hand, hyperthyroidism can occur if the patient is overtreated with L-T4.
- Acute adverse effects: Nausea, vomiting, sialadenitis, and mouth dryness.
- Radiation-induced effects include the following:
  - Thyroiditis.
  - In metastatic cases, radiation-induced fibrosis of the lung when large doses of ^{131} I (>150 mCi) are administered at short intervals.
  - Mild pancytopenia observed after repeated ^{131} I therapy, particularly in patients with bone metastases who also have received external radiotherapy.
  - Genetic defects and infertility may include the following:
  - Transient reduction in spermatogenesis.

- Transient ovarian failure and menstrual disturbances (usually resolve within the first year of treatment).
- Increased frequency of miscarriages.
- Increased risk of secondary carcinoma or leukemia, only in patients who have received a high cumulative dose of ^{131}I (>500 mCi) and those who also receive external radiation therapy.

12.9.8 Patient Education

The need for life-long L-T4 treatment should be explained to all patients. Radiation precautions should be explained clearly and in detail to patients who will be receiving RAI treatment. Women of childbearing age should be advised not to become pregnant for at least 1 year after treatment with ^{131}I.

References

1. Shawky M, Sakr M. Hurthle cell lesion: controversies, challenges, and debates. Indian J Surg. 2016;78(1):41–8.
2. Lloyd RV, Osamura RY, Klöppel G, Rosai J. WHO classification of tumours of endocrine organs. 4th ed. Lyon: IARC Press; 2017.
3. Wei S, LiVolsi VA, Montone KT, Morrissette JJ, Baloch ZW. PTEN and TP53 mutations in oncocytic follicular carcinoma. Endocr Pathol. 2015;26:365–9.
4. Cooper DS, Doherty GM, Haugen BR, Kloos RT, Lee SL, Mandel SJ, et al. Revised American Thyroid Association management guidelines for patients with thyroid nodules and differentiated thyroid cancer. Thyroid. 2009;19(11):1167–214.
5. Siegel RL, Miller KD, Jemal A. Cancer statistics 2016. CA Cancer J Clin. 2016;66(1):7–30.
6. Matsuura D, Yuan A, Wang L, Ranganath R, Adilbay D, Harries V, et al. Follicular and Hurthle cell carcinoma: comparison of Clinicopathological features and clinical outcomes. Thyroid. 2022;32(3):245–54.
7. Jin M, Kim ES, Kim BH, Kim HK, Kang YE, Jeon MJ, et al. Clinicopathological characteristics and disease-free survival in patients with Hürthle cell carcinoma: a multicenter cohort study in South Korea. Endocrinol Metab. 2021;36(5):1078–85.
8. Chindris AM, Casler JD, Bernet VJ, Rivera M, Thomas C, Kachergus JM, et al. Clinical and molecular features of Hürthle cell carcinoma of the thyroid. J Clin Endocrinol Metab. 2015;100(1):55–62.
9. Haigh PI, Urbach DR. The treatment and prognosis of Hurthle cell follicular thyroid carcinoma compared with its non-Hurthle cell counterpart. Surgery. 2005;138:1152–7.
10. Oluic B, Paunovic I, Loncar Z, Djukic V, Diklic A, Jovanovic M, et al. Survival and prognostic factors for survival, cancer specific survival and disease free interval in 239 patients with Hurthle cell carcinoma: a single center experience. BMC Cancer. 2017;17:371.
11. Santana NO, Freitas RMC, Marcos VN, Chammas MC, Camargo RYA, Schmerling CK, et al. Diagnostic performance of thyroid ultrasound in Hürthle cell carcinomas. Arch Endocrinol Metab. 2019;63(3):300–5.
12. Goffredo P, Roman SA, Sosa JA. Hurthle cell carcinoma: a population-level analysis of 3311 patients. Cancer. 2013;119:504–11.
13. Sugino K, Kameyama K, Ito K, Nagahama M, Kitagawa W, Shibuya H, et al. Does Hurthle cell carcinoma of the thyroid have a poorer prognosis than ordinary follicular thyroid carcinoma? Ann Surg Oncol. 2013;20:2944–50.

14. Petric R, Gazic B, Besic N. Prognostic factors for disease-specific survival in 108 patients with Hürthle cell thyroid carcinoma: a single-institution experience. BMC Cancer. 2014;14:777.
15. Zhou X, Zheng Z, Chen C, Zhao B, Cao H, Li T, et al. Clinical characteristics and prognostic factors of Hurthle cell carcinoma: a population based study. BMC Cancer. 2020;20(1):407.
16. Zito G, Richiusa P, Bommarito A, Carissimi E, Russo L, Coppola A, et al. In vitro identification and characterization of CD133(pos) cancer stem-like cells in anaplastic thyroid carcinoma cell lines. PLoS One. 2008;3(10):e3544.
17. Hardin H, Montemayor-Garcia C, Lloyd RV. Thyroid cancer stem-like cells and epithelial-mesenchymal transition in thyroid cancers. Hum Pathol. 2013;44:1707–13.
18. Todaro M, Iovino F, Eterno V, Cammareri P, Gambara G, Espina V, et al. Tumorigenic and metastatic activity of human thyroid cancer stem cells. Cancer Res. 2010;70(21):8874–85.
19. Zheng X, Cui D, Xu S, Brabant G, Derwahl M. Doxorubicin fails to eradicate cancer stem cells derived from anaplastic thyroid carcinoma cells: characterization of resistant cells. Int J Oncol. 2010;37:307–15.
20. Ohashi R, Kawahara K, Namimatsu S, Okamura R, Igarashi T, Sugitani I, et al. Expression of MRP1 and ABCG2 is associated with adverse clinical outcomes of papillary thyroid carcinoma with a solid component. Hum Pathol. 2017;67:11–7.
21. Mitsutake N, Iwao A, Nagai K, Namba H, Ohtsuru A, Saenko V, et al. Characterization of side population in thyroid cancer cell lines: cancer stem-like cells are enriched partly but not exclusively. Endocrinology. 2007;148:1797–803.
22. Li W, Reeb AN, Sewell WA, Elhomsy G, Lin RY. Phenotypic characterization of metastatic anaplastic thyroid cancer stem cells. PLoS One. 2013;8:e65095.
23. Corver WE, Ruano D, Weijers K, den Hartog WCE, Nieuwenhuizen MP, de Miranda N, et al. Genome haploidisation with chromosome 7 retention in oncocytic follicular thyroid carcinoma. PLoS One. 2012;7(6):e38287.
24. Doerfler WR, Nikitski AV, Morariu EM, Paul Ohori N, Chiosea SI, Landau MS, et al. Molecular alterations in Hurthle cell nodules and preoperative cancer risk. Endocr Relat Cancer. 2021;28(5):301–9.
25. Gopal RK, Kübler K, Calvo SE, Polak P, Livitz D, Rosebrock D, et al. Widespread chromosomal losses and mitochondrial DNA alterations as genetic drivers in Hurthle cell carcinoma. Cancer Cell. 2018;34(2):242–55.
26. Ganly I, Filho JR, Eng S, Ghossein R, Morris LGT, Liang Y, et al. Genomic dissection of Hurthle cell carcinoma reveals a unique class of thyroid malignancy. J Clin Endocrinol Metab. 2013;98(5):E962–72.
27. Maxwell EL, Palme CE, Freeman J. Hürthle cell tumors: applying molecular markers to define a new management algorithm. Arch Otolaryngol Head Neck Surg. 2006;132(1):54–8.
28. Asa SL. My approach to oncocytic tumours of the thyroid. J Clin Pathol. 2004;57(3):225–32.
29. Troncone G, Iaccarino A, Russo M, Palmieri EA, Volante M, Papotti M, et al. Accumulation of p27(kip1) is associated with cyclin D3 overexpression in the oxyphilic (Hurthle cell) variant of follicular thyroid carcinoma. J Clin Pathol. 2007;60(4):377–81.
30. Máximo V, Botelho T, Capela J, Soares P, Lima J, Taveira A, et al. Somatic and germline mutation in GRIM-19, a dual function gene involved in mitochondrial metabolism and cell death, is linked to mitochondrion-rich (Hurthle cell) tumours of the thyroid. Br J Cancer. 2005;92(10):1892–8.
31. Wasvary H, Czako P, Poulik J, Lucas R. Unilateral lobectomy for Hurthle cell adenoma. Am Surg. 1998;64:729–32.
32. Lopez-Penabad L, Chiu AC, Hoff AO, Schultz P, Gaztambide S, Ordoñez NG, et al. Prognostic factors in patients with Hürthle cell neoplasms of the thyroid. Cancer. 2003;97(5):1186–94.
33. Ito Y. Diagnosis and surgical indications of oxyphilic follicular tumors in Japan: surgical specimens and cytology. Endocr J. 2016;63:977–82.
34. Chiapponi C, Hartmann MJM, Schmidt M, Faust M, Burns CJ, Schulteis AM, et al. Hürthle cell carcinoma: single center analysis and considerations for surgical management based on the recent literature. Front Endocrinol. 2022;13:904986.

35. Coca-Pelaz A, Rodrigo JP, Shah JP, Sanabria A, Al Ghuzlan A, Silver CE, et al. Hürthle cell carcinoma of the thyroid gland: systematic review and meta-analysis. Adv Ther. 2021;38(10):5144–64.
36. Barnabei A, Ferretti E, Baldelli R, Procaccini A, Spriano G, Appetecchia M. Hurthle cell tumours of the thyroid. Personal experience and review of the literature. Acta Otorhinolaryngol Ital. 2009;29(6):305–11.
37. Shaha AR, Ferlito A, Rinaldo A. Distant metastases from thyroid and parathyroid cancer. ORL J Otorhinolaryngol Relat Spec. 2001;63(4):243–9.
38. Heimann A, Moll U. Spinal metastasis of a thyroglobulin-rich Hürthle cell carcinoma detected by fine needle aspiration. Light and electron microscopic study of an unusual case. Acta Cytol. 1989;33:639–44.
39. Musholt PB, Musholt TJ, Morgenstern SC, Worm K, Sheu SY, Schmid KW. Follicular histotypes of oncocytic thyroid carcinomas do not carry mutations of the BRAF hot-spot. World J Surg. 2008;32(5):722–8.
40. Montone KT, Baloch ZW, LiVolsi VA. The thyroid Hürthle (oncocytic) cell and its associated pathologic conditions: a surgical pathology and cytopathology review. Arch Pathol Lab Med. 2008;132:1241–50.
41. Kure S, Ohashi R. Thyroid Hürthle cell carcinoma: clinical, pathological, and molecular features. Cancer. 2021;13(1):26.
42. Petric R, Besic H, Besic N. Preoperative serum thyroglobulin concentration as a predictive factor of malignancy in small follicular and Hürthle cell neoplasms of the thyroid gland. World J Surg Oncol. 2014;12:282.
43. Vini L, Harmer C. Radioiodine treatment for differentiated thyroid cancer. Clin Oncol. 2000;12:365–72.
44. Christian J, Cook G, Harmer C. Indium-111-labelled octreotide scintigraphy in the diagnosis and management of non-iodine avid metastatic carcinoma of the thyroid. Br J Cancer. 2003;89:258–61.
45. Haslinghuis LM, Krenning EP, De Herder WW, Reijs AE, Kwekkeboom DJ. Somatostatin receptor scintigraphy in the follow-up of patients with differentiated thyroid cancer. J Endocrinol Investig. 2001;24:415–22.
46. Gulec SA, Serafini AN, Sridhar KS, Peker KR, Gupta A, Goodwin WJ, et al. Somatostatin receptor expression in Hurthle cell cancer of the thyroid. J Nucl Med. 1998;39:243–5.
47. Gorges R, Kahaly G, Muller-Brand J, Macke H, Walgenbach S, Bruns C, et al. Somatostatin receptor status in non-medullary thyroid carcinoma. Nuklearmedizin. 1999;38:15–23.
48. Tisell LE, Ahlman H, Wängberg B, Kölby L, Fjälling M, Forssell-Aronsson E, Mölne J, Nilsson O. Expression of somatostatin receptors in oncocytic (Hürthle cell) neoplasia of the thyroid. Br J Cancer. 1999;79(9–10):1579–82.
49. Kostoglou-Athanassiou I, Pappas A, Gogou L, Kaldrymides P. Scintigraphy with [111In]octreotide and 201Tl in a Hürthle cell thyroid carcinoma without detectable radioiodine uptake. Report of a case and review of the literature. Horm Res. 2003;60(4):205–8.
50. Jahanpanah P, Shakeri S, Kiamanesh Z, Nasiri Z, Aryana K. Detection of solitary bone metastasis by 99mTc-octreotide scintigraphy in a patient with Hurthle cell carcinoma: a case report. Iran J Nucl Med. 2020;28(1):48–50.
51. Maizlin ZV, Wiseman SM, Vora P, Kirby JM, Mason AC, Filipenko D, et al. Hurthle cell neoplasms of the thyroid: sonographic appearance and histologic characteristics. J Ultrasound Med. 2008;27(5):751–7.
52. Ito Y, Amino N, Yokozawa T, Ota H, Ohshita M, Murata N, et al. Ultrasonographic evaluation of thyroid nodules in 900 patients: comparison among ultrasonographic, cytological, and histological findings. Thyroid. 2007;17(12):1269–76.
53. Kim MJ, Shin JH, Hahn SY, Lyun OY, Wook Kim S, Kim TH, et al. Ultrasonographic characteristics of Hurthle cell neoplasms: prediction of malignancy. Ultrasonography. 2022;41(4):689–97.
54. Parikh PP, Allan BJ, Lew JI. Surgeon-performed ultrasound predictors of malignancy in patients with Hurthle cell neoplasms of the thyroid. J Surg Res. 2013;184(1):247–52.

55. Haugen BR, Alexander EK, Bible KC, Doherty GM, Mandel SJ, Nikiforov YE, et al. 2015 American Thyroid Association management guidelines for adult patients with thyroid nodules and differentiated thyroid cancer: the American Thyroid Association guidelines task force on thyroid nodules and differentiated thyroid cancer. Thyroid. 2016;26(1):1–133.
56. Jeh SK, So LJ, Bum SK, Yoen SL. Evaluating the degree of conformity of papillary carcinoma and follicular carcinoma to the reported ultrasonographic findings of malignant thyroid tumor. Korean J Radiol. 2007;8(3):192–7.
57. Wiesner W, Engel H, von Schulthess GK, Krestin GP, Bicik I. FDG PET negative liver metastases of a malignant melanoma and FDG PET-positive Hurthle cell tumor of the thyroid. Eur Radiol. 1999;9:975–8.
58. Grunwald F, Menzel C, Bender H, et al. Comparison of 18FDG-PET with 131iodine and 99mTc-sestamibi scintigraphy in differentiated thyroid cancer. Thyroid. 1997;7:327–35.
59. Blount CL, Dworkin HJ. F-18 FDG uptake by recurrent Hurthle cell carcinoma of the thyroid using high-energy planar scintigraphy. Clin Nucl Med. 1996;21:831–3.
60. Plotkin M, Hautzel H, Krause BJ, et al. Implication of 2-18fluor-2-deoxyglucose positron emission tomography in the follow-up of Hurthle cell thyroid cancer. Thyroid. 2002;12:155–61.
61. Lowe VJ, Mullan BP, Hay ID, McIver B, Kasperbauer JL. 18F-FDG PET of patients with Hurthle cell carcinoma. J Nuc Med. 2003;44(9):1402–6.
62. Plotkin M, Hautzel H, Krause BJ, Schmidt D, Larisch R, Mottaghy FM, et al. Implication of 2-18fluor-2-deoxyglucose positron emission tomography in the follow-up of Hurthle cell thyroid cancer. Thyroid. 2002;12:155–61.
63. Pryma DA, Schoder H, Gonen M, Robbins RJ, Larson SM, Yeung HW, et al. Diagnostic accuracy and prognostic value of 18F-FDG PET in Hurthle cell thyroid cancer patients. J Nucl Med. 2006;47(8):1260–6.
64. Pathak KA, Klonisch T, et al. FDG-PeTcharacteristics of Hürthle cell and follicular adenomas. Ann Nucl Med. 2016;30(7):506–9.
65. Zandieh S, Pokieser W, Knoll P, Sonneck-Koenne C, Kudlace KM, Mirzaei S. Oncocytic adenomas of thyroid-mimicking benign ormetastatic disease on 18F-FDG-Pe T scan. Acta Radiol. 2015;56(6):709–13.
66. Prestwich RJ, Viner S, Gerrard G, Patel CN, Scarsbrook AF. Increasing the yield of recombinant thyroid-stimulatinghormone-stimulated 2-(18-fluoride)-flu-2-deoxy-D-glucose positron emission tomography-CT in patients with differentiated thyroid carcinoma. Br J Radiol. 2012;85(1018):e805–13.
67. Palaniswamy SS, Subramanyam P. Diagnostic utility of PeT/CT in thyroid malignancies: an update. Ann Nucl Med. 2013;27(8):681–93.
68. Lowhagen T, Willems JS, Lundell G, Sundblad R, Granberg PO. Aspiration biopsy cytology in diagnosis of thyroid cancer. World J Surg. 1981;5:61–73.
69. Frates MC, Benson CB, Charboneau JW, Cibas ES, Clark OH, Coleman BG, et al. Management of thyroid nodules detected at US: society of radiologists in ultrasound consensus conference statement. Radiology. 2005;237:794–800.
70. Cibas ES, Ali SZ. The Bethesda system for reporting thyroid cytopathology. Thyroid. 2009;19:1159–65.
71. Cannon J. The significance of hurthle cells in thyroid disease. Oncologist. 2011;16:1380–7.
72. Mete O, Asa SL. Oncocytes, oxyphils, Hurthle, and Askanazy cells: morphological and molecular features of oncocytic thyroid nodules. Endocr Pathol. 2010;21:16–24.
73. Pu RT, Yang J, Wasserman PG, Bhuiya T, Griffith KA, Michael CW. Does Hurthle cell lesion/neoplasm predict malignancy more than follicular lesion/neoplasm on thyroid fine-needle aspiration? Diagn Cytopathol. 2006;34:330–4.
74. Ren Y, Kyriazidis N, Faquin WC, Soylu S, Kamani D, Saade R, Torchia N, et al. The presence of Hürthle cells does not increase the risk of malignancy in most Bethesda categories in thyroid fine-needle aspirates. Thyroid. 2020;30(3):425–31.
75. Faquin WC, Michael CW, Renshaw AA, Vielh P. Follicular neoplasm, Hürthle cell (oncocytic) type/suspicious for a follicular neoplasm, Hürthle cell (oncocytic) type. In: Ali SZ,

Cibas ES, editors. The Bethesda system for reporting thyroid cytopathology: definitions, criteria and explanatory notes. 2nd ed. New York: Springer; 2017. p. 81–100.
76. DeLellis R, Lloyd RVHP, Eng C. Pathology and genetics of tumours of endocrine organs. WHO classification of Tumours, vol. 8. 3rd ed. Lyon: IARC Press; 2017.
77. Sorrenti S, Trimboli P, Catania A, Ulisse S, De Antoni E, D'Armiento M. Comparison of malignancy rate in thyroid nodules with cytology of indeterminate follicular or indeterminate Hurthle cell neoplasm. Thyroid. 2009;19:355–60.
78. Auger M. Hurthle cells in fine-needle aspirates of the thyroid: a review of their diagnostic criteria and significance. Cancer Cytopathol. 2014;122:241–9.
79. Mathur A, Najafian A, Schneider EB, Zeiger MA, Olson MT. Malignancy risk and reproducibility associated with atypia ofundetermined significance on thyroid cytology. Surgery. 2014;156(6):1471–6.
80. van den Bussche CJ, Adams C, Ali SZ, Olson MT. Cytotechnologist performance for screening Hürthle cell atypia in indeterminate thyroid fine-needle aspirates. Acta Cytol. 2015;59(5):377–83.
81. McKee S, Wu H, Wang X, Cramer H, Lin J, Chen S. Hürthlecell neoplasms diagnosed by fine needle aspiration are not associated with an increased risk of malignancy. Acta Cytol. 2014;58(3):235–8.
82. Ali SZ, Cibas ES. The Bethesda system for reporting thyroidcytopathology II. Acta Cytol. 2016;60(5):397–8.
83. Caleo A, Landolfi L, et al. The diagnostic accuracy of fine-needle cytology of Hurthle cell lesions: a comprehensive cytological, clinical and ultrasonographic experience. Int J Surg. 2016;28(Suppl 1):S65–9.
84. Ferris RL, Baloch Z, Bernet V, Chen A, Fahey TJ 3rd, Ganly I, et al. American Thyroid Association statement on surgicalapplication of molecular profiling for thyroid nodules: Currentimpact on perioperative decision making. Thyroid. 2015;25(7):760–8.
85. Zakerkish M, Rajaei E, Dargahi M, Bahadoram M. A rare constellation of Hurthle cell thyroid carcinoma and parathyroid carcinoma. J Clin Diagn Res. 2015;9(12):8–10.
86. Sinno S, Choucair M, Nasrallah M, Wadi L, Jabbour MN, Nassif S. Activating BRAF mutations detected in mixed Hurthle cell carcinoma and multifocal papillary carcinoma of the thyroid gland: report of an unusual case and review of the literature. Int J Surg Pathol. 2016;24(6):519–24.
87. Sriphrapradang C, Sornmayura P, Chanplakorn N, Trachoo O, Sae-Chew P, Aroonroch R. Fine-needle aspiration cytology of parathyroid carcinoma mimic Hürthle cell thyroid neoplasm. Case Rep Endocrinol. 2014;2014:680876.
88. Silva de Morais N, Stuart J, Guan H, Wang Z, Cibas ES, Frates MC, et al. The impact of Hashimoto thyroiditis on thyroid nodule cytology and risk of thyroid cancer. J Endocr Soc. 2019;3:791–800.
89. Jankovic B, Le KT, Hershman JM. Clinical review: Hashimoto's thyroiditis and papillary thyroid carcinoma: is there a correlation? J Clin Endocrinol Metab. 2013;98:474–82.
90. Radetti G, Loche S, D'Antonio V, Salerno M, Guzzetti C, Aversa T, et al. Influence of Hashimoto thyroiditis on the development of thyroid nodules and cancer in children and adolescents. J Endocr Soc. 2019;3:607–16.
91. Elliott DD, Pitman MB, Bloom L, Faquin WC. Fine-needle aspiration biopsy of Hurthle cell lesions of the thyroid gland: a cytomorphologic study of 139 cases with statistical analysis. Cancer. 2006;108(2):102–9.
92. Doria MI Jr, Attal H, Wang HH, Jensen JA, DeMay RM. Fine needle aspiration cytology of the oxyphil variant of papillary carcinoma of the thyroid. A report of three cases. Acta Cytol. 1996;40(5):1007–11.
93. Renshaw AA. Fine-needle aspirations of papillary carcinoma with oncocytic features: an expanded cytologic and histologic profile. Cancer Cytopathol. 2011;119:247–53.
94. Kaushal S, Iyer VK, Mathur SR, Ray R. Fine needle aspiration cytology of medullary carcinoma of the thyroid with a focus on rare variants: a review of 78 cases. Cytopathology. 2011;22:95–105.

95. Sams SB, Tompkins KD, Mayson S, Raeburn CD, Mehrotra S. Oncocytic variant of medullary thyroid carcinoma; a rare tumor with numerous diagnostic mimics by fine needle aspiration. Diagn Cytopathol. 2017;45:1148–52.
96. Canberk S. Oncocytic variant of medullary thyroid carcinoma. Endocr Pathol. 2015;26:320–3.
97. Harach HR, Bergholm U. Medullary (C cell) carcinoma of the thyroid with features of follicular oxyphilic cell tumours. Histopathology. 1988;13:645–56.
98. Renshaw AA. Hurthle cell carcinoma is a better gold standard than Hurthle cell neoplasm for fine-needle aspiration of the thyroid: defining more consistent and specific cytologic criteria. Cancer. 2002;96:261–6.
99. Wu HH, Clouse J, Ren R. Fine-needle aspiration cytology of Hurthle cell carcinoma of the thyroid. Diagn Cytopathol. 2008;36:149–54.
100. Grani G, Lamartina L, Durante C, Filetti S, Cooper DS. Follicular thyroid cancer and Hürthle cell carcinoma: challenges in diagnosis, treatment, and clinical management. Lancet Diabetes Endocrinol. 2018;6(6):500–14.
101. Cibas ES, Ali SZ. The Bethesda system for reporting thyroid cytopathology. 2nd ed. Berlin/Heidelberg: Springer International Publishing; 2018.
102. Cibas ES, Ali SZ. The 2017 Bethesda system for reporting thyroid cytopathology. Thyroid Off J Am Thyroid Assoc. 2017;27:1341–6.
103. Jacques C, Guillotin D, Fontaine JF, et al. DNA microarray and miRNA analyses reinforce the classification of follicular thyroid tumors. J Clin Endocrinol Metab. 2013;98(5):E981–9.
104. Alexander EK, Kennedy GC, Baloch ZW, Cibas ES, Chudova D, Diggans J, et al. Preoperative diagnosis of benign thyroid nodules with indeterminate cytology. N Engl J Med. 2012;367(8):705–15.
105. Donatini G, Beaulieu A, Castagnet M, Kraimps JL, Levillain P, Fromont G. Thyroid Hürthle cell tumors: research of potential markers of malignancy. J Endocrinol Investig. 2016;39(2):153–8.
106. Máximo V, Sobrinho-Simões M. Hürthle cell tumours of the thyroid. A review with emphasis on mitochondrial abnormalities with clinical relevance. Virchows Arch Int J Pathol. 2000;437:107–15.
107. Nesland JM, Sobrinho-Simões MA, Holm R, Sambade MC, Johannessen JV. Hürthle-cell lesions of the thyroid: a combined study using transmission electron microscopy, scanning electron microscopy, and immunocytochemistry. Ultrastruct Pathol. 1985;8(4):269–90.
108. Wang D, Feng JF, Zeng P, Yang YH, Luo J, Yang YW. Total oxidant/antioxidant status in sera of patients with thyroid cancers. Endocr Relat Cancer. 2011;18(6):773–82.
109. Xing M. Oxidative stress: a new risk factor for thyroid cancer. Endocr Relat Cancer. 2012;19:C7–C11.
110. Wallace DC. Mitochondrial diseases in man and mouse. Science (NY). 1999;283:1482–8.
111. Maximo V, Lima J, Prazeres H, Soares P, Sobrinho-Simoes M. The biology and the genetics of Hurthle cell tumors of the thyroid. Endocr Relat Cancer. 2012;19:R131–47.
112. Müller-Höcker J. Immunoreactivity of p53, Ki-67, and Bcl-2 in oncocytic adenomas and carcinomas of the thyroid gland. Hum Pathol. 1999;30:926–33.
113. Conti L, Vatrano S, Bertero L, Masu L, Pacchioni D, Daniele L, De Rosa G, et al. Mitochondrial DNA "common deletion" in post–fine needle aspiration infarcted oncocytic thyroid tumors. Hum Pathol. 2017;69:23–30.
114. Volante M, Bozzalla-Cassione F, DePompa R, Saggiorato E, Bartolazzi A, Orlandi F, et al. Galectin-3 and HBME-1 expression in oncocytic cell tumors of the thyroid. Virchows Arch. 2004;445(2):183–8.
115. Okoń K, Wierzchowski W, Jabłońska E, Wójcik P, Steczko A. Anaplastic, sarcomatoid carcinoma of the thyroid originating from a Hürthle cell tumor. Pol J Pathol. 2003;54(4):277–81.
116. Papotti M, Torchio B, Grassi L, Favero A, Bussolati G. Poorly differentiated oxyphilic (Hurthle cell) carcinomas of the thyroid. Am J Surg Pathol. 1996;20(6):686–94.
117. Hunt JL, Tometsko M, LiVolsi VA, Swalsky P, Finkelstein SD, Barnes EL. Molecular evidence of anaplastic transformation in coexisting well-differentiated and anaplastic carcinomas of the thyroid. Am J Surg Pathol. 2003;27(12):1559–64.

118. Coca-Pelaz A, Vivanco-Allende B, Alvarez-Marcos C, Suarez-Nieto C. Multifocal papillary thyroid carcinoma associated with primary amyloid goiter. Auris Nasus Larynx. 2012;39(5):549–51.
119. Munitiz V, Martinez-Barba E, Riquelme J, Rodriguez JM, Piñero A, Parrilla P. Elevated basal calcitonin levels in a patient with a hurthle-cell carcinoma of the thyroid and neuroendocrine differentiation: report of a case. Surg Today. 2005;35(5):404–6.
120. Spaulding SL, Ho R, Everest S, Chai RL. The role of molecular testing in the diagnosis of medullary thyroid cancer: a case report of oncocytic medullary thyroid carcinoma and review of the literature. Am J Otolaryngol. 2020;41:102312.
121. Donatini G, Beaulieu A, Castagnet M, Kraimps JL, Levillain P, Fromont G. Thyroid Hürthle cell tumors: research of potential markers of malignancy. J Endocrinol Investig. 2016;39:153–8.
122. Ding L, Jiang Y, Yang W. Approach the invasive potential with Hurthle cell tumors of thyroid. Pathol Oncol Res. 2019;25:697–701.
123. Erickson LA, Jin L, Goellner JR, Lohse C, Pankratz VS, Zukerberg LR, et al. Pathologic features, proliferative activity, and cyclin D1 expression in Hurthle cell neoplasms of the thyroid. Mod Pathol. 2000;13(2):186–92.
124. Sobrinho-Simões M, Máximo V, Castro IV, Fonseca E, Soares P, Garcia-Rostan G, et al. Hürthle (oncocytic) cell tumors of thyroid: etiopathogenesis, diagnosis and clinical significance. Int J Surg Pathol. 2005;13(1):29–35.
125. Ambu R, Riva A, Lai ML, Loffredo F, Riva FT, Tandler B. Scanning electron microscopy of the interior of cells in Hürthle cell tumors. Ultrastruct Pathol. 2000;24(4):211–9.
126. Tallini G. Oncocytic tumours. Virchows Arch Int J Pathol. 1998;433:5–12.
127. Matias C, Nunes JF, Sobrinho LG, Soares J. Giant mitochondria and intramitochondrial inclusions in benign thyroid lesions. Ultrastruct Pathol. 1991;15:221–9.
128. Ganly I, Ricarte Filho J, Eng S, Ghossein R, Morris LG, Liang Y, et al. Genomic dissection of Hurthle cell carcinoma reveals a unique class of thyroid malignancy. J Clin Endocrinol Metab. 2013;98(5):E962–72.
129. Masood S, Auguste LJ, Westerband A, Belluco C, Valderama E, Attie J. Differential oncogenic expression in thyroid follicular and Hürthle cell carcinomas. Am J Surg. 1993;166(4):366–8.
130. Kuo EJ, Roman SA, Sosa JA. Patients with follicular and Hurthle cell microcarcinomas have compromised survival: a population level study of 22,738 patients. Surgery. 2013;154(6):1246–53.
131. McHenry CR, Sandoval BA. Management of follicular and Hürthle cell neoplasms of the thyroid gland. Surg Oncol Clin N Am. 1998;7(4):893–910.
132. Padovani RP, Kasamatsu TS, Nakabashi CC, Camacho CP, Andreoni DM, Malouf EZ, et al. One month is sufficient for urinary iodine to return to its baseline value after the use of water-soluble iodinated contrast agents in post-thyroidectomy patients requiring radioiodine therapy. Thyroid. 2012;22(9):926–30.
133. Stojadinovic A, Hoos A, Ghossein RA, Urist MJ, Leung DH, Spiro RH, et al. Hurthle cell carcinoma: a 60-year experience. Ann Surg Oncol. 2002;9(2):197–203.
134. Ahmadi S, Stang M, Jiang XS, Sosa JA. Hürthle cell carcinoma: current perspectives. Onco Targets Ther. 2016;9:6873–84.
135. Paphavasit A, Thompson GB, Hay ID, Grant CS, van Heerden JA, Ilstrup DM, et al. Follicular and Hürthle cell thyroid neoplasms is frozen-section evaluation worthwhile? Arch Surg. 1997;132(6):674–80.
136. Dralle H, Musholt TJ, Schabram J, Steinmüller T, Frilling A, Simon D, et al. German Association of Endocrine Surgeons Practice Guideline for the surgical management of malignant thyroid tumors. Langenbeck's Arch Surg. 2013;398(3):347–75.
137. Carcangiu ML. Hürthle cell carcinoma: clinic-pathological and biological aspects. Tumori. 2003;89(5):529–32.
138. Kushchayeva Y, Duh QY, Kebebew E, Clark OH. Prognostic indications for Hürthle cell cancer. World J Surg. 2004;28(12):1266–70.

139. Carling T, Udelsman R. Follicular neoplasms of the thyroid: what to recommend. Thyroid. 2005;15(6):583–7.
140. Besic N, Hocevar M, Zgajnar J, Petric R, Pilko G. Aggressiveness of therapy and prognosis of patients with Hürthle cell papillary thyroid carcinoma. Thyroid. 2006;16(1):67–72.
141. Guerrero MA, Suh I, Vriens MR, Shen WT, Gosnell J, Kebebew E, et al. Age and tumor size predicts lymph node involvement in Hürthle cell carcinoma. J Cancer. 2010;1:23–6.
142. Sanders LE, Silverman M. Follicular and Hürthle cell carcinoma: predicting outcome and directing therapy. Surgery. 1998;124(6):967–74.
143. McDonald MP, Sanders LE, Silverman ML, Chan HS, Buyske J. Hürthle cell carcinoma of the thyroid gland: prognostic factors and results of surgical treatment. Surgery. 1996;120(6):1000–4.
144. Fernández CA, Puig-Domingo M, Lomeña F, Estorch M, Camacho Martí V, Bittini AL, et al. Effectiveness of retinoic acid treatment for redifferentiation of thyroid cancer in relation to recovery of radioiodine uptake. J Endocrinol Investig. 2009;32(3):228–33.
145. Kim WG, Kim EY, Kim TY, Ryu JS, Hong SJ, Kim WB, et al. Redifferentiation therapy with 13-cis retinoic acids in radioiodine-resistant thyroid cancer. Endocr J. 2009;56(1):105–12.
146. Besic N, Vidergar-Kralj B, Frkovic-Grazio S, Movrin-Stanovnik T, Auersperg M. The role of radioactive iodine in the treatment of Hurthle cell carcinoma of the thyroid. Thyroid. 2003;13(6):577–84.
147. Besic N, Schwarzbartl-Pevec A, Vidergar-Kralj B, Crnic T, Gazic B, Marolt MM. Treatment and outcome of 32 patients with distant metastases of Hurthle cell thyroid carcinoma: a single-institution experience. BMC Cancer. 2016;16:162–9.
148. Jillard CL, Youngwirth L, Scheri RP, Roman S, Sosa JA. Radioactive iodine treatment is associated with improved survival for patients with Hurthle cell carcinoma. Thyroid. 2016;26(7):959–64.
149. Foote RL, Brown PD, Garces YI, McIver B, Kasperbauer JL. Is there a role for radiation therapy in the management of Hürthle cell carcinoma? Int J Radiat Oncol Biol Phys. 2003;56(4):1067–72.
150. Tuttle RM, Rondeau G, Lee NY. A risk-adapted approach to the use of radioactive iodine and external beam radiation in the treatment of well-differentiated thyroid cancer. Cancer Control. 2011;18(2):89–95.
151. Romesser PB, Sherman EJ, Shaha AR, Lian M, Wong RJ, Sabra M, et al. External beam radiotherapy with or without concurrent chemotherapy in advanced or recurrent non-anaplastic non-medullary thyroid cancer. J Surg Oncol. 2014;110(4):375–82.
152. Servagi Vernat S, Khalifa J, Sun XS, Kammerer E, Blais E, Faivre JC, et al. 10-year Locoregional control with postoperative external beam radiotherapy in patients with locally advanced high-risk non-anaplastic thyroid carcinoma de novo or at relapse, a propensity score analysis. Cancers (Basel). 2019;11(6):849.
153. Schlumberger M, Challeton C, De Vathaire F, Travagli JP, Gardet P, Lumbroso JD, et al. Radioactive iodine treatment and external radiotherapy for lung and bone metastases from thyroid carcinoma. J Nucl Med. 1996;37(4):598–605.
154. Goffredo P, Robinson TJ, Youngwirth LM, Roman SA, Sosa JA. Intensity-modulated radiation therapy use for the localized treatment of thyroid cancer: nationwide practice patterns and outcomes. Endocrine. 2016;53(3):761–73.
155. Farahati J, Reiners C, Stuschke M, Müller SP, Stüben G, Sauerwein W, et al. Differentiated thyroid cancer. Impact of adjuvant external radiotherapy in patients with perithyroidal tumor infiltration (stage pT4). Cancer. 1996;77(1):172–80.
156. O'Connell ME, A'Hern RP, Harmer CL. Results of external beam radiotherapy in differentiated thyroid carcinoma: a retrospective study from the Royal Marsden Hospital. Eur J Cancer. 1994;30A(6):733–9.
157. Philips P, Hanzen C, Andry G, Van Houtte P, Früuling J. Postoperative irradiation for thyroid cancer. Eur J Surg Oncol. 1993;19(5):399–404.
158. Kim TH, Yang DS, Jung KY, Kim CY, Choi MS. Value of external irradiation for locally advanced papillary thyroid cancer. Int J Radiat Oncol Biol Phys. 2003;55(4):1006–12.

159. Keum KC, Suh YG, Koom WS, Cho JH, Shim SJ, Lee CG, et al. The role of postoperative external-beam radiotherapy in the management of patients with papillary thyroid cancer invading the trachea. Int J Radiat Oncol Biol Phys. 2006;65(2):474–80.
160. Farooki A, Leung V, Tala H, Tuttle RM. Skeletal-related events due to bone metastases from differentiated thyroid cancer. J Clin Endocrinol Metab. 2012;97(7):2433–9.
161. Bernier MO, Leenhardt L, Hoang C, Aurengo A, Mary JY, Menegaux F, et al. Survival and therapeutic modalities in patients with bone metastases of differentiated thyroid carcinomas. J Clin Endocrinol Metab. 2001;86(4):1568–73.
162. Sandri A, Carbognin G, Regis D, Gaspari D, Calciolari C, Girardi V, et al. Combined radiofrequency and kyphoplasty in painful osteolytic metastases to vertebral bodies. Radiol Med. 2010;115(2):261–71.
163. Toyota N, Naito A, Kakizawa H, Hieda M, Hirai N, Tachikake T, et al. Radiofrequency ablation therapy combined with cementoplasty for painful bone metastases: initial experience. Cardiovasc Intervent Radiol. 2005;28(5):578–83.
164. Monchik JM, Donatini G, Iannuccilli J, Dupuy DE. Radiofrequency ablation and percutaneous ethanol injection treatment for recurrent local and distant well-differentiated thyroid carcinoma. Ann Surg. 2006;244(2):296–304.
165. Henriques de Figueiredo B, Godbert Y, Soubeyran I, Carrat X, Lagarde P, Cazeau AL, et al. Brain metastases from thyroid carcinoma: a retrospective study of 21 patients. Thyroid. 2014;24(2):270–6.
166. Chiu AC, Delpassand ES, Sherman SI. Prognosis and treatment of brain metastases in thyroid carcinoma. J Clin Endocrinol Metab. 1997;82(11):3637–42.
167. McWilliams RR, Giannini C, Hay ID, Atkinson JL, Stafford SL, Buckner JC. Management of brain metastases from thyroid carcinoma: a study of 16 pathologically confirmed cases over 25 years. Cancer. 2003;98(2):356–62.
168. Bernad DM, Sperduto PW, Souhami L, Jensen AW, Roberge D. Stereotactic radiosurgery in the management of brain metastases from primary thyroid cancers. J Neuro-Oncol. 2010;98(2):249–52.
169. Kim IY, Kondziolka D, Niranjan A, Flickinger JC, Lunsford LD. Gamma knife radiosurgery for metastatic brain tumors from thyroid cancer. J Neuro-Oncol. 2009;93(3):355–9.
170. McFadden DG, Sadow PM. Genetics, diagnosis, and management of Hürthle cell thyroid neoplasms. Front Endocrinol (Lausanne). 2021;12:696386.
171. Santana NO, Lerario AM, Schmerling CK, Marui S, Alves VAF, Hoff AO, et al. Molecular profile of Hürthle cell carcinomas: recurrent mutations in the Wnt/β-catenin pathway. Eur J Endocrinol. 2020;183(6):647–56.
172. Dong Y, Gong Y, Kuo F, Makarov V, Reznik E, Nanjangud GJ, et al. Targeting the Mtor pathway in Hurthle cell carcinoma results in potent antitumor activity. Mol Cancer Ther. 2022;21(2):382–94.
173. Haugen BR, Sherman SI. Evolving approaches to patients with advanced differentiated thyroid cancer. Endocr Rev. 2013;34(3):439–55.
174. Younes MN, Yigitbasi OG, Park YW, Kim SJ, Jasser SA, Hawthorne VS, et al. Antivascular therapy of human follicular thyroid cancer experimental bone metastasis by blockade of epidermal growth factor receptor and vascular growth factor receptor phosphorylation. Cancer Res. 2005;65(11):4716–27.
175. Younes MN, Yazici YD, Kim S, Jasser SA, El-Naggar AK, Myers JN. Dual epidermal growth factor receptor and vascular endothelial growth factor receptor inhibition with NVP-AEE788 for the treatment of aggressive follicular thyroid cancer. Clin Cancer Res. 2006;12:3425–34.
176. Schlumberger M, Tahara M, Wirth LJ, Robinson B, Brose MS, Elisei R, et al. Lenvatinib versus placebo in radioiodine-refractory thyroid cancer. N Engl J Med. 2015;372(7):621–30.
177. Brose MS, Nutting CM, Jarzab B, Elisei R, Siena S, Bastholt L, et al. Sorafenib in radioactive iodine-refractory, locally advanced or metastatic differentiated thyroid cancer: a randomised, double-blind, phase 3 trial. Lancet. 2014;384(9940):319–28.

178. Leboulleux S, Bastholt L, Krause T, de la Fouchardiere C, Tennvall J, Awada A, et al. Vandetanib in locally advanced or metastatic differentiated thyroid cancer: a randomised, double-blind, phase 2 trial. Lancet Oncol. 2012;13(9):897–905.
179. Locati LD, Licitra L, Agate L, Ou SH, Boucher A, Jarzab B, et al. Treatment of advanced thyroid cancer with axitinib: phase 2 study with pharmacokinetic/pharmacodynamic and quality-of-life assessments. Cancer. 2014;120(17):2694–703.
180. NCCN. Clinical Practice Guidelines in Oncology (NCCN Guidelines); 2015. (Thyroid Carcinoma, Version 2.2015).
181. Drilon A, Laetsch TW, Kummar S, DuBois SG, Lassen UN, Demetri GD, et al. Efficacy of Larotrectinib in TRK fusion-positive cancers in adults and children. N Engl J Med. 2018;378(8):731–9.
182. Drilon A, Siena S, Dziadziuszko R, Barlesi F, Krebs MG, Shaw AT, et al. Entrectinib in ROS1 fusion-positive non-small-cell lung cancer: integrated analysis of three phase 1-2 trials. Lancet Oncol. 2020;21(2):261–70.
183. Wirth LJ, Sherman E, Robinson B, Solomon B, Kang H, Lorch J, et al. Efficacy of selpercatinib in *RET*-altered thyroid cancers. N Engl J Med. 2020;383(9):825–35.
184. Li AY, McCusker MG, Russo A, Scilla KA, Gittens A, Arensmeyer K, Mehra R, Adamo V, Rolfo C. RET fusions in solid tumors. Cancer Treat Rev. 2019;81:101911.
185. Drilon A, Oxnard GR, Tan DSW, Loong HHF, Johnson M, Gainor J, et al. Efficacy of Selpercatinib in *RET* fusion-positive non-small-cell lung cancer. N Engl J Med. 2020;383(9):813–24.
186. Marabelle A, Le DT, Ascierto PA, Di Giacomo AM, De Jesus-Acosta A, Delord JP, et al. Efficacy of Pembrolizumab in patients with noncolorectal high microsatellite instability/mismatch repair-deficient cancer: results from the phase II KEYNOTE-158 study. J Clin Oncol. 2020;38(1):1–10.
187. Bishop JA, Wu G, Tufano RP, Westra WH. Histological patterns of Locoregional recurrence in Hürthle cell carcinoma of the thyroid gland. Thyroid. 2012;22(7):690–4.
188. Wertenbroek MW, Links TP, Prins TR, Plukker JT, van der Jagt EJ, de Jong KP. Radiofrequency ablation of hepatic metastases from thyroid carcinoma. Thyroid. 2008;18(10):1105–10.
189. Segkos K, Schmidt C, Nabhan F. Isolated liver metastasis in Hürthle cell thyroid cancer treated with microwave ablation. Case Rep Endocrinol. 2017;2017:2790741.
190. Lee GM, You JY, Kim HY, Chai YJ, Kim HK, Dionigi G, et al. Successful radiofrequency ablation strategies for benign thyroid nodules. Endocrine. 2019;64(2):316–21.
191. Aydemirli MD, Corver W, Beuk R, Roepman P, Solleveld-Westerink N, van Wezel T, et al. Targeted treatment options of recurrent radioactive iodine refractory Hürthle cell cancer. Cancers (Basel). 2019;11(8):1185.
192. Wenter V, Albert NL, et al. Clinical impact of follicular oncocytic (Hürthle cell) carcinoma in comparison with corresponding classical follicular thyroid carcinoma. Eur J Nucl Med Mol Imaging. 2021;48:449–60.
193. Crombé A, Buy X, Godbert Y, Alberti N, Kind M, Bonichon F, et al. 23 lung metastases treated by radiofrequency ablation over 10 years in a single patient: successful oncological outcome of a metastatic cancer without altered respiratory function. Cardiovasc Intervent Radiol. 2016;39:1779–84.
194. Paz-Fumagalli R, Li X, Smallridge RC. Ethanol ablation of neck metastases from differentiated thyroid carcinoma. Semina Intervent Radiol. 2019;36(5):381–5.
195. Solbiati L, Giangrande A, De Pra L, Bellotti E, Cantù P, Ravetto C. Percutaneous ethanol injection of parathyroid tumors under US guidance: treatment for secondary hyperparathyroidism. Radiology. 1985;155(03):607–10.
196. Charboneau JW, Hay ID, van Heerden JA. Persistent primary hyperparathyroidism: successful ultrasound-guided percutaneous ethanol ablation of an occult adenoma. Mayo Clin Proc. 1988;63(09):913–7.

197. Lewis BD, Hay ID, Charboneau JW, McIver B, Reading CC, Goellner JR. Percutaneous ethanol injection for treatment of cervical lymph node metastases in patients with papillary thyroid carcinoma. Am J Roentgenol. 2002;178(03):699–704.
198. NCCN. Clinical Practice Guidelines in Oncology: Thyroid Carcinoma. National Comprehensive Cancer Network. Version3; 2022.
199. Hay ID, Lee RA, Davidge-Pitts C, Reading CC, Charboneau JW. Long-term outcome of ultrasound-guided percutaneous ethanol ablation of selected "recurrent" neck nodal metastases in 25 patients with TNM stages III or IVA papillary thyroid carcinoma previously treated by surgery and ^{131}I therapy. Surgery. 2013;154(6):1448–54.
200. Ford D, Giridharan S, McConkey C, Hartley A, Brammer C, Watkinson JC, et al. External beam radiotherapy in the management of differentiated thyroid cancer. Clin Oncol (R Coll Radiol). 2003;15(6):337–41.

Oncocytic (Hürthle Cell) Carcinoma: Updates in Genetic and Molecular Diagnostics

13

13.1 Introduction

The genetic profile of oncocytic carcinoma of the thyroid (Hürthle cell carcinoma—HCC) differs from that of papillary thyroid carcinoma (PTC) and follicular thyroid carcinoma (FTC). Molecular pathways that differentiate oncocytic adenoma (Hürthle cell adenoma—HCA) from widely invasive HCC (wiHCC) include the PIK3CA-Akt-mTOR and Wnt β-catenin pathways, providing rationale toward new targets of this type of malignancy in the future [1]. Testing for genetic alteration in oncocytic/Hürthle cell neoplasms (HCNs) shows aneuploidy, *H-RAS* mutations, allelic alterations, mitochondrial genetics, and PCR-based microsatellite polymorphism analysis [2].

Despite having a common origin in the follicular cell, follicular thyroid carcinoma and oncocytic/HCC should be considered as two separate entities due to the significant difference in oncogene expression between both [3]. Changes in both nuclear DNA and mitochondrial DNA (mtDNA) suggest the diagnosis of oncocytic/HCC. "Molecular" changes in nuclear DNA involve several signaling pathways and mitochondrial functions. "Mitochondrial genetic" changes involve interaction between mutations in the mitochondrial and nuclear genomes [4].

The World Health Organization classification of follicular-derived differentiated thyroid carcinomas (and their subtypes) (fifth edition, 2022) and their morphological characteristics and molecular markers are summarized in Table 13.1 [5].

M. Sakr, *Oncocytic (Hürthle Cell) Thyroid Lesions*,
https://doi.org/10.1007/978-3-032-03115-0_13

Table 13.1 WHO classification of differentiated follicular-derived thyroid carcinomas: morphological parameters and molecular markers

Tumor type	Morphology	Molecular markers
NIFTP	Encapsulated, clear nuclei, no papillae	*RAS, BRAF K601E*
Papillary thyroid carcinoma (PTC)		
Classical	Papillae and clear nuclei	*BRAF V600E, RET/PTC fus, NTRK fus, ALK fus*, 1q amp
Follicular variant (subtype)	Follicles and clear nuclei	*BRAF K601E, RAS, PAX8/PPARγ, EIF1AX, THADA fus*, 22q del
Tall, columnar, solid, hobnail variants (subtypes)	Special structural and cell features	*BRAF V600E*, 1q amp, *TERT* promoter, *TP53, PIK3CA, CTNNB1*
Follicular thyroid carcinoma (FTC)	Capsular invasion (MI), vascular invasion >4 blood vessels (angioinvasive), extra-thyroidal invasion (WI)	*RAS, PAX8/PPARγ, PTEN, PIK3CA, TSHR, TERT* promoter, *CNA*
Oncocytic carcinoma (Hürthle cell carcinoma—HCC)	Capsular invasion (MI), vascular invasion >4 blood vessels (WI)	*RAS, EIF1AX, PTEN, TP53, CNA, mtDNA*
Poorly differentiated thyroid carcinoma (PDTC)	Invasion, mitoses >3, necrosis, convoluted nuclei	*RAS, TERT* promoter, *TP53, PIK3CA, PTEN, CTNNB1, AKT1, EIF1AX, ALK* fus, histone methyltransferases, SWI/SNF chromatin remodeling complex

Amp amplification, *PTC* papillary thyroid carcinoma, *FTC* follicular thyroid carcinoma, *HCC* Hürthle cell carcinoma, *PDTC* poorly differentiated thyroid carcinoma, *CNA* copy number alteration, *del* deletion, *fus* fusion, *MI* minimally invasive, *NIFTP* noninvasive follicular thyroid neoplasm with papillary-like nuclear features, *SWI/SNF* switch/sucrose non-fermentable, *WHO* World Health Organization, *WI* widely invasive

13.2 Genetic Change in Genes Involved in *RAS/RAF/MAPK* and *PIK3/AKT/MTOR* Pathways

The *RAS* proteins are small GTPases that play a central role in transducing signals that regulate cell proliferation, survival, and differentiation. Approximately, 30% of human cancers, including solid tumors and hematologic malignancies, are associated with mutations in *RAS* genes. Interestingly, mutations in different *RAS* isoforms are preferentially associated with cancers of different organs [6]. Mutation or translocation of the *RAS* oncogene is common in both follicular adenomas and follicular thyroid carcinomas (FTCs) (approximately 40%). Such *RAS* oncogene mutations are *not* specific for follicular tumors as they also occur in papillary thyroid carcinoma (PTC). The *RAS* oncogene is frequently involved in the pathogenesis of oncocytic/Hürthle cell neoplasms (HCNs). ThyroSeq v2 complete next-generation sequencing assay on thyroid cytology specimens were performed by researchers from the University of Pittsburgh, Pennsylvania, USA [7]. "Point mutations" involved the *NRAS*, followed by the *KRAS*, the *TERT* gene, and the *TSHR* gene. The identified "fusions" involved the thyroid adenoma-associated (*THADA*) gene, the peroxisome proliferator-activated receptor γ (*PPARG*) gene, and the neurotrophic tyrosine kinase receptor, type 3 (*NTRK3*) gene.

Oncogenic point mutations in the three human *RAS* genes (*NRAS*, *KRAS*, *HRAS*) have been detected in a wide variety of human cancers, with carcinomas of the pancreas, colon, thyroid, and lung showing the highest incidence [7]. More recently, activating mutations in the *RAS* effector protein *BRAF* were identified as frequent genetic aberrations in malignant melanomas [8, 9] and in different types of carcinomas [10–12]. *RAS* family mutations—*NRAS*, *KRAS*, and *HRAS*—are identified in nearly 45% of follicular tumors as compared to only 10–15% in oncocytic/HCC [1, 13–15]. The exact mechanism for *RAS* gene mutation to cause oncocytic/HCC progression is unknown [16]. *BRAF* mutations are the predominant genetic changes in PTC, but the incidence of *BRAF* mutation in oncocytic/HCC is not common [17].

The *BRAF* gene produces *RAF* proteins (*ARAF*, *BRAF*, and *CRAF*), which are essential serine/threonine protein kinases [18]. The mutation *PIK3CA* gene (the product that binds specifically with *RAS* and activates the *PIK3/AKT* signaling pathway) also has an important role in the thyroid tumorigenesis [19]. Ganly et al. reported in 2013 [1] and later in 2019 [13] that they identified genetic mutations associated with *RAS/RAF/MAPK* and *PIK3/AKT/mTOR* pathways in oncytic/HCCs. These genes included *PTEN*, *PIK3*, *PTEN*, *TSC1*, *TSC2*, and *RAS* family. In the literature, *PTEN* was observed in approximately 5% of cases overall [13, 20] and in 25% of *TP53* mutation positive cases [21].

13.3 Genetic Rearrangements

Rearrangement of the *RET* gene, also known as *RET*/PTC rearrangement, is the most common genetic alteration identified to date in papillary thyroid carcinomas (PTCs). The prevalence of *RET*/PTC in PTCs shows significant geographic variation reaching approximately 35% in North America. *RET*/PTC is more common in tumors in children and young adults, and in PTCs associated with radiation exposure. There are at least ten different types of *RET*/PTC, all resulting from the fusion of the tyrosine kinase domain of *RET* to the 5′ portion of different genes. *RET*/PTC1 and *RET*/PTC3 are the most common types, accounting for more than 90% of all rearrangements. There is some evidence that different types of *RET*/PTC may be associated with distinct biological properties of PTCs. *RET*/PTC1 tends to be more common in tumors with typical papillary growth and micro-carcinomas and to have a more benign clinical course, whereas *RET*/PTC3 in some populations shows a strong correlation with the solid variant of PTC and more aggressive tumor behavior [22]. *RET*/PTC has also been found in hyalinizing trabecular adenomas of the thyroid gland, providing molecular evidence in favor of this tumor to be a variant of PTC [23, 24]. The occurrence of *RET*/PTC in benign thyroid lesions such as follicular adenomas [25, 26], chronic lymphocytic thyroiditis (Hashimoto's thyroiditis) [27, 28], and hyperplastic nodules [29–31], reported in several studies, has *not* been confirmed in other studies and remains controversial.

Along with the point mutations, chromosomal rearrangements are also common mutational mechanisms in thyroid cancers [32]. However, several researchers reported that genetic rearrangements of *PAX8/PPAR*, *RET/PTC*, *EML4/ALK*, and *ETV6/NTRK3* are infrequently observed in oncocytic/HCC [15, 17, 33].

13.4 Tumor Protein 53 (TP53) Gene Mutation

The tumor protein 53 (*TP53*) gene provides instructions for making a protein called "tumor protein p53," which acts as a tumor suppressor by regulating cell division, keeping cells from growing and proliferating too fast or in an uncontrolled way. Mutation of this gene is known to occur with increasing frequency in dedifferentiated thyroid tumors rather than well-differentiated tumors. *TP53* mutations were found in 22% of thyroid cancer overall [20], and in 42% [21] of oncocytic/HCC cases. All the mutations are in the DNA-binding domain [20].

13.5 Telomerase Reverse Transcriptase (*TERT*) Promoter Mutations

Telomerase reverse transcriptase (*TERT*) serves as the pivotal catalytic subunit of telomerase, a crucial enzyme responsible for telomere maintenance and human genome stability. The high activation of human *TERT* (*hTERT*), observed in over 90% of tumors, plays a significant role in tumor initiation and progression [34].

The *hTERT* is detected by immunohistochemistry (IHC), and the telomere length can be determined by tissue quantitative fluorescence in situ hybridization. The *hTERT* protein expression is observed in 86% of FTCs and 49% of follicular adenomas. All oncocytic/Hürthle cell neoplasms (HCNs) express *hTERT* protein, but oncocytic/HCCs have significantly very shortened telomeres than oncocytic adenomas (Hürthle cell adenomas—HCAs) [35]. The common *TERT C228T* promoter mutation is detected in both wiHCC and miHCCs [36]. This "promotor" mutation is very common in advanced cancers, especially those with *BRAF* or *RAS* mutation [37].

The *TERT/hTERT* promoter mutations are associated with unfavorable prognosis in various cancers. Major *TERT* promoter mutations are *C228T* and *C250T*. *TERT* promoter mutations are found in 32% of wiHCCs and in only 5% of miHCCs [15, 36]. In a recent study by Tanaka et al. (2019), some thyroid tumors showed increased *TERT mRNA* expression even in the absence of *TERT* promoter mutations, which has a significantly high recurrence rate [38]. In oncocytic/HCCs, increased *TERT mRNA* expression has *not* been observed [36].

13.6 Tumor Mutational Burden (*TMB*) and Global Copy Number Diversity

Tumor mutational burden (TMB) refers to the number of mutations that exist within a tumor [39]. Ganly et al. (2018) reported that oncocytic/HCCs contain an average of 2.6 mutations/Mb, which was sixfold greater than that reported in The Cancer Genome Atlas (TCGA) of PTC (0.41 mutations/Mb) [15]. High TMB has been associated with responses to immune checkpoint inhibitors in several tumors, such as non-small cell lung cancer, and can be a promising biomarker. Still, its cutoff and clinical relevance for thyroid tumors have *not* yet been elucidated.

Regions of "chromosomal gain and loss" are observed in oncocytic/HCCs. Large regions of amplification are observed on chromosomes *5*, *7*, *12*, and *17*. These chromosomal amplifications potentially lead to activation of *RAS-RAF-MEK* and *PI3K-Akt-mTOR* pathways [1]. Chromosome *7* and *12* potentially activate the *RAS-RAF-MEK* pathway. Chromosomal regions of gain and loss in oncocytic/HCC differ from PTC and FTC [1]. Through amplification of chromosome *7*, *BRAF* was found to be significantly overexpressed in oncocytic/HCC, which is involved in the *mTOR* pathway. According to clustering analysis of the copy number data, three groups of oncocytic/Hürthle cell neoplasms were observed—deletions predominant type, amplification predominant type, and mixed type. Among these, the mixed type was mostly attributed in aggressive oncocytic/HCC [1]. On the other hand, loss of heterogeneity (LOH) has been reported in oncocytic/HCC and was found to be associated with more aggressive diseases. However, the reason why LOH leads to a worsened course is unknown [15, 40].

13.7 Mutations in Mitochondrial DNA (*mtDNA*) and Related Genes

The mitochondrial DNA (mtDNA) is small, and incorporates a sequence of 16,569 bp, encoding 13 essential components in cellular energy production [41]. It is more susceptible than nuclear DNA to mutagen-induced damage. As in other types of cancers [42, 43], alterations of mtDNA in oncocytic/HCC have been revealed. The so-called common deletion is the most common mitochondrial alteration. It is a large-scale deletion of 4977 base pairs (bp) of mtDNA residing between two 13-bp direct repeats in the mtDNA sequence at nucleotide positions 13,447–13,459 and 8470–8484. Common deletion was significantly higher in oncocytic/HCCs than in non-Hürthle cell neoplasms [44].

Disruptive mutations in mtDNA are found in complex-I subunit genes in oncocytic/HCNs. Usually, mutations of mtDNA are hetero-plasmic, but homoplasmy in the oncocytic/Hürthle cell tumors is frequently observed. Gasparre et al. (2007) sequenced the entire mtDNA in thyroid oncocytic tumors and controls and reported that 26% of the analyzed thyroid oncocytic tumors showed disruptive mutations (nonsense or frameshift) [45]. This was observed in complex-I subunit genes, and the association between these mutations and the oncocytic phenotype was statistically significant [45]. Attributing a causal role to single mitochondrial mutation is difficult, and a more-than-one-hit hypothesis is more plausible. The authors concluded that mitochondrial mutations may play a part as one of many factors leading to tumor development [45].

The genes associated with Retinoid-interferon-induced Mortality-19 (*GRIM-19*), one of the *IFN/RA* inducible *GRIM* products, is a 552-base pair cDNA mapped to human chromosome *19p13.2* [46], which encodes a *16-kDa* protein. It was originally identified as a potential tumor suppressor associated with growth inhibition or cell apoptosis. Subsequently, it was identified as an essential subunit of the mitochondrial respiratory chain complex-I [47, 48]. It also represses *STAT3* and serves as a negative regulator of cell growth [46, 49]. Somatic missense mutation in *GRIM-19* has been found in approximately 11% of oncocytic/HCCs [50]. *GRIM-19* may potentially aid as a cytological marker of malignancy in oncocytic/Hürthle cell neoplasms (HCNs) [51].

Variations in the inner mitochondrial membrane transporter have been also reported. Mitochondrial protein is mostly encoded by the nuclear genome. These are imported from cytosol into mitochondria via translocator, translocase of inner mitochondrial membrane 44 homolog (*TRMM44*) [52]. Variations in the inner mitochondrial membrane transporter *TIMM44* have been observed in patients with oncocytic thyroid tumors. Details of how these variation cause or affect oncocytic/HCC is still not known.

13.8 Other Molecular Changes

Differences between of miHCC and wiHCC could be demonstrated by "gene expression analysis." Among these differences, beta-catenin (*CTNNB1*) was a significant gene set that was enriched [1]. In wiHCC, beta-catenin is involved in processes regulating vascular invasion [1].

Sheu et al. (2007) reported that oncocytic thyroid tumors, including both oncocytic/HCA and oncocytic/HCC, showed a statistically significant increase in C-allele frequency of *GNB3 C825T* polymorphism of the G protein beta3-subunit compared to all non-oncocytic tumors [53]. *GNB3 C825T* has been reported to contribute to increased risk of cancer, especially thyroid carcinoma [54]. This polymorphism may thus be a cofactor favoring the development of oncocytic thyroid tumors, but the biological mechanism remains unclear. Whether this is somehow related to the mitochondrial DNA (mtDNA) changes seen in oncocytic thyroid tumors also remains to be seen [41].

Kasaian et al. (2015) found multiple endocrine neoplasia (*MEN-1*) gene mutation in 4% of oncocytic/HCC [55]. At the cellular level, common functional polymorphisms in antioxidant gene *GPX1* have been found to be associated with occurrence of *recurrent* oncocytic (Hürthle) cell malignant disease [56].

In 2018, Ganly et al. [15] reported that oncocytic/HCCs can be divided into three groups according to the combination of *TERT* promoter mutation, widespread LOH, and whole-chromosome duplication of chromosome *7* assigns The first group shows

TERT alterations, major LOH, and whole-chromosome duplication (WCD) of chromosome *7* and is observed in wiHCC. The second group shows major LOH and WCD of chromosome *7*, without *TERT* alteration. The third group does not show these genetic changes, which are observed in miHCC and nonrecurrent oncocytic/HCCs [15].

A micro-ribonucleic acid (*miRNA*) is a small noncoding RNA molecule (containing about 22 nucleotides) found in plants, animals, and some viruses, which functions in RNA-silencing and posttranscriptional regulation of gene expression. Petric et al. (2016) investigated the expression of *miRNAs* in 39 patients with oncocytic/HCCs (22 with nonmetastatic and 17 with regional or distant metastatic disease). They reported that the expression of *miRNA* (*miR-183*, *miR-221*, and *miR-885-5p*) in tumor tissue is correlated with the risk of distant metastases in patients with oncocytic/HCC [57].

Somatic mutations in cancer database for oncocytic/Hürthle cell carcinoma (HCC) in addition to the possible mechanism of action of each, are summarized in Table 13.2.

Table 13.2 Genetic mutations in oncocytic/Hürthle cell carcinoma (HCC)

Gene [reference number]	Possible mechanism
MEN1, multiple endocrine neoplasia [55]	Loss of function to produce the tumor suppressor protein, called menin, which is required for apoptosis
TERT, telomerase reverse transcriptase [35, 36]	*TERT* encodes the reverse transcriptase component of telomerase, which is required for cell immortalization HRAS
RAS, Harvey rat sarcoma viral oncogene homolog [16, 57]	Encodes transforming protein 21. Point mutations affect production of proteins that convey signals originating from tyrosine kinase membrane receptors to a cascade of mitogen-activated protein kinases
MAPK, mitogen-activated protein kinases [37]	This activates the transcription of target genes involved in cell proliferation, survival, and apoptosis
PIK3CA, phosphatidylinositol-3-kinase catalytic alpha polypeptide [19]	The product binds specifically with *RAS* and activates the phosphoinositide-3-kinase/AKT (*PI3K/AKT*) signaling pathway
NRAS, neuroblastoma RAS [52]	Encodes the protein *N-RAS* that is involved primarily in regulating cell division
BRAF, murine sarcoma viral oncogene homolog B1A [7]	Potent activator of the *MAPK* pathway
KRAS, Kirsten RAS [37]	Encodes the protein *K-RAS* that is involved primarily in regulating cell division
AKT1, AKT serine/threonine kinase 1 [18, 58]	Encodes a protein called *AKT1* kinase, which is found in various cell types throughout the body, where it plays a critical role in many signaling pathways
IDH1, isocitrate dehydrogenase 1 [59, 60]	Produces 2-hydroxyglutarate (2HG), which induces histone- and DNA-hypermethylation through inhibition of epigenetic regulators

(continued)

Table 13.2 (continued)

Gene [reference number]	Possible mechanism
GNAS, guanine nucleotide stimulatory protein [61]	Encodes the alpha subunit of the stimulatory G protein, activating mutation of this potent tumor suppressor
SMAD4 [62] gene promotor's mutation	*SMAD4* is a tumor suppressor
TSHR, thyroid-stimulating hormone receptor [63]	Promotes growth and progression of thyroid cancer once initiated by oncogenic alterations
SETD2, SET domain containing 2 (enzyme) [64]	Required for DNA double-strand break repair and activation of the p53-mediated checkpoint
ARID1B (AT-rich interactive domain-containing protein 1B) [65]	Encodes the largest subunit of the *SwI/SNF* chromatin remodeling complex, which has tumor suppressor activity
DAXX, probable ATP-dependent RNA helicase DDX6 [66]	Telomere maintenance
EWSR1 Ewing sarcoma [67]	A member of the *TET* family of genes (detailed mechanism unknown)
DDX6, DEAD-box helicase 6 [68]	Increases messenger ribonucleic acid production
MLLT4, mixed lineage leukemia [69, 70]	The *AF-6/MLLT4* gene encodes the Afadin scaffold protein essential for epithelial integrity. Depletion of the protein markedly promotes proliferation and metastasis
SEPT6, Septin 6 [71]	Membrane-interacting proteins with a highly conserved domain structure involved in various cellular processes, including cytoskeleton organization, cytokinesis, and membrane dynamics
CACNA1D, calcium voltage-gated channel subunit alpha1 D [72]	Proteins involved in calcium signaling unstimulated Tg <5–10 ng/mL

References

1. Ganly I, Ricarte Filho J, Eng S, Ghossein R, Morris LG, Liang Y, et al. Genomic dissection of Hurthle cell carcinoma reveals a unique class of thyroid malignancy. J Clin Endocrinol Metab. 2013;98(5):E962–72.
2. Dettori T, Frau DV, Lai ML, Mariotti S, Uccheddu A, Daniele GM, et al. Aneuploidy in oncocytic lesions of the thyroid gland: diffuse accumulation of mitochondria within the cell is associated with trisomy 7 and progressive numerical chromosomal alterations. Genes Chromosomes Cancer. 2003;38(1):22–31.
3. Masood S, Auguste LJ, Westerband A, Belluco C, Valderama E, Attie J. Differential oncogenic expression in thyroid follicular and Hürthle cell carcinomas. Am J Surg. 1993;166(4):366–8.
4. Wallace DC. Mitochondrial diseases in man and mouse. Science (NY). 1999;283:1482–8.
5. Baloch ZW, Asa SL, Barletta JA, Ghossein RA, Juhlin CC, Jung CK, et al. Overview of the 2022 WHO classification of thyroid neoplasms. Endocr Pathol. 2022;33(1):27–63.
6. Bos JL. Ras oncogenes in human cancer: a review. Cancer Res. 1989;49:4682–9.
7. Nikiforov YE, Carty SE, Chiosea SI, Coyne C, Duvvuri U, et al. Highly accurate diagnosis of cancer in thyroid nodules with follicular neoplasm/suspicious for a follicular neoplasmcytology by ThyroSeq v2 next-generation sequencing assay. Cancer. 2014;120(23):3627–34.
8. Davies H, Bignell GR, Cox C, Stephens P, Edkins S, Clegg S, et al. Mutations of the BRAF gene in human cancer. Nature. 2002;417(6892):949–54.

9. Reifenberger J, Knobbe CB, Sterzinger AA, Blaschke B, Schulte KW, Ruzicka T, Reifenberger G. Frequent alterations of Ras signaling pathway genes in sporadic malignant melanomas. Int J Cancer. 2004;109:377–84.
10. Cohen Y, Xing M, Mambo E, Guo Z, Wu G, Trink B, Beller U, Westra WH, Ladenson PW, Sidransky D. *BRAF* mutation in papillary thyroid carcinoma. J Natl Cancer Inst. 2003;95:625–7.
11. Kimura ET, Nikiforova MN, Zhu Z, Knauf JA, Nikiforov YE, Fagin JA. High prevalence of *BRAF* mutations in thyroid cancer: genetic evidence for constitutive activation of the RET/PTC-RAS-BRAF signaling pathway in papillary thyroid carcinoma. Cancer Res. 2003;63:1454–7.
12. Rajagopalan H, Bardelli A, Lengauer C, Kinzler KW, Vogelstein B, Velculescu VE. Tumorigenesis: *RAF/RAS* oncogenes and mismatch-repair status. Nature. 2002;418:934.
13. Ganly I, McFadden DG. Short review: genomic alterations in Hurthle cell carcinoma. Thyroid. 2019;29:471–9.
14. Tallini G, Hsueh A, Liu S, Garcia-Rostan G, Speicher MR, Ward DC. Frequent chromosomal DNA unbalance in thyroid oncocytic (Hürthle cell) neoplasms detected by comparative genomic hybridization. Lab Investig. 1999;79(5):547–55.
15. Ganly I, Makarov V, Deraje S, Dong Y, Reznik E, Seshan V, et al. Integrated genomic analysis of Hürthle cell cancer reveals oncogenic drivers, recurrent mitochondrial mutations, and unique chromosomal landscapes. Cancer Cell. 2018;34(2):256–270.e5.
16. Barbacid M. Ras genes. Annu Rev Biochem. 1987;56:779–827.
17. Musholt PB, Musholt TJ, Morgenstern SC, Worm K, Sheu SY, Schmid KW. Follicular histotypes of oncocytic thyroid carcinomas do not carry mutations of the BRAF hot-spot. World J Surg. 2008;32(5):722–8.
18. Valerio L, Pieruzzi L, Giani C, Agate L, Bottici V, et al. Targeted therapy in thyroid cancer: state of the art. Clin Oncol (R Coll Radiol). 2017;29(5):316–24.
19. Hou P, Liu D, Shan Y, Hu S, Studeman K, et al. Genetic alterations and their relationship in the phosphatidylinositol3-kinase/Akt pathway in thyroid cancer. Clin Cancer Res. 2007;13(4):1161–70.
20. Nikiforova MN, Wald AI, Roy S, Durso MB, Nikiforov YE. Targeted next-generation sequencing panel (ThyroSeq) for detection of mutations in thyroid cancer. J Clin Endocrinol Metab. 2013;98(11):E1852–60.
21. Wei S, LiVolsi VA, Montone KT, Morrissette JJD, Baloch ZW. PTEN and TP53 mutations in oncocytic follicular carcinoma. Endocr Pathol. 2015;26:365–9.
22. Nikiforov YE. RET/PTC rearrangement in thyroid tumors. Endocr Pathol. 2002;13:3–16.
23. Papotti M, Volante M, Giuliano A, Fassina A, Fusco A, Bussolati G, Santoro M, et al. RET/PTC activation in hyalinizing trabecular tumors of the thyroid. Am J Surg Pathol. 2000;24:1615–21.
24. Cheung CC, Boerner SL, MacMillan CM, Ramyar L, Asa SL. Hyalinizing trabecular tumor of the thyroid: a variant of papillary carcinoma proved by molecular genetics. Am J Surg Pathol. 2000;24:1622–6.
25. Santoro M, Carlomagno F, Hay ID, Herrmann MA, Grieco M, Melillo R, et al. Ret oncogene activation in human thyroid neoplasms is restricted to the papillary cancer subtype. J Clin Invest. 1992;89:1517–22.
26. Cinti R, Yin L, Ilc K, Berger N, Basolo F, Cuccato S, et al. RET rearrangements in papillary thyroid carcinomas and adenomas detected by interphase FISH. Cytogenet Cell Genet. 2000;88:56–61.
27. Wirtschafter A, Schmidt R, Rosen D, Kundu N, Santoro M, Fusco A, et al. Expression of the RET/PTC fusion gene as a marker for papillary carcinoma in Hashimoto's thyroiditis. Laryngoscope. 1997;107:95–100.
28. Sheils OM, O'Eary JJ, Uhlmann V, Lättich K, Sweeney EC. ret/PTC-1 activation in Hashimoto thyroiditis. Int J Surg Pathol. 2000;8:185–9.
29. Ishizaka Y, Kobayashi S, Ushijima T, Hirohashi S, Sugimura T, Nagao M. Detection of retTPC/PTC transcripts in thyroid adenomas and adenomatous goiter by an RT-PCR method. Oncogene. 1991;6:1667–72.

30. Bounacer A, Wicker R, Caillou B, Cailleux AF, Sarasin A, Schlumberger M, et al. High prevalence of activating ret proto-oncogene rearrangements, in thyroid tumors from patients who had received external radiation. Oncogene. 1997;15:1263–73.
31. Elisei R, Romei C, Vorontsova T, Cosci B, Veremeychik V, Kuchinskaya E, et al. RET/PTC rearrangements in thyroid nodules: studies in irradiated and not irradiated, malignant and benign thyroid lesions in children and adults. J Clin Endocrinol Metab. 2001;86(7):3211–6.
32. Nikiforov YE, Nikiforova MN. Molecular genetics and diagnosis of thyroid cancer. Nat Rev Endocrinol. 2011;7:569–80.
33. Musholt PB, Imkamp F, von Wasielewski R, Schmid KW, Musholt TJ. RET rearrangements in archival oxyphilic thyroid tumors: new insights in tumorigenesis and classification of Hurthle cell carcinomas? Surgery. 2003;134:881–9.
34. Yang R, Han Y, Guan X, Hong Y, Meng J, Ding S, et al. Regulation and clinical potential of telomerase reverse transcriptase (TERT/hTERT) in brest cancer. Cell Commun Signal. 2023;21:218.
35. Sugishita Y, Kammori M, Yamada O, Yamazaki K, Ito K, et al. Biological differential diagnosis of follicular thyroid tumor and Hürthle cell tumor on the basis of telomere length and hTeRT expression. Ann Surg Oncol. 2014;21(7):2318–25.
36. Chindris AM, Casler JD, Bernet VJ, Rivera M, Thomas C, et al. Clinical and molecular features of Hürthle cell carcinoma of the thyroid. J Clin Endocrinol Metab. 2015;100(1):55–62.
37. Landa I, Ganly I, Chan TA, Mitsutake N, Matsuse M, et al. Frequent somatic TeRT promoter mutations in thyroid cancer: higher prevalence in advanced forms of the disease. J Clinendocrinol Metab. 2013;98(9):e1562–6.
38. Tanaka A, Matsuse M, Saenko V, Nakao T, Yamanouchi K, Sakimura C, et al. TERT mRNA expression as a novel prognostic marker in papillary thyroid carcinomas. Thyroid. 2019;29:1105–14.
39. Ritterhouse LL. Tumor mutational burden. Cancer Cytopathol. 2019;127:735–6.
40. Gopal RK, Kübler K, Calvo SE, Polak P, Livitz D, Rosebrock D, et al. Widespread chromosomal losses and mitochondrial DNA alterations as genetic drivers in Hürthle cell carcinoma. Cancer Cell. 2018;34(2):242–255.e5.
41. Máximo V, Sobrinho-Simões M. Hürthle cell tumours of the thyroid. A review with emphasis on mitochondrial abnormalities with clinical relevance. Virchows Arch Int J Pathol. 2000;437:107–15.
42. Chen K, Lu P, Beeraka NM, Sukocheva OA, Madhunapantula SRV, Mikhail JLY, et al. Mitochondrial mutations and mitoepigenetics: focus on regulation of oxidative stress-induced responses in breast cancers. Semin Cancer Biol. 2022;83:556–69.
43. Ni J, Wang Y, Cheng X, Teng F, Wang C, Han S, et al. Pathogenic heteroplasmic somatic mitochondrial DNA mutation confers platinum-resistance and recurrence of high-grade serous ovarian cancer. Cancer Manag Res. 2020;12:11085–93.
44. Máximo V, Soares P, Lima J, Cameselle-Teijeiro J, Sobrinho-Simões M. Mitochondrial DNA somatic mutations (point mutations and large deletions) and mitochondrial DNA variants in human thyroid pathology: a study with emphasis on Hürthle cell tumors. Am J Pathol. 2002;160(5):1857–65.
45. Gasparre G, Porcelli AM, Bonora E, Pennisi LF, Toller M, Iommarini L, et al. Disruptive mitochondrial DNA mutations in complex I subunits are markers of oncocytic phenotype in thyroid tumors. Proc Natl Acad Sci USA. 2007;104(21):9001–6.
46. Lufei C, Ma J, Huang G, Zhang T, Novotny-Diermayr V, Ong CT, et al. GRIM-19, a death-regulatory gene product, suppresses Stat3 activity via functional interaction. EMBO J. 2003;22(6):1325–35.
47. Liu X, Kim CN, Yang J, Jemmerson R, Wang X. Induction of apoptotic program in cell-free extracts: requirement for dATP and cytochrome c. Cell. 1996;86:147–57.
48. Angell JE, Lindner DJ, Shapiro PS, Hofmann ER, Kalvakolanu DV. Identification of GRIM-19, a novel cell death-regulatory gene induced by the interferon-beta and retinoic acid combination, using a genetic approach. J Biol Chem. 2000;275(43):33416–26.

49. Huang Y, Yang M, Hu H, Zhao X, Bao L, Huang D, et al. Mitochondrial GRIM-19 as a potential therapeutic target for STAT3-dependent carcinogenesis of gastric cancer. Oncotarget. 2016;7(27):41404–20.
50. Máximo V, Botelho T, Capela J, Soares P, Lima J, Taveira A, et al. Somatic and germline mutation in GRIM-19, a dual function gene involved in mitochondrial metabolism and cell death, is linked to mitochondrion-rich (Hurthle cell) tumours of the thyroid. Br J Cancer. 2005;92(10):1892–8.
51. Donatini G, Beaulieu A, Castagnet M, Kraimps JL, Levillain P, Fromont G. Thyroid Hürthle cell tumors: research of potential markers of malignancy. J Endocrinol Investig. 2016;39:153–8.
52. Rehling P, Brandner K, Pfanner N. Mitochondrial import and the twin-pore translocase. Nat Rev Mol Cell Biol. 2004;5:519–30.
53. Sheu SY, Handke S, Bröcker-Preuss M, Görges R, Frey UH, Ensinger C, et al. The C allele of the GNB3 C825T polymorphism of the G protein beta3-subunit is associated with an increased risk for the development of oncocytic thyroid tumours. J Pathol. 2007;211(1):60–6.
54. Wang Y, Zhang S. Quantitative assessment of the association between GNB3 C825T polymorphism and cancer risk. J BUON. 2014;19:1092–5.
55. Kasaian K, Chindris AM, Wiseman SM, Mungall KL, Zeng T, et al. MEN1 mutations in Hürthle cell (oncocytic) thyroid carcinoma. J Clin Endocrinol Metab. 2015;100(4):e611–5.
56. Krhin B, Goricar K, Gazic B, Dolzan V, Besic N. Functional polymorphisms in antioxidant genes in Hurthle cell thyroid neoplasm: an association of GPX1 polymorphism and recurrent Hurthle cell thyroid carcinoma. Radiol Oncol. 2016;50(3):289–96.
57. Petric R, Gazic B, Goricar K, Dolzan V, Dzodic R, et al. Expression of miRNA and occurrence of distant metastases inpatients with Hürthle cell carcinoma. Int J Endocrinol. 2016;2016:8945247.
58. Carpten JD, Faber AL, Horn C, Donoho GP, Briggs SL, Robbins CM, et al. A transforming mutation in the pleckstrin homology domain of AKT1 in cancer. Nature. 2007;448(7152):439–44.
59. Yoo SK, Lee S, Kim SJ, Jee HG, Kim BA, Cho H, et al. Comprehensive analysis of the transcriptional and mutational landscape of follicular and papillary thyroid cancers. PLoS Genet. 2016;12(8):e1006239.
60. Santos JC, Bastos AU, Cerutti JM, Ribeiro ML. Correlation of MLH1 and MGMT expression and promoter methylation with genomic instability in patients with thyroid carcinoma. BMC Cancer. 2013;13:79.
61. Campo C, Köhler A, Figlioli G, Elisei R, Romei C, et al. Inherited variants in genes somatically mutated in thyroid cancer. PLoS One. 2017;12(4):e0174995.
62. Nikolic A, Ristanovic M, Zivaljevic V, Rankov AD, Radojkovic D, et al. SMAD4 gene promoter mutations in patients with thyroid tumors. Exp Mol Pathol. 2015;99(1):100–3.
63. Xing M. Molecular pathogenesis and mechanisms of thyroid cancer. Nat Rev Cancer. 2013;13(3):184–99.
64. Carvalho S, Vítor AC, Sridhara SC, Martins FB, Raposo AC, et al. SeTD2 is required for DNA double-strand break repair and activation of the p53-mediated checkpoint. elife. 2014;3:e02482.
65. Vengoechea J, Carpenter L, Zárate YA. Papillary thyroid cancer in a patient with interstitial 6q25 deletion including ARID1B. Am J Med Genet A. 2014;164A(7):1857–9.
66. Nasirden A, Saito T, Fukumura Y, Hara K, Akaike K. In Japanese patients with papillary thyroid carcinoma, TeRT promoter mutation is associated with poor prognosis, in contrast to BRAF (v600e) mutation. Virchows Arch. 2016;469(6):687–96.
67. Oliveira G, Polónia A, Cameselle-Teijeiro JM, Leitão D, Sapia S, et al. ewSR1 rearrangement is a frequent event in papillary thyroid carcinoma and in carcinoma of the thyroid with Ewing family tumor elements (CeFTe). Virchows Arch. 2017;470(5):517–25.
68. Mück F, Bracharz S, Marschalek R. DDX6 transfers P-TEFbkinase to the AF4/AF4N (AFF1) super elongation complex. Am J Blood Res. 2016;6(3):28–45.

69. Lim JH, Jang S, Park CJ, Chi HS, Lee JO, et al. FISH analysis of MLL gene rearrangements: detection of the concurrent loss or gain of the 3′ signal and its prognostic significance. Int J Lab Hematol. 2014;36(5):571–9.
70. Vargas C, Radziwill G, Krause G, Diehl A, Keller S, et al. Small-molecule inhibitors of AF6 PDZ-mediated protein-protein interactions. Chem Med Chem. 2014;9(7):1458–62.
71. Heasley LR, McMurray MA. Small molecule perturbations of septins. Methods Cell Biol. 2016;136:311–9.
72. Danecek P, Nellåker C, McIntyre RE, Buendia-Buendia JE, Bumpstead S, et al. High levels of RNA-editing site conservation amongst 15 laboratory mouse strains. Genome Biol. 2012;13(4):26.

Oncocytic (Hürthle Cell) Carcinoma: Guidelines and Decision-Making

14

14.1 Introduction

The aim of clinical practice guidelines is to provide physicians with the best available evidence on particular issues and recommendations for the best standards of care. They help health professionals weigh the benefits and the risks of available diagnostic or therapeutic options. With specifically tailored treatments becoming commonplace, it is important to consider each patient with thyroid cancer individually. Additionally, it is important to note that while a number of different groups have put forth guidelines for the management of thyroid surveillance and cancer therapy [1–7], there is some controversy among guidelines regarding certain situations, which has raised concerns about the effects on patient management and outcome [8].

For the sake of simplification and clarity, this chapter will largely refer to guidelines for diagnosis and management of thyroid cancer including oncocytic carcinoma of the thyroid (Hürthle cell carcinoma—HCC), from the following organizations and classification systems:

- American Thyroid Association (ATA) [1, 9–12]
- National Comprehensive Cancer Network (NCCN) [2]
- European Society for Medical Oncology (ESMO) [3]
- American Association of Clinical Endocrinologists/Associazione Medici Endocrinologi (AACE/AME) [13] (diagnosis only)
- European Thyroid Association (ETA) [14]
- Bethesda System for Cytopathology [15]
- American College of Radiology (ACR) Thyroid Imaging, Reporting and Data System (TI-RADS) [16]
- The fifth edition (2022) of the WHO Classification of Thyroid Neoplasms [17]

M. Sakr, *Oncocytic (Hürthle Cell) Thyroid Lesions*,
https://doi.org/10.1007/978-3-032-03115-0_14

14.2 Diagnostic Guidelines

14.2.1 Initial Evaluation

Evaluation of any thyroid complaint begins with a thorough history-taking and a physical examination that includes examination of cervical lymph nodes (LNs). Important historical factors include age, gender, family history (e.g., thyroid cancer), environmental exposures, and radiation exposure.

When a thyroid "nodule" is discovered, either incidentally on imaging or on physical exam, all the guidelines [1–4] advocate ultrasound (US) evaluation of thyroid nodules and cervical lymph nodes (LNs) along with measurement of serum thyroid-stimulating hormone (TSH) levels to determine whether a fine needle aspiration biopsy (FNAB) is indicated. A routine measurement of serum thyroglobulin (Tg) for the initial evaluation of thyroid nodules is *not* recommended because Tg levels are elevated in most benign thyroid conditions and are an insensitive and nonspecific test for thyroid cancer [1–4].

The AACE/AME guideline has an algorithm that comprises data from clinical assessment, imaging, cytology, and molecular markers and incorporates both TI-RADS [16] and the 2023 Bethesda classification [15] to help guide clinical decisions regarding nodule evaluation and workup [18].

14.2.2 Ultrasonography (US)

14.2.2.1 ATA Guidelines [1]

Certain features found on ultrasound examination are predictive of malignancy and may guide FNAB decision-making (Table 14.1) [1].

Ultrasound-guided FNA of sonographically suspicious LNs ≥8–10 mm in the smallest diameter should be performed to confirm malignancy. The addition of FNA-Tg washout in the evaluation of suspicious cervical LNs is appropriate in selected patients, but interpretation may be difficult in patients with an intact thyroid gland.

Table 14.1 Ultrasound features of thyroid neoplasms according to ATA guidelines

Thyroid neoplasms	Characteristic ultrasound features
Papillary thyroid carcinoma (PTC)	Solid or predominantly solid Hypo-echoic Micro-calcifications (highly specific) Infiltrative irregular margins (common) Increased nodular vascularity
Follicular thyroid carcinoma (FTC)/ Oncocytic (Hürthle cell) carcinoma (HCC)	Iso- to hyper-echoic Thick irregular halo
Benign thyroid nodule	Purely cystic nodule Spongiform appearance (aggregation of multiple microcystic components >50% volume)

14.2.2.2 AACE/AME Guidelines [4]

Ultrasound (US) features are used to categorize risk of malignancy and classify nodules as low-risk (US1), intermediate-risk (US2), or high-risk (US3) [18]. Table 14.2 summarizes the US features of US1, US2, and US3, where presence of one or more of the features categorizes the nodule.

14.2.2.3 ETA Guidelines [14]

- Neck US, including the thyroid gland and the central and lateral cervical compartments, should be performed in all patients suspected of nodular thyroid disease. Nodule size, location, US features, and expected risk of malignancy (TIRADS) should be described.
- Doppler imaging, elasto-sonography, and contrast-enhanced US (CEUS) may be considered as ancillary techniques. CEUS may be considered for defining the size and boundaries of the ablated area after minimally invasive procedures.

14.2.3 Non-ultrasound Imaging Modalities

14.2.3.1 Thyroid Scintigraphy

Thyroid scintigraphy allows the assessment of regional thyroid function and the detection of functioning nodules [19, 20]. Radionuclide thyroid scanning may be considered in patients with low TSH or, in patients with multiple nodules, to determine the functional status of the nodules; hyperfunctional nodules are less commonly associated with malignancy [1].

Table 14.2 AACE/AME categories of risk of malignancy (ROM) by ultrasound (US) features

Ultrasound category	Characteristic features
US1 (low-risk)	Spongiform composition (uniformly microcystic) Margins: smooth, ill-defined, or unable to be determined Oval or round shape Nodule cystic and anechoic Nodule solid or mixed and marked hyper-echoic Nodule solid or mixed and hyper-echoic Nodule solid or mixed and isoechoic and <20 mm and lacking any US2 or US3 features
US2 (intermediate risk)	Echogenic foci that include intra-modular macro-calcifications, peripheral rim calcifications, those difficult to characterize Irregular margin with protrusion into adjacent thyroid tissue Nodule solid or mixed and solid component is hypoechoic Nodule is solid or mixed and isoechoic and either >20 mm or displaying ≥1 intermediate-risk feature and lacking any US3 features
US3 (high risk)	Margin: spiculated or with sharp angles Profoundly hypoechoic Microcalcifications Shape: taller than wide

US ultrasound

For routine use, most often ^{99m}Tc is used, based on a combination of low cost, wide availability, and low radiation burden. However, in a minority, this approach may lead to the misclassification of hypofunctioning as hyperfunctioning nodules [19].

ATA [1], NCCN [2], AACE/AME [4], and ETA [14] Guidelines

- Radionuclide imaging is recommended if the cytology report documents a follicular neoplasm, especially in patients with a low TSH level or in the low-normal range.
- No radionuclide scan is needed for a reading of "suspicious of PTC" or "Hürthle cell neoplasm," as either lobectomy or total thyroidectomy (TT) is recommended, depending on the nodule size and risk factors [1].

ETA Guidelines [14]

- Thyroid scintigraphy should be performed when serum TSH is suppressed or at the lower normal limits. Of note, in areas of current or previous iodine deficiency, hyperfunctioning nodules may also be seen in individuals with normal TSH, meriting the use of thyroid scintigraphy [21, 22].
- Thyroid scintigraphy provides useful information in (1) solitary hyperfunctioning nodules, to avoid FNAB, as hyperfunctioning nodules are rarely malignant, and (2) multinodular goiter (MNG), to differentiate hypofunctioning nodules suitable for FNA from hyperfunctioning lesions that do not need cytological evaluation; to determine the eligibility for radioactive iodine (RAI) therapy.

14.2.3.2 Other Non-ultrasound Imaging Modalities

ATA Guidelines [1]

- Preoperative computed tomography (CT) scan or magnetic resonance imaging (MRI) with IV contrast is recommended as an adjunct to US for patients with clinical suspicion for advanced disease, including invasive primary tumor, or clinically apparent multiple or bulky LN involvement.
- Routine preoperative ^{18}FDG-PET scanning is *not* recommended.

ETA Guidelines [14]

- While there is no indication for initial evaluation of nodular thyroid disease using cross-sectional (i.e., contrast-enhanced CT and magnetic resonance imaging (MRI)) or functional (e.g., [^{18}F]FDG-PET/CT) studies, incidentally detected thyroid lesions do have a risk of malignancy (ROM) of 5–13% when using CT scan and MRI and of about 35% of high activity lesions when using [^{18}F]FDG-PET/CT [23].
- Neck and upper mediastinal CT scan should be performed in case of US or clinical suspicion of substernal extension. If using contrast media, the risk of thyrotoxicosis should be considered. The aim is to assess the extension into the upper mediastinum, the location and dimensions of the trachea, and the anatomical relation of the goiter to the esophagus [24].

ESMO Guidelines [3]

- In addition to ultrasonography, other imaging studies should be ordered if locoregional and/or distant metastases are known to be present or suspected [1].
- A whole body scan (WBS) can be carried out after the administration of diagnostic or therapeutic doses of radioactive iodine (RAI). Because its sensitivity is low (27–55%), diagnostic WBS is *not* indicated during follow-up [25]. Uptake is highly specific (91–100%) for the presence of thyroid tissue, but false-positive results are possible. In these cases, single-photon emission computed tomography or computed tomography (CT) scan offers better anatomical resolution [25].
- FDG–PET combined with CT is useful for assessing the extent of disease and defining the prognosis [26, 27]. Its sensitivity is around 94%, and specificity is between 80% and 84%. FDG–PET is more sensitive than therapeutic WBS for detecting persistent disease in patients with negative cross-sectional imaging studies, serum Tg levels >10 ng/dL, and/or aggressive histotypes (e.g., wiHCC) [28]. FDG–PET is the first-line isotopic imaging technique for patients with RAI-refractory disease.
- Cross-sectional imaging modalities should be chosen on the basis of the anatomical region to be explored. The best for neck and chest imaging is CT scan. Contrast enhancement is used for studies of the neck and mediastinal LNs, but *not* for the lungs. Contrast-enhanced MRI is appropriate for exploring the neck, liver, bones, and brain [25]. MRI of the neck is subject to substantial image degradation due to respiratory motion, and a CT scan is often a better alternative. Suspected aero-digestive-tract involvement should always be assessed endoscopically.

14.2.4 Thyroid Biopsy

14.2.4.1 Ultrasound Guidance

ATA Guidelines [1]

ATA guidelines state that FNAB provides the most economical and accurate methodology for diagnosing differentiated thyroid cancer (DTCs). Due to potential false negatives or sampling error, it is recommended that FNAB procedures be performed under ultrasound (US) guidance. US guidance is particularly important for nodules located posteriorly and for those that are difficult to palpate.

ETA Guidelines [14]

Ultrasound guidance and the use of either capillary action or suction is recommended when performing thyroid nodule FNA.

14.2.4.2 Clinical Indications of FNA

AACE/AME Guidelines [4]

The AACE/AME guidelines use clinical criteria to guide consideration of fine needle aspiration (FNA). Features that argue against performing FNA are termed clinical 1; those that favor FNA are termed clinical 2 as shown in Table 14.3 [18].

14.2.4.3 Nodular Size

Decisions to aspirate thyroid nodules should be guided by lesion size and sonographic appearance [1]. Although all the guidelines recommend FNAB as the procedure of choice in the evaluation of solid thyroid nodules, there is variance in the size of the nodule as an indication for FNAB [1–4].

Recommended indications of FNAB according to size of the thyroid nodule are listed in Table 14.4.

14.2.4.4 Cytological Results and Risk of Malignancy

Cytology findings are classified into diagnostic categories associated with different risks of malignancy [29]. The most appropriate cytological evaluation and classification of malignancy risk is "The Bethesda System for Reporting Thyroid Cytopathology" (TBSRTC 2023), which comprises the following categories with the risk of malignancy (ROM) represented as "mean" percentage [15] (Table 14.5).

Table 14.3 Clinical features that argue against or favor fine-needle aspiration (FNA)

Clinical category	Feature(s) (one or more)
Clinical 1 (features arguing against performing FNA)	Low thyrotropin level in a patient not taking thyroid hormone Autonomous nodule on imaging Prior benign FNA of the same nodule Other medical conditions that take precedence History of prior lobectomy with vocal cord paralysis Significant comorbidity making thyroid surgery a high risk of complications Limited life expectancy (<1 year)
Clinical 2 (features favoring performing FNA)	History of head and neck radiation Compressive symptoms such as dysphonia, dysphagia, or dyspnea without another cause Nodule position posterior or adjacent to the thyroid capsule or trachea History of documented nodule growth History of progressive growth (i.e., ≥50% increase in volume in ≤1 year, especially of the solid component, or 20% increase in one dimension) History of sudden enlargement Planned thyroid or parathyroid surgery Cosmetic concerns Patient preference or anxiety Protocol requiring documentation of cancer

FNA fine-needle aspiration

Table 14.4 Indications of FNAB according to the size of the thyroid nodule

Association/organization	Nodular size
American Thyroid Association (ATA) [1]	>0.5 cm in diameter
European Society for Medical Oncology (ESMO) [3]	>1 cm in diameter
National Comprehensive Cancer Network (NCCN) [2]	Nodules ≥1 cm if suspicious sonographic features are present Nodules ≥1.5 cm for moderately suspicious nodules Nodules ≥2.5 cm for mildly suspicious nodules
European Thyroid Association (ETA) [4]	Lesions ≥10 mm with high-risk US features (EU-TIRADS 5) Lesions ≥20 mm with intermediate-risk US features (EU-TIRADS 4) Lesions >20 mm with low-risk US features, but that are increasing in size or associated with a risk history and before thyroid surgery or minimally invasive ablation therapy (EU-TIRADS 3)

FNAB fine-needle aspiration biopsy, *US* ultrasound, *EU-TIRADS* European Union-Thyroid Imaging, Reporting and Data System

Table 14.5 Categories of The Bethesda System for Reporting Thyroid Cytopathology and the risk of malignancy (ROM)

Category	Description (nomenclature)	Mean ROM
I	Nondiagnostic	13%
II	Benign	4%
III	Atypia of unknown significance (AUS)	22%
IV	Follicular neoplasm	30%
V	Suspicious for malignancy	74%
VI	Malignant	97%

ROM risk of malignancy

14.2.4.5 Other Recommendations

ATA Guidelines [1]

- For cytology "diagnostic of" or "suspicious of" PTC cancer, surgery is recommended.
- If FNAB cytology is "indeterminate," the use of molecular markers such as *BRAF, RAS, RET/PTC, Pax8-PPARγ,* or *galectin-3* may be considered to guide management.
- An iodine-123 (^{123}I) thyroid scan may be considered if the cytology report documents a "follicular neoplasm" (Bethesda IV), especially if serum TSH is in the low-normal range. No radionuclide scan is needed for a reading of "suspicious of PTC" or "oncocytic/Hürthle cell neoplasm," as either lobectomy or total thyroidectomy is recommended depending on the nodule size and risk factors.

NCCN Guidelines [2]

The NCCN recommends FNAB as the primary test for differentiated thyroid cancer (DTC). If FNAB reveals PTC, follicular neoplasm, or oncocytic/HCC, the following diagnostic recommendations should be undertaken for oncocytic/HCC:

- Thyroid and neck US (including central and lateral compartments) if *not* previously done
- CT/MRI with contrast for fixed, bulky, or sub-sternal lesions
- Consider evaluation of vocal cord mobility
- Consider molecular diagnostics such as *BRAF, RAS, RET/PTC, Pax8-PPARγ*, or *galectin-3*
- Screen for personal and/or family history suggestive of inherited cancer risk

ESMO Guidelines [3]

Diagnosis with FNA can be facilitated by assessment of "malignancy markers" (including proteins commonly over-expressed in tumors, e.g., *HBME1* or *galectin-3*) and molecular alterations specifically associated with malignancy such as BRAF mutations, *RET* fusions, and other novel gene alterations. Specifically designed gene panels are reportedly useful for identifying malignancy when cytology samples are morphologically indeterminate [30].

ETA Guidelines [14]

- Combine clinical factors, laboratory evaluation, and US risk stratification when defining the indication for FNA, in a shared decision with the patient.
- FNA should be repeated in case of (1) a first nondiagnostic sample [31], (2) a Bethesda class III cytology (AUS) [32], and (3) discrepancy between US risk score (i.e., high risk) and cytological findings (i.e., benign cytology).
- FNA is recommended in suspicious LNs, with thyroglobulin (Tg) or calcitonin washout dependent on phenotype.
- Core-needle biopsy (CNB), performed with a large bore spring-activated device, may provide a micro-histological sample from thyroid lesions. There are no clear advantages of using CNB, a more invasive and expensive procedure compared to FNA, based on cost and risk–benefit analysis [33]. Thus, CNB should *not* be used as a first-line tool to assess thyroid nodules after US, but could be considered a second-line procedure for specific conditions as follows; (1) repeat inadequate FNA as an alternative to diagnostic surgery [34], repeat Bethesda class III cytology (AUS) [35], and (3) when histological assessment can improve preoperative diagnosis (e.g., suspicion of poorly differentiated thyroid cancer (PDTC), anaplastic thyroid cancer (ATC), thyroid lymphoma, or thyroid metastases) [36].

14.3 Therapeutic Guidelines

14.3.1 Clinical Surveillance

14.3.1.1 NCCN Guidelines [2]

As per the NCCN guidelines, when "molecular testing" is performed on thyroid lesions, (i.e., low-suspicion Bethesda III or IV), those lesions that show benign characteristics can be followed-up with surveillance. If the molecular diagnostics are not informative, or the sample is insufficient or degraded, then nodule surveillance, lobectomy in select situations, or repeat biopsy may be considered.

14.3.1.2 ETA Guidelines [14]

The majority of benign thyroid nodules are asymptomatic and diagnosed incidentally [37]. In the absence of elevated TSH, the use of thyroid hormone in order to decrease TSH level should be discouraged not only to limit the increased morbidity and mortality seen with such therapy [38, 39], but mainly because of its inefficacy in adequately decreasing size in symptomatic nodules [40].

Deficiency of iodine and selenium is associated with increased goiter prevalence. However, neither iodine [4] nor selenium supplementation [41] is recommended in iodine and selenium replete populations.

During 1 year, significant growth, defined as an increase ≥20% in at least two nodule diameters with a minimum increase of 2 mm, or nodule volume increase >50%, occur only in a minority of cases reaching 16% over a period of 5 years [42]. Thus, "asymptomatic" nodules should be followed based on the sonographic pattern and cytological assessment.

14.3.2 Surgery

14.3.2.1 ATA Guidelines [1]

Recommendations According to FNA Results

The ATA does *not* have comprehensive guidelines for the treatment of FTC and oncocytic/HCC as separate entities from PTC; however, there are several individual recommendations that apply decision-making principles to these conditions [1].

The ATA recommends that if cytology readings report a follicular neoplasm (Bethesda IV), an ^{123}I thyroid scan may be considered, especially if serum TSH is in a low-normal range. If a concordant autonomously functioning nodule is not seen, lobectomy or total thyroidectomy (TT) should be considered.

If the cytology report indicates "oncocytic/HCN" or "suspicious for PTC," the ATA recommends a lobectomy or thyroidectomy, depending on nodule size and other risk factors. For patients with an isolated "indeterminate" ("follicular neoplasm" or "oncocytic/HCN") solitary nodule, a more limited approach is preferred; the ATA recommends an initial lobectomy.

The ATA recommends a total thyroidectomy (TT) for patients with "indeterminate nodules" in any of the following situations:

- The tumor exceeds 4 cm.
- Marked atypia is observed.
- Biopsy result is reported as "suspicious for PTC" (Bethesda V).
- The patient has a family history of thyroid carcinoma.
- The patient has a history of radiation exposure.

The ATA recommends that patients with "indeterminate nodules" who have bilateral nodular disease or who wish to avoid future surgery should undergo TT or near-TT [1].

Operative Approach Recommendations of ATA

- For patients with thyroid cancer >4 cm, or with gross extra-thyroidal extension (ETE) (cT4), or clinically apparent metastatic disease to nodes (cN1) or distant sites (cM1), the initial surgical procedure should be total thyroidectomy (TT).
- For patients with thyroid cancer >1 and <4 cm without ETE, and without clinical evidence of any LN metastases (cN0), the initial surgical procedure can be either a bilateral procedure (near-total or TT) or a unilateral procedure (lobectomy). Thyroid lobectomy alone may be sufficient initial treatment for low-risk PTC and FTC; however, the treatment team may choose TT to enable RAI therapy or to enhance follow-up based upon disease features and/or patient preferences.
- If surgery is chosen for patients with thyroid cancer <1 cm without ETE and cN0, the initial surgical procedure should be a "thyroid lobectomy" unless there are clear indications to remove the contralateral lobe. Thyroid lobectomy alone is sufficient treatment for small, unifocal, intrathyroidal carcinomas in the absence of prior head and neck radiation, familial thyroid carcinoma, or clinically detectable cervical nodal metastases.
- "Therapeutic" central-compartment (level VI) neck dissection for patients with clinically involved central LNs should accompany TT to provide clearance of disease from the central neck.
- "Prophylactic" central-compartment neck dissection (ipsilateral or bilateral) should be considered in patients with PTC with clinically uninvolved central neck LNs (cN0) who have advanced primary tumors (T3 or T4) or clinically involved lateral neck nodes (cN1b).
- Thyroidectomy *without* prophylactic central neck dissection is appropriate for small (T1 or T2), noninvasive, clinically node-negative PTC (cN0) and for most follicular cancers.
- Therapeutic lateral neck compartmental LN dissection should be performed for patients with biopsy-proven metastatic lateral cervical lymphadenopathy.

Completion Thyroidectomy

- Completion thyroidectomy should be offered to patients for whom a bilateral thyroidectomy would have been recommended had the diagnosis been available

before the initial surgery. Therapeutic central neck LN dissection should be included if the LNs are clinically involved. Thyroid lobectomy alone may be sufficient treatment for low-risk PTCs and FTCs.
- Radioactive iodine (RAI) ablation in lieu of completion thyroidectomy is *not* recommended routinely; however, it may be used to ablate the remnant lobe in selected cases.

14.3.2.2 NCCN Guidelines [2]

According to the NCCN guidelines, the treatment of choice of primary DTC is surgery, whenever possible, followed by RAI (^{131}I) in selected patients and thyrotropin suppression in most patients [2, 43].

The NCCN guidelines recommend lobectomy plus isthmusectomy as the initial surgery for patients with follicular neoplasms and oncocytic/HCCs, with prompt completion of thyroidectomy if pathology reports widely invasive cancer or encapsulated angioinvasive disease involving ≥4 vessels. Therapeutic neck dissection of involved compartments is recommended for clinically apparent/biopsy-proven disease [2].

The NCCN recommends total thyroidectomy (TT) as the initial procedure only if invasive cancer or metastatic disease is apparent at the time or surgery, or if the patient wishes to avoid a second, completion thyroidectomy should the pathological review reveal cancer [2].

14.3.2.3 ESMO Guidelines [3]

While ESMO guidelines consider thyroidectomy to be standard of care for other thyroid tumors, they recommend proposing active ultrasound surveillance of every 6–12 months for unifocal papillary micro-carcinomas (≤10 mm) with no evidence of extracapsular extension (ETE) or LN involvement. Lobectomy (instead of TT) may be proposed for selected low-risk (T1a–T1b–T2, N0) tumors [3].

14.3.2.4 ETA Guidelines [14]

Surgery for thyroid nodules may be appropriate in the following situation [13, 44–46]:

- Symptomatic nodular thyroid disease, as an alternative option to minimally invasive techniques (MITs) and RAI therapy.
- Nodules that have been classified as benign at cytology and/or low risk at US (i.e., EU-TIRADS 2 or 3) and become symptomatic over time.
- Nodules with indeterminate cytology (Bethesda classes III and IV) that are *not* suitable for active surveillance (i.e., large size, high suspicion of malignancy on US, symptomatology).
- Nodules with a Bethesda class V and VI cytology.

For nodules of uncertain malignant potential (Bethesda class III–V cytology), surgery allows for a definitive diagnosis [13]. Molecular test results (if available) should be considered prior to operation [47]. For diseases limited to one lobe, lobectomy/hemithyroidectomy is recommended. If such a disease is diagnosed in a nodular goiter, near-total thyroidectomy or total thyroidectomy (TT) should be considered.

In benign lesions (Bethesda II), even if asymptomatic, surgical treatment may be considered for nodules ≥4 cm (due to the risk of malignancy (ROM) and increased probability of a false negative FNA) [48, 49], symptomatic nodules (airway or esophagus compression), in case of cosmetic concern, and retro-clavicular and mediastinal extension. Surgery is one of the available therapeutic options, besides RAI and MIT, for hyperfunctioning nodules and toxic multinodular goiter (MNG) [50].

14.3.3 Minimally Invasive Techniques

14.3.3.1 ETA Guidelines [14]

Minimally invasive techniques (MITs) are out-patient procedures, performed under Ultrasound guidance, for "non-surgical" management of thyroid lesions that cause local pressure symptoms or esthetic concerns [51, 52]. They include ethanol ablation (EA), based on the direct injection of ethanol into a cystic cavity, and thermal ablation (TA) techniques, which use various energy sources; namely, laser, radio frequency, micro-waves, or high-intensity focused ultrasound [51]. MITs result in a relevant and long-lasting decrease of nodule volume (57–77% at 5 years) that is paralleled by improvement of local symptoms [53, 54] and disease-related quality of life [55]. These treatments do *not* require general anesthesia, rarely cause complications, and even more rarely thyroid dysfunction [51].

While ethanol ablation (EA) is preferred as an effective, safe, and inexpensive treatment for cystic (or predominantly cystic) symptomatic thyroid nodules [56], thermal ablation (TA) procedures, due to their geometric and predictable volume of tissue destruction, are the first-line treatment for solid thyroid lesions [51]. Thermal ablation treatments should aim at a balance between nearly complete nodule destruction, to prevent late regrowth, and sparing of at-risk areas, to minimize the risk of complications. TA is an alternative to RAI and surgery in small hyperfunctioning nodules (<10 mL), while it performs poorer in larger nodules [57]. In such cases, TA may be considered for patients who decline or are not candidates for RAI therapy or surgery. Currently, a major limitation of TA procedure use is their limited availability and lack of long-term data [58].

14.3.4 Radioactive Iodine (RAI) Therapy

RAI is administered after TT for several reasons: (1) to eliminate the normal thyroid remnant, thereby ensuring undetectable serum Tg levels (in the absence of neoplastic tissue), which facilitate follow-up (remnant ablation), (2) to irradiate presumed foci of neoplastic cells, thereby reducing the recurrence risk (adjuvant therapy); and/or (3) to treat persistent or recurrent disease (treatment of known disease) [1].

In all three cases, RAI administration must be followed by an iodine-131 (^{131}I) whole-body scan (WBS) to stage the disease and document the ^{131}I avidity of any structural lesion. The expected benefits of a given RAI dose should outweigh the risks associated with its administration, which include adverse events and diminished quality of life [59].

14.3.4.1 ATA Guidelines [1]

Indications of Radioactive Iodine (RAI) Therapy

Radioactive Iodine RAI remnant ablation is *not* routinely recommended after thyroidectomy for ATA *low-risk* DTC patients. The ATA recommendations of RAI therapy are as follows:

RAI is recommended for "all patients" if any of the following is present:

- Distant metastases
- Extra-thyroid extension (ETE) of the tumor regardless of tumor size
- Primary tumor size >4 cm even in the absence of other higher-risk features.

RAI therapy is "selectively" recommended for the following:

- Patients with 1–4 cm thyroid cancers confined to the thyroid who have documented LN metastases or other higher risk features
- When the combination of age, tumor size, LN status, and individual histology predicts an intermediate to high risk of recurrence or death from thyroid cancer.

RAI therapy is "not" recommended for the following:

- Patients with unifocal cancer <1 cm without other higher-risk features
- Patients with multifocal cancer when all foci are <1 cm in the absence of other higher-risk features.

Role of Adjunctive External Beam Radiation Therapy (EBRT) or Chemotherapy

- There is *no* role for routine adjuvant EBRT to the neck in patients with DTC after initial complete surgical removal of the tumor.
- There is *no* role for routine systemic adjuvant therapy in patients with DTC (beyond RAI and/or TSH suppressive therapy using LT_4).

14.3.4.2 NCCN Guidelines [2]

If RAI imaging shows no uptake, the NCCN recommends monitoring disease versus external beam radiation therapy (EBRT)/Intensity-modulated radiation therapy (IMRT). Radiation therapy can be considered upfront for patients with viscerally invasive or rapid progression. If RAI uptake is present, RAI treatment is preferred, followed by posttreatment ^{131}I whole body imaging.

NCCN guidelines recommend RAI (^{131}I) therapy if *any* of the following criteria are present [2]:

- Extra-thyroidal extension (ETE)
- Tumor >4 cm in diameter
- Postoperative unstimulated thyroglobulin (Tg) level >5–10 ng/mL

RAI therapy is "not" recommended if *all* of the following are present [2]:

- Classic PTC
- Primary tumor <1 cm
- Intrathyroidal tumor
- Unifocal or multifocal tumor
- No detectable anti-Tg antibodies
- Postoperative unstimulated Tg < 1 ng/mL

RAI therapy is "selectively" recommended if *any* of the following is present when the combination of clinical factors predicts a significant risk of recurrence [2]:

- Primary tumor 1–4 cm in size
- High-risk histology
- Lympho vascular invasion
- Cervical LN metastases
- Macroscopic multifocality (one focus >1 cm)
- Presence of anti-Tg antibodies
- Postoperative unstimulated Tg < 5–10 ng/mL

14.3.4.3 ESMO Guidelines [3]

- The estimated level of risk for persistent/recurrent disease will determine whether and how much RAI is given. According to ESMO guidelines, low activities are usually given for remnant ablation (30 mCi, 1.1 GBq); high activities (≥100 mCi, 3.7 GBq) are used for treatment purposes. To optimize isotope uptake, RAI should be given after TSH stimulation, which can be achieved by withdrawing levothyroxine for 4–5 weeks, ideally until serum TSH levels reach ≥30 μIU/mL. Alternatively, recombinant human TSH (rhTSH) can be given (two daily injections of 0.9 mg of rhTSH followed by RAI on day 3). The resulting TSH level is not usually measured (unless doubts arise as to whether the injections have been properly administered). Levothyroxine withdrawal is preferred if distant metastases are present. The use of rhTSH is associated with superior short-term quality of life [60].
- Practice guidelines unanimously recommend treatment with high RAI activities (≥100 mCi, 3.7 GBq) for patients with high-risk of recurrence [1, 7, 61–63]. RAI administration is *not* recommended for certain low-risk patients [i.e., those with a small (≤1 cm) intrathyroidal DTC and no evidence of locoregional metastases]

[59]. The term "very low-risk" is often applied to these patients in the literature [61, 64]. There is less consensus regarding other low-risk DTC patients.
– Repeat RAI administrations every 6–12 months as long as RAI uptake is present. Carry out cross-sectional imaging between RAI administrations to insure RAI efficacy. Repeating RAI administrations after a cumulative activity of 600 mCi should be given on a per-patient basis [3].

14.3.4.4 ETA Guidelines [14]

Approximately 5–10% of solitary/dominant thyroid nodules are functioning on thyroid scintigraphy, with suppression of the peri-nodular thyroid tissue. Such nodules are, with extremely rare exceptions, benign, should not be biopsied, and are eligible for RAI treatment. Most patients are euthyroid or subclinically hyperthyroid at the time of diagnosis [65]. Unless severely hyperthyroid or with cardiac comorbidity, individuals rarely need pretreatment with antithyroid drugs (ATDs). RAI is most often given as a fixed activity (e.g., 185–370 MBq), most often achieves euthyroidism, may cause hypothyroidism, and reduces nodule size by 30–50% in 12 months [66]. Life-long follow-up is recommended.

Symptomatic and benign thyroid nodules may, as an alternative to surgery, be eligible for RAI, especially in case of patients at surgical risk. Most patients are offered fixed activity RAI, dependent on local regulations. Hypothyroidism is rare (10–20% after 10 years), but life-long follow-up is recommended. Thyroid volume is typically reduced by 40% within 12 months and alleviates symptoms in most. In case of low RAI uptake and/or a large goiter, pre-stimulation with rhTSH has been demonstrated to augment thyroid volume reduction by 35% [67] and increases the smallest cross-sectional area of the trachea, improves pulmonary function, and reduces pressure symptoms [68].

14.3.5 Levothyroxine Therapy

14.3.5.1 ATA [1] and NCCN Guidelines [2]

The ATA [1] and NCCN [2] Guidelines recommend postoperative treatment with levothyroxine to suppress TSH level maintaining normal or low TSH, and to measure Tg and anti-Tg antibodies 6–12 weeks postoperatively. In patients with gross residual disease, TSH suppression therapy should be delayed until completion of RAI workup and treatment if indicated. The degree of suppression is based on risk of "recurrence," as follows [1, 2]:

– Low-risk: Maintenance of TSH at or slightly below the lower limit of normal (0.1–0.5 mU/L).
– Intermediate-risk: Initial TSH suppression to <0.1 mU/L.
– High-risk: Initial TSH suppression to <0.1 mU/L.

The NCCN Guidelines [2] recommend that in patients who remain disease-free for several years, TSH levels can probably be maintained within the reference range

(0.5–2 mU/L). For gross residual disease, patients can undergo measurement of TSH, Tg, and anti-Tg antibodies at 6–12 weeks or undergo ^{123}I or ^{131}I total body imaging with TSH stimulation. The latter is preferred for viscerally invasive or rapidly progressing disease.

14.3.6 Follow-Up Strategies

14.3.6.1 ATA Guidelines [1]

For patients whose recurrence risk is initially classified as high, a more in-depth imaging workup may be advisable even if serum Tg levels remain or become undetectable, as the absence of the circulating Tg may simply reflect the dedifferentiation of any residual tumor tissue that might be present [1]. Serum TSH levels should be suppressed in all patients with biochemical incomplete or indeterminate responses to treatment (0.1–0.5 μIU/ml) [1]. Patients with structural incomplete responses can be placed on active surveillance or referred for local or systemic treatments.

14.3.6.2 ESMO Guidelines [3]

All patients with DTC including oncocytic/Hürthle cell carcinoma (HCC) should have a neck US and serum Tg and TgAb assays 6–18 months after primary treatment (surgery ± RAI therapy). The subsequent follow-up schedule will depend on the initially estimated risk of persistent/recurrent disease and responses to therapy.

In patients with wiHCC (or high-risk PTCs, or PDTC), serum Tg and TgAb levels should be assessed every 6–12 months if the response to therapy is excellent or biochemical indeterminate/incomplete. Cross-sectional or functional imaging studies should be repeated if detectable Tg levels persist [69, 70].

14.3.7 Treatment of Recurrent/Metastatic Disease

14.3.7.1 ATA Guidelines [1]

Distant metastases occur in fewer than 10% of patients with DTC. Approximately, 50% are present when the tumor is first discovered; the others are found later, sometimes decades after initial treatment. Metastases are observed most frequently in patients with aggressive histological subtypes, vascular invasion, large primary tumors, macroscopic ETE, and bulky locoregional nodal disease [1]. The most common sites are lungs and bones (49% and 25% of all cases, respectively), and in 15% of cases, both are affected [71]. The overall mortality rates 5 and 10 years after diagnosis of distant metastases are 65% and 75%, respectively [72].

Distant metastases are usually diagnosed because of clinical symptoms or suspicious imaging/laboratory findings (abnormal uptake on a post-ablation WBS, or a positive finding on an FDG–PET-CT scan or a cross-sectional study prompted by elevated Tg levels in patients whose post-ablation WBS is negative).

According to the ATA Guidelines [1], radioactive iodine (RAI) therapy is recommended for "all patients" with metastatic disease. EBRT and systemic therapy are considered in selected cases.

14.3.7.2 NCCN Guidelines [2]

The NCCN recommendations for treatment of recurrent or metastatic thyroid disease include EBRT, with consideration of systemic therapy for tumors that have all the following characteristics [2]:

- Not resectable
- Not responsive to RAI therapy
- Not amenable to EBRT
- Showing significant disease progression

Oral kinase inhibitors (e.g., vandetanib) are associated with longer progression-free survival, but are *not* curative; adverse effects that may have a significant effect on quality of life should be considered. Kinase inhibitor therapy may *not* be appropriate for symptomatic patients with indolent disease [2].

For recurrent disease and widely metastatic disease, the tumor should be evaluated for actionable mutations such as*ALK, NTRK, RET* gene fusions, DNA mismatch repair (dMMR), micro-satellite instability (MSI), and tumor mutational burden (TMB). This may guide use of targeted therapy [2].

14.3.7.3 ESMO Guidelines [3]

The ESMO recommendations for treatment of recurrent or metastatic thyroid disease include RAI, EBRT, with the consideration of systemic therapy [3].

RAI Therapy

ESMO guidelines recommend that patients with distant metastases should receive 100–200 mCi (3.7–7.4 GBq) of ^{131}I after TSH stimulation with levothyroxine withdrawal (or with injections of rhTSH) [71]. If the distant metastases are RAI-avid, ^{131}I is administered every 6 months for 2 years and less frequently thereafter. Between treatments, suppressive doses of levothyroxine are given to maintain serum TSH levels below 0.1 μIU/mL [73–75].

Systemic Therapy

The treatment strategy should be based on multiple factors, including symptoms, tumor burden, lesion characteristics, and disease progression. Temporal trends in the levels of serum tumor markers (e.g., Tg doubling time) can be used to support and help decision-making [76]. Importantly, however, an increase in serum Tg levels in the absence of radiologically evident disease progression should not be used to select patients requiring systemic therapy. A complete cross-sectional imaging assessment of the extent of the disease is mandatory for any treatment decisions.

The imaging assessment should be repeated every 3–12 weeks during treatment. Reductions in serum Tg are expected in responders, but clinical decisions cannot be based on this parameter alone.

14.3.8 Treatment of Thyroid Nodules and Cancer During Pregnancy

14.3.8.1 ATA Guidelines [1]

During pregnancy and the postpartum, ATA Guidelines include the following recommendations on thyroid nodules and cancer in these patients [77]:

- For women with suppressed serum TSH levels that persist beyond 16 weeks gestation, FNA of a clinically relevant thyroid nodule may be deferred until after pregnancy. At that time, if serum TSH remains suppressed, a radionuclide scan to evaluate nodule function can be performed if the woman is not breastfeeding.
- There is insufficient evidence to recommend for or against routine measurement of serum calcitonin in pregnant women with thyroid nodules.
- Thyroid nodule FNA, based on the nodule's sonographic pattern, is generally recommended for newly detected nodules in pregnant women with a non-suppressed TSH. The decision whether to perform FNA during gestation or early postpartum may be influenced by the clinical assessment of cancer risk or by patient preference.
- Radionuclide scintigraphy or RAI uptake determination should *not* be performed during pregnancy.
- Pregnant women with cytologically benign thyroid nodules do *not* require special surveillance strategies during pregnancy and should be managed according to the ATA guidelines for adults with thyroid nodules and DTC.
- Pregnant women with cytologically "indeterminate" nodules, in the absence of cytologically malignant LNs or other signs of metastatic disease, do not routinely require surgery while pregnant.
- Surgery may be considered during pregnancy if there is clinical suspicion of an aggressive behavior in cytologically indeterminate nodules.
- Molecular testing is *not* recommended for evaluation of cytologically indeterminate nodules during pregnancy.
- Pregnancy should be deferred for 6 months after a woman has received therapeutic RAI treatment.
- In women with thyroid cancer who become pregnant, the TSH goal should remain the same as determined preconception. TSH should be monitored approximately every 4 weeks until 16–20 weeks of gestation, and at least once between 26 and 32 weeks of gestation.

14.4 Concluding Remarks and Future Perspectives

Although very few thyroid nodules are malignant, the possibility of cancer represents the overriding concern when thyroid gland lesions are brought to attention. Neck ultrasound (US) is the central hub in the diagnostic algorithm aimed at stratifying the risk of malignancy (ROM), allowing US-guided FNA, and promoting the individualized management currently advocated. For the vast majority of patients, both tools provide a reliable foundation for defining the initial management strategy, whether follow-up, surgery or nonsurgical treatment with minimally invasive techniques (MITs). However, in a number of cases, the estimates of the ROM will remain uncertain and the subsequent choices unsettled. In such cases, the clinicians' experience and individualized choices based on patient-related factors and preferences represent the way forward. New tools are emerging in clinical practice, such as molecular testing, which are not yet generally available in Europe. While the analytical and clinical validity have been extensively studied, the ability of the molecular analysis to improve patient outcomes sufficiently to justify its incorporation into real-world clinical practice has yet to be proven. Such studies are warranted for years to come.

References

1. Haugen BR, Alexander EK, Bible KC, Doherty GM, Mandel SJ, Nikiforov YE, et al. 2015 American Thyroid Association management guidelines for adult patients with thyroid nodules and differentiated thyroid cancer: the American Thyroid Association guidelines task force on thyroid nodules and differentiated thyroid cancer. Thyroid. 2016;26(1):1–133.
2. NCCN. Clinical practice guidelines in oncology: thyroid carcinoma. National Comprehensive Cancer Network Version 2.2024.
3. Filetti S, Durante C, Hartl D, Leboulleux S, Locati LD, Newbold K, et al. Thyroid cancer: ESMO clinical practice guidelines for diagnosis, treatment and follow-up. Ann Oncol. 2019;30(12):1856–83.
4. Gharib H, Papini E, Garber JR, Duick DS, Harrell RM, Hegedüs L, et al. American Association of Clinical Endocrinologists, American College of Endocrinology, and Associazione Medici Endocrinologi medical guidelines for clinical practice for the diagnosis and management of thyroid nodules—2016 update. Endocr Pract. 2016;5:622–39.
5. Perros P, Boelaert K, Colley S, Evans C, Evans RM, Gerrard Ba G, et al. Guidelines for the management of thyroid cancer. Clin Endocrinol. 2014;Suppl 1:1–122.
6. Trigo JM, Capdevila J, Grande E, Grau J, Lianes P, Spanish Society for Medical Oncology. Thyroid cancer: SEOM clinical guidelines. Clin Transl Oncol. 2014;12:1035–42.
7. Mitchell AL, Gandhi A, Scott-Coombes D, Perros P. Management of thyroid cancer: United Kingdom national multidisciplinary guidelines. J Laryngol Otol. 2016;130(S2):S150–60.
8. Nabhan F, Ringel MD. Thyroid nodules and cancer management guidelines: comparisons and controversies. Endocr Relat Cancer. 2017;24(2):R13–26.
9. Wells SA Jr, Asa SL, Dralle H, Elisei R, Evans DB, Gagel RF, et al. Revised American Thyroid Association guidelines for the management of medullary thyroid carcinoma. Thyroid. 2015;25(6):567–610.

10. Stagnaro-Green A, Abalovich M, Alexander E, Azizi F, Mestman J, Negro R, et al. Guidelines of the American Thyroid Association for the diagnosis and management of thyroid disease during pregnancy and postpartum. Thyroid. 2011;21(10):1081–125.
11. Haugen BR. 2015 American Thyroid Association management guidelines for adult patients with thyroid nodules and differentiated thyroid cancer: what is new and what has changed? Cancer. 2017;123(3):372–81.
12. Bible KC, Kebebew E, Brierley J, Brito JP, Cabanillas ME, Clark TJ Jr, et al. 2021 American Thyroid Association guidelines for management of patients with anaplastic thyroid cancer. Thyroid. 2021;31(3):337–86.
13. Schneider DF, Cherney Stafford LM, Brys N, Greenberg CC, Balentine CJ, Elfenbein DM. Gauging the extent of thyroidectomy for indeterminate thyroid nodules: an oncologic perspective. Endocr Pract. 2017;23(4):442–50.
14. Durante C, Hegedus L, Czarniecka A, Paschke R, Russ G, Schmitt F. 2023 European Thyroid Association clinical practice guidelines for thyroid nodule management. Eur Thyroid J. 2023;12(5):e230067.
15. Ali SZ, Baloch ZW, Cochand-Priollet B, Schmitt FC, Vielh P, VanderLann PA. The 2023 Bethesda system for reporting thyroid cytopathology. Thyroid. 2023;23(9):1039–44.
16. Tessler FN, Middleton WD, Grant EG, Hoang JK, Berland LL, Teefey SA, et al. ACR thyroid imaging, reporting and data system (TI-RADS): white paper of the ACR TI-RADS Committee. J Am Coll Radiol. 2017;14(5):587–95.
17. Baloch ZW, Asa SL, Barletta JA, Ghossein RA, Juhlin CC, Jung CK, et al. Overview of the 2022 WHO classification of thyroid neoplasms. Endocr Pathol. 2022;33(1):27–63.
18. Garber JR, Papini E, Frasoldati A, Lupo MA, Harrell RM, Parangi S, et al. American Association of Clinical Endocrinology and Associazione Medici Endocrinologi thyroid nodule algorithmic tool. Endocr Pract. 2021;27(7):649–60.
19. Giovanella L, Avram AM, Iakovou I, Kwak J, Lawson SA, Lulaj E, et al. EANM practice guideline/SNMMI procedure standard for RAIU and thyroid scintigraphy. Eur J Nucl Med Mol Imaging. 2019;46(12):2514–25.
20. Schenke SA, Görges R, Seifert P, Zimny M, Kreissl MC. Update on diagnosis and treatment of hyperthyroidism: ultrasonography and functional imaging. Q J Nucl Med Mol Imaging. 2021;65(2):102–12.
21. Treglia G, Trimboli P, Verburg FA, Luster M, Giovanella L. Prevalence of normal TSH value among patients with autonomously functioning thyroid nodule. Eur J Clin Investig. 2015;45(7):739–44.
22. Schenke SA, Kreissl MC, Grunert M, Hach A, Haghghi S, Kandror T, et al. Distribution of functional status of thyroid nodules and malignancy rates of hyperfunctioning and hypofunctioning thyroid nodules in Germany. Nuklearmedizin/Nucl Med. 2022;61:376–84.
23. Soelberg KK, Bonnema SJ, Brix TH, Hegedüs L. Risk of malignancy in thyroid incidentalomas detected by 18F-fluorodeoxyglucose positron emission tomography: a systematic review. Thyroid. 2012;22:918–25.
24. Hegedüs L, Bonnema SJ. Approach to management of the patient with primary or secondary intrathoracic goiter. J Clin Endocrinol Metab. 2010;95:5155–62.
25. Lamartina L, Deandreis D, Durante C, Filetti S. Endocrine Tumours: imaging in the follow-up of differentiated thyroid cancer: current evidence and future perspectives for a risk-adapted approach. Eur J Endocrinol. 2016;175(5):R185–202.
26. Leboulleux S, Schroeder PR, Schlumberger M, Ladenson PW. The role of PET in follow-up of patients treated for differentiated epithelial thyroid cancers. Nat Clin Pract Endocrinol Metab. 2007;3(2):112–21.
27. Robbins RJ, Wan Q, Grewal RK, Reibke R, Gonen M, Strauss HW, et al. Real-time prognosis for metastatic thyroid carcinoma based on 2-[18F]fluoro-2-deoxy-D-glucose-positron emission tomography scanning. J Clin Endocrinol Metab. 2006;91(2):498–505.
28. Nascimento C, Borget I, Al Ghuzlan A, Deandreis D, Hartl D, Lumbroso J, et al. Postoperative fluorine-18-fluorodeoxyglucose positron emission tomography/computed tomography: an

important imaging modality in patients with aggressive histology of differentiated thyroid cancer. Thyroid. 2015;25(4):437–44.
29. Cibas ES, Ali SZ, NCI Thyroid FNA State of the Science Conference. The Bethesda system for reporting thyroid cytopathology. Am J Clin Pathol. 2009;132(5):658–65.
30. Nikiforova MN, Mercurio S, Wald AI, Barbi de Moura M, Callenberg K, Santana-Santos L, et al. Analytical performance of the ThyroSeq v3 genomic classifier for cancer diagnosis in thyroid nodules. Cancer. 2018;124(8):1682–90.
31. Ferreira MA, Gerhard R, Schmitt F. Analysis of nondiagnostic results in a large series of thyroid fine-needle aspiration cytology performed over 9 years in a single center. Acta Cytol. 2014;58:229–34.
32. Bayona A, Benavent P, Muriel A, Abuchaibe C, Sharpe SC, Tarasova V, et al. Outcomes of repeat fineneedle aspiration biopsy for AUS/FLUS thyroid nodules. Eur J Endocrinol. 2021;185:497–506.
33. Appukutty SJ, Paterson A, Patel NS, Duckworth A, Chan J, O'Donovan M, et al. Thyroid diagnostic modalities (fine needle aspiration and core needle biopsy) with histology correlation: a tertiary centre experience. J Clin Pathol. 2022;75:620–6.
34. Wolinski K, Stangierski A, Ruchala M. Comparison of diagnostic yield of core-needle and fine-needle aspiration biopsies of thyroid lesions: systematic review and meta-analysis. Eur Radiol. 2017;27:431–6.
35. Choi YJ, Baek JH, Suh CH, Shim WH, Jeong B, Kim JK, et al. Core-needle biopsy versus repeat fine-needle aspiration for thyroid nodules initially read as atypia/follicular lesion of undetermined significance. Head Neck. 2017;39:361–9.
36. Matrone A, De Napoli L, Torregrossa L, Aghababyan A, Papini P, Ambrosini CE, et al. Core needle biopsy can early and precisely identify large thyroid masses. Front Oncol. 2022;12:854755.
37. Grani G, Sponziello M, Pecce V, Ramundo V, Durante C. Contemporary thyroid nodule evaluation and management. J Clin Endocrinol Metab. 2020;105:2869–83.
38. Lillevang-Johansen M, Abrahamsen B, Jørgensen HL, Brix TH, Hegedüs L. Excess mortality in treated and untreated hyperthyroidism is related to cumulative periods of low serum TSH. J Clin Endocrinol Metab. 2017;102:2301–9.
39. Lillevang-Johansen M, Abrahamsen B, Jørgensen HL, Brix TH, Hegedüs L. Duration of over- and under-treatment of hypothyroidism is associated with increased cardiovascular risk. Eur J Endocrinol. 2019;180:407–16.
40. Bennedbæk FN, Nielsen LK, Hegedüs L. Effect of percutaneous ethanol injection therapy versus suppressive doses of L-thyroxine on benign solitary solid cold thyroid nodules: a randomized trial. J Clin Endocrinol Metab. 1998;83:830–5.
41. Winther KH, Rayman MP, Bonnema SJ, Hegedüs L. Selenium in thyroid disorders – essential knowledge for clinicians. Nat Rev Endocrinol. 2020;16:165–76.
42. Durante C, Costante G, Lucisano G, Bruno R, Meringolo D, Paciaroni A, et al. The natural history of benign thyroid nodules. JAMA. 2015;313:926–35.
43. Stojadinovic A, Ghossein RA, Hoos A, Urist MJ, Spiro RH, Shah JP. Hürthle cell carcinoma: a critical histopathologic appraisal. J Clin Oncol. 2001;19(10):2616–25.
44. Guan SH, Wang H, Teng DK. Comparison of ultrasound-guided thermal ablation and conventional thyroidectomy for benign thyroid nodules: a systematic review and meta-analysis. Int J Hyperth. 2020;37(1):442–9.
45. Jin H, Lin W, Lu L, Cui M. Conventional thyroidectomy vs thyroid thermal ablation on postoperative quality of life and satisfaction for patients with benign thyroid nodules. Eur J Endocrinol. 2021;184:131–41.
46. Paparodis RD, Karvounis E, Bantouna D, Chourpiliadis C, Hourpiliadi H, Livadas S, et al. Large, slowly growing, benign thyroid nodules frequently coexist with synchronous thyroid cancers. J Clin Endocrinol Metab. 2022;107:e3474–8.
47. Krasner JR, Alyouha N, Pusztaszeri M, Forest VI, Hier MP, Avior G, et al. Molecular mutations as a possible factor for determining extent of thyroid surgery. J Otolaryngol Head Neck Surg. 2019;48:51.

48. Angell TE, Maurer R, Wang Z, Kim MI, Alexander CA, Barletta JA, et al. A cohort analysis of clinical and ultrasound variables predicting cancer risk in 20,001 consecutive thyroid nodules. J Clin Endocrinol Metab. 2019;104:5665–72.
49. Cipriani NA, White MG, Angelos P, Grogan RH. Large cytologically benign thyroid nodules do not have high rates of malignancy or false-negative rates and clinical observation should be considered: a meta-analysis. Thyroid. 2018;28:1595–608.
50. Mu L, Ren C, Xu J, Guo C, Huang J, Ding K. Total versus near-total thyroidectomy in Graves' disease: a systematic review and meta-analysis of comparative studies. Gland Surg. 2021;10:729–38.
51. Papini E, Monpeyssen H, Frasoldati A, Hegedüs L. 2020 European Thyroid Association clinical practice guideline for the use of image-guided ablation in benign thyroid nodules. Eur Thyroid J. 2020;9:172–85.
52. Mauri G, Hegedüs L, Bandula S, Cazzato RL, Czarniecka A, Dudeck O, et al. Clinical practice guideline for the use of minimally invasive treatments in malignant thyroid lesions. Eur Thyroid J. 2021;10:185–97.
53. Døssing H, Bennedbæk FN, Hegedüs L. Long-term outcome following interstitial laser photocoagulation of benign cold thyroid nodules. Eur J Endocrinol. 2011;165:123–8.
54. Bernardi S, Giudici F, Cesareo R, Antonelli G, Cavallaro M, Deandrea M, et al. Five-year results of radiofrequency and laser ablation of benign thyroid nodules: a multicenter study from the Italian minimally invasive treatments of the thyroid group. Thyroid. 2020;30:1759–70.
55. Sorensen JR, Døssing H, Watt T, Cramon P, Hegedüs L, Bonnema SJ, et al. The effect of laser thermal ablation on quality of life: improvements in patients with solid-cystic thyroid nodules. Thyroid. 2022;32:917–25.
56. Bennedbaek FN, Hegedüs L. Treatment of recurrent thyroid cysts with ethanol: a randomized double-blind controlled trial. J Clin Endocrinol Metab. 2003;88:5773–7.
57. Mauri G, Papini E, Bernardi S, Barbaro D, Cesareo R, De Feo P, et al. Image-guided thermal ablation in autonomously functioning thyroid nodules. A retrospective multicenter three-year follow-up study from the Italian Minimally Invasive Treatment of the Thyroid (MITT) Group. Eur Radiol. 2022;32:1738–46.
58. Hegedüs L, Frasoldati A, Negro R, Papini E. European Thyroid Association survey on use of minimally invasive techniques for thyroid nodules. Eur Thyroid J. 2020;9:194–204.
59. Lamartina L, Durante C, Filetti S, Cooper DS. Low-risk differentiated thyroid cancer and radioiodine remnant ablation: a systematic review of the literature. J Clin Endocrinol Metab. 2015;100(5):1748–61.
60. Pacini F, Ladenson PW, Schlumberger M, Driedger A, Luster M, Kloos RT, et al. Radioiodine ablation of thyroid remnants after preparation with recombinant human thyrotropin in differentiated thyroid carcinoma: results of an international, randomized, controlled study. J Clin Endocrinol Metab. 2006;91(3):926–32.
61. Pacini F, Schlumberger M, Dralle H, Elisei R, Smit JW, Wiersinga W, European Thyroid Cancer Taskforce. European consensus for the management of patients with differentiated thyroid carcinoma of the follicular epithelium. Eur J Endocrinol. 2006;154(6):787–803.
62. Pacini F, Basolo F, Bellantone R, Boni G, Cannizzaro MA, De Palma M, et al. Italian consensus on diagnosis and treatment of differentiated thyroid cancer: joint statements of six Italian societies. J Endocrinol Investig. 2018;41(7):849–76.
63. Luster M, Clarke SE, Dietlein M, Lassmann M, Lind P, Oyen WJ, et al. Guidelines for radioiodine therapy of differentiated thyroid cancer. Eur J Nucl Med Mol Imaging. 2008;35(10):1941–59.
64. Durante C, Attard M, Torlontano M, Ronga G, Monzani F, Costante G, et al. Identification and optimal postsurgical follow-up of patients with very low-risk papillary thyroid microcarcinomas. J Clin Endocrinol Metab. 2010;95(11):4882–8.
65. Bonnema SJ, Hegedüs L. Radioiodine therapy in benign thyroid diseases: effects, side effects, and factors affecting therapeutic outcome. Endocr Rev. 2012;33:920–80.
66. Nygaard B, Hegedüs L, Nielsen KG, Ulriksen P, Hansen JM. Long-term effect of radioactive iodine on thyroid function and size in patients with solitary autonomously functioning toxic thyroid nodules. Clin Endocrinol. 1999;50:197–202.

67. Nielsen VE, Bonnema SJ, Boel-Jørgensen H, Grupe P, Hegedüs L. Stimulation with 0.3-mg recombinant human thyrotropin prior to iodine 131 therapy to improve the size reduction of benign nontoxic nodular goiter: a prospective randomized double-blind trial. Arch Int Med. 2006;166:1476–82.
68. Bonnema SJ, Nielsen VE, BoelJørgensen H, Grupe P, Andersen PB, Bastholt L, et al. Recombinant human thyrotropin-stimulated radioiodine therapy of large nodular goiters facilitates tracheal decompression and improves inspiration. J Clin Endocrinol Metab. 2008;93:3981–4.
69. Castagna MG, Maino F, Cipri C, Belardini V, Theodoropoulou A, Cevenini G, et al. Delayed risk stratification, to include the response to initial treatment (surgery and radioiodine ablation), has better outcome predictivity in differentiated thyroid cancer patients. Eur J Endocrinol. 2011;165(3):441–6.
70. Tuttle RM, Tala H, Shah J, Leboeuf R, Ghossein R, Gonen M, et al. Estimating risk of recurrence in differentiated thyroid cancer after total thyroidectomy and radioactive iodine remnant ablation: using response to therapy variables to modify the initial risk estimates predicted by the new American Thyroid Association staging system. Thyroid. 2010;20(12):1341–9.
71. Durante C, Haddy N, Baudin E, Leboulleux S, Hartl D, Travagli JP, et al. Long-term outcome of 444 patients with distant metastases from papillary and follicular thyroid carcinoma: benefits and limits of radioiodine therapy. J Clin Endocrinol Metab. 2006;91(8):2892–9.
72. Ruegemer JJ, Hay ID, Bergstralh EJ, Ryan JJ, Offord KP, Gorman CA. Distant metastases in differentiated thyroid carcinoma: a multivariate analysis of prognostic variables. J Clin Endocrinol Metab. 1988;67(3):501–8.
73. McGriff NJ, Csako G, Gourgiotis L, Lori CG, Pucino F, Sarlis NJ. Effects of thyroid hormone suppression therapy on adverse clinical outcomes in thyroid cancer. Ann Med. 2002;34(7–8):554–64.
74. Sugitani I, Fujimoto Y. Does postoperative thyrotropin suppression therapy truly decrease recurrence in papillary thyroid carcinoma? A randomized controlled trial. J Clin Endocrinol Metab. 2010;95(10):4576–83.
75. Carhill AA, Litofsky DR, Ross DS, Jonklaas J, Cooper DS, Brierley JD, et al. Long-term outcomes following therapy in differentiated thyroid carcinoma: NTCTCS registry analysis 1987–2012. J Clin Endocrinol Metab. 2015;100(9):3270–9.
76. Sabra MM, Sherman EJ, Tuttle RM. Tumor volume doubling time of pulmonary metastases predicts overall survival and can guide the initiation of multikinase inhibitor therapy in patients with metastatic, follicular cell-derived thyroid carcinoma. Cancer. 2017;123(15):2955–64.
77. Alexander EK, Pearce EN, Brent GA, Brown RS, Chen H, Dosiou C, et al. 2017 guidelines of the American Thyroid Association for the Diagnosis and Management of Thyroid Disease during Pregnancy and the postpartum. Thyroid. 2017;27(3):315–89.

15 Oncocytic (Hürthle Cell) Carcinoma: Controversy of Prognosis

15.1 Survival

Prognostic factors for "survival" include old age, gender, mitotic rate, and depth of invasion, while multifocal disease, size of the primary tumor, nodal involvement, distant metastases, stage of the neoplasm, microscopic residual disease, extrathyroid extension (ETE), and degree of invasion are prognostic factors for both "survival" and "recurrence." Older age, larger tumor size at diagnosis, ETE, and higher stage (AMES prognostic index) at diagnosis are considered by many authors as poor prognostic features with lower survival rates for oncocytic carcinoma of the thyroid (Hürthle cell carcinoma—HCC) [1, 2]. With the exception of few studies [3–5], nodal metastasis was correlated with an adverse prognosis [6–8], while distant metastasis always resulted in a poor prognosis with dismal outcome [7, 8]. Extensive surgery, external beam radiation therapy (EBRT), and chemotherapy were also reported by Lopez-Penabad et al. (2003) as factors that were associated with decreased survival [1]. Zavitsanos et al. (2017) from the University of Florida, USA, reported a patient with cervical oncocytic/HCC "recurrence" who was successfully treated with further surgery, RAI ablation, EBRT, and alive 9 years later [9].

In the Surveillance, epidemiology, and end Results (SEER)-9 database (1975–2009), 10-year survival rates of oncocytic/HCC improved dramatically over time; 75% in1975–1979, 81% 1995–1999, and 91% in 2000–2004 [10]. The improvement in survival occurred in both genders, age ≥45 years, local and regional disease, tumors >4 cm, and Caucasian race. It is not certain if this is related to improvement in diagnosis (e.g., positron emission tomography scan) or treatment (more extensive surgery, and increased use of EBRT and radioactive iodine ablation). Both the SEER database [10] and a Japanese study [11] reported that the outcome of oncocytic/HCC approaches that of follicular thyroid carcinoma (FTC), which has a stable survival over the recent decades.

M. Sakr, *Oncocytic (Hürthle Cell) Thyroid Lesions*,
https://doi.org/10.1007/978-3-032-03115-0_15

15.2 Distant Metastases

Oncocytic/Hürthle cell carcinoma (HCC) is associated with a more aggressive clinical behavior compared to other differentiated thyroid cancers (DTC); for example, it is more often seen with a higher rate of distant metastases [1, 12–15]. The most common site of distant metastases is the lung, followed by bone. Compared to follicular thyroid carcinoma (FTC), oncocytic/HCCs are considered in case reviews to be more aggressive and carry a higher rate of metastases and lower overall survival [1, 16–18].

In a retrospective study of 32 patients with metastatic oncocytic/HCC, Besic et al. (2016) reported estimated 5- and 10-year disease-specific survival rates of 81% and 60%, respectively [6]. On average, patients with metastatic oncocytic/HCC have a 10-year cause-specific survival rate of 60% and live a median of 77 months after developing metastases as reported by Nagar et al. (2013) [10].

In a large retrospective study that analyzed the Surveillance, Epidemiology, and End Results (SEER) database from 1988 to 2009, 3311 patients with oncocytic/Hürthle cell cancer (HCC) were identified and compared with 59,585 patients with differentiated thyroid cancer (DTC). Accordingly, Goffredo et al. (2013) found that oncocytic/HCC has a tendency to higher frequency of metastasis and higher mortality rates. Overall disease-specific survival rates were lower for patients with oncocytic/HCC ($p < 0.001$), confirming that oncocytic/HCC has a more aggressive behavior and compromises survival more than other DTCs [12].

15.3 Locoregional Recurrence

Overall recurrence rates and average time to relapse reported in the literature are 12–33% and 90.74 months, respectively [19, 20]. Average time without symptoms of disease is 222.4 months [19, 20]. Other researchers reported a wider range of 3–50% for locoregional recurrence on follow-up [21–24]. It should be noted that oncocytic/HCC recurrence may occur without detectable serum thyroglobulin (Tg).

Extra-thyroid extension (ETE) was reported by several authors to significantly compromise survival [6, 8]. In these studies, which were done at Memorial Sloan-Kettering Cancer center, the outcome of 56 patients with oncocytic/HCC was analyzed and recurrence was found to be a significant predictor of tumor-related mortality, and the most significant predictor of outcome was the extent of invasion. However, this was found to be insignificant in a more recent study by Barnabei et al. (2009) [4]. Presence of mitosis and a solid/trabecular tumor growth pattern also correlated with higher risk of recurrence [6, 8]. Recurrent oncocytic/HCCs are considered by some to be "incurable."

Recurrence of HCC may involve the lymph nodes (LNs) or other soft tissues in the neck (Fig. 15.1) such as paratracheal implants in the central compartment, jugular tumors in the lateral compartment, supraclavicular tumor ventral of the sternocleidomastoid (SCM) muscle [24].

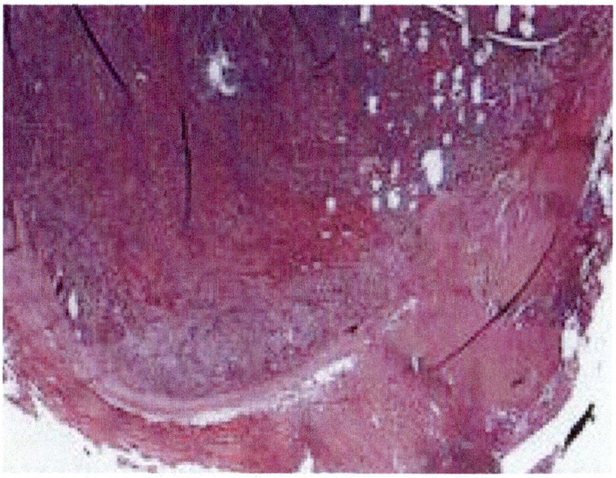

Fig. 15.1 Soft tissue implant from oncocytic/Hürthle cell carcinoma after total thyroidectomy showing a well-circumscribed tumor nodule partially surrounded by a fibrous capsule, clinically and radiologically mimicking lymph node metastasis

Chiapponi et al. (2022) [25] retrospectively studied 51 patients with oncocytic/HCC treated at the "Interdisciplinary Endocrine Center of the University Hospital of Cologne, Germany" between 2005 and 2020. The aim of this study was to describe the clinicopathological features and outcomes of patients with oncocytic/HCC in order to adapt the surgical management. Patients' median age was 63 years (range 29–78 years) with 64.7% of cases being female. Primary treatment included surgery (total thyroidectomy in all cases and additional central lymphadenectomy in 90.2% of cases) and postoperative radioactive iodine (RAI) therapy with 3.7 GBq in all patients. The median number of harvested lymph nodes (LNs) was 11 (range 2–31). Involvement of LNs was found in two (4.3%) pT4a tumors. In all other cases (95.7%), central lymphadenectomy was prophylactic and LNs were free of metastasis in final histopathology. Regular follow-up examination was scheduled every 6 months for 5 years and yearly thereafter. Twelve (23.5%) patients with incomplete biochemical response to primary treatment were diagnosed with structural relapse (persistence/recurrence) during the course of disease, for which seven (58.4%) underwent resection of isolated cervical metastasis. Histopathology revealed soft tissue implants in all cases and cervical surgery led to biochemical and radiological cure in only two (28.5%) cases. Five (41.6%) patients developed metastatic disease, followed by systemic therapy in two patients. Vascular invasion of the primary tumor was significantly associated with relapse ($p < 0.01$). They concluded that recurrence of oncocytic/HCC was rather common in their study and given the low rate of LN metastases compared to soft tissue metastasis, the benefit of routine prophylactic central LN dissection for oncocytic/HCC remains controversial as it does *not* avoid recurrence, especially in the absence of vascular invasion from the primary tumor [25].

As reported by Chiapponi et al. in 2022 [25], despite initial surgery (total thyroidectomy and prophylactic central LN dissection) and radioactive iodine (RAI) treatment, recurrence rate was as high as 23.5%, which is similar to that previously reported with follicular thyroid cancer (FTC) [26], but higher than that reported in some recent studies reported in the literature [27, 28]. The reasons underlying these differences are unclear and might be of demographic, ethnic, or environmental nature.

There is an increasing number of recent studies questioning the reported aggressiveness of oncocytic/HCC. Jin et al. (2021) [27] reported persistence/recurrence rates of 8% and no death in a follow-up of 8.5 years in South Korea, a region with a good iodine intake. Matsuura et al. (2022) [28] compared oncocytic/HCC to FTC in a US American population and reported that oncocytic/HCC patients were more likely to recur, but they had shown no significant different overall survival. Vascular invasion was a critical prognostic parameter for predicting recurrence in their study [28].

15.4 Age, Metastases, Extra-thyroid Extension, Stage [AMES]

Age, metastasis, extra-thyroid extension (ETE), and size (AMES) prognostic index, which has been long used to predict outcome of differentiated thyroid carcinoma (DTC), was also validated to stratify oncocytic/HCC into high- and low-risk groups and was subsequently found to correlate significantly with survival and to predict recurrence risk [3, 29]. However, as with other aspects of this tumor, controversy exists.

Older age, larger tumor size at diagnosis, ETE, and higher stage at diagnosis are considered poor prognostic features with lower survival rates for oncocytic/Hürthle cell carcinomas (HCCs) [1, 2]. These factors (male gender and older age at diagnosis) have been associated with worse prognosis in oncocytic/HCC, along with larger tumor size, the presence of extra-thyroidal extension (ETE), and higher stage at diagnosis [12, 16, 17, 30].

15.4.1 Old Age [A]

Several authors reported that advancing age is significantly correlated with poor outcome [16]; Goffredo et al. (2013) identified 3311 patients with oncocytic/HCC above the age of 18 years and 59,585 patients with PTC and FTC from the Surveillance, Epidemiology and End Result (SEER) database from 1988 to 2009 and determined that older age, larger tumor size, extra-thyroidal tumor extension, and not undergoing surgery were independently associated with reduced overall survival among patients with oncocytic/HCC. Hürthle cell carcinoma was more common in older men, and it appeared to be more aggressive compared to other differentiated thyroid cancers [12]. Contradictory findings regarding the impact of older age on prognosis of patients with HCC were concluded by many other authors [6–8, 31].

15.4.2 Metastases [M]

With the exception of few studies [3–5], "nodal" metastasis was correlated with an adverse prognosis [6–8], while distant metastasis always caused a dismal outcome [7, 8]. Metastatic disease is reported at the time of initial diagnosis in 10–20% of patients and in 34% of the patients overall. Overall survival rates reportedly are similar or worse in patients with oncocytic/HCC compared with rates for persons with FTC. In a case series of oncocytic/HCC, mortality rates at 5, 10, and 20 years were 8%, 18%, and 33%, respectively. Two other case series confirmed a 20-year cause-specific mortality rate of 20–35%. One study showed that when "distant" metastases were present, the 5-year mortality rate was 65% [32]. Another study involving 33 patients showed that disease-free survival was 65% in 5 years and 40.5% in 10 years [17]. In a study of 108 patients with metastatic oncocytic/HCC, Besic et al., in 2016 [33], reported that sites of metastasis, in decreasing order of frequency, were lung, bone, mediastinum, kidney, and liver. Overall 10-year disease-specific survival was 60%. Median disease-specific survival after the diagnosis of metastatic disease was 72 months for patients with pulmonary metastases and 138 months for patients with metastases at other sites.

In a retrospective review of all patients treated with oncocytic/HCC at their institution between 1946 and 2003 ($n = 62$), Mills et al. (2009) reported that independent predictors of disease-free survival were lymph node (LN) status ($p = 0.008$), presence of metastases at diagnosis ($p = 0.005$), and tumor stage ($p = 0.009$). These authors suggest that radical surgery may improve outcome. On multivariate analysis, extent of surgery ($p < 0.001$) was the only independent factor that affected cause-specific survival [20].

15.4.3 Extra-thyroid Extension [E]

The extent of invasion has also been found to be prognostic in oncocytic/HCC. Extrathyroid extension (ETE) was reported by Stojadinovic and colleagues in 2001 [6] and 2002 [8] to significantly increase the recurrence rate and compromise survival. However, ETE was found to be an insignificant predictor of tumor-related mortality in a more recent study by Barnabei et al. (2009) [4].

Similar to FTC, patients who have oncocytic/HCC with focal capsular invasion (CI) have improved prognosis compared with patients with angioinvasion, while the worst outcomes are seen in patients who have widely invasive tumors [34–38]. The College of American Pathologists (CAP) therefore recommends reporting oncocytic/HCC as (1) minimally invasive, (2) encapsulated angioinvasive, or (3) widely invasive [39]. Additionally, the extent of vascular invasion (VI) has been shown to be prognostic in FTC and oncocytic/HCC [34, 35, 38]. Tumors with focal (<4 foci) of vascular invasion have better outcomes compared to those with extensive vascular invasion (≥4 foci) [34, 38]. Ghossein et al. (2006) [34] reported that the 5-year recurrence-free survival in oncocytic/HCC with "focal" vascular invasion was 100% compared with only 20% for those with "extensive" vascular invasion. For this reason, the CAP also recommends documenting the extent of vascular invasion in these tumors [39]. In the recent American Thyroid Association (ATA) guidelines for differentiated thyroid cancers, FTCs (and by extension oncocytic/HCCs) with focal capsular or vascular invasion are categorized as low-risk for recurrence, while tumors with extensive vascular invasion are considered high risk [40].

15.4.4 Stage [S]

The 5-year cumulative probability of recurrence or mortality among patients with TNM stage I–II among female and male patients were 0% and 17%, respectively. Among patients with TNM stage III–IV, the 5-year cumulative probability of recurrence or mortality for female and male patients were 74% and 91%, respectively [30].

Likewise, larger tumor size (T) was found by some authors to adversely impact the outcome [7, 8, 16] while others found no significant association [6, 31]. Stage (TNM) of the tumor at diagnosis was found to be the most important prognostic factor by Chindris et al. (2015) [30]; although the 5-year survival among all oncocytic/HCCs in their cohort was 85%, it was only 24% in patients who were M1 (distant metastasis present) at diagnosis compared with 91% in patients who were M0 (no distant metastasis).

Mortality rates vary in different series, based on the staging systems used, which consider the patient's age, tumor size, extra-thyroidal tumor spread, pathological classification of the neoplasm (carcinoma versus adenoma), and the therapeutic approach. Morbidity depends on the behavior of the oncocytic/HCC.

15.5 Effect of Gender/Stage

Similar to the effect of age on prognosis in patients with oncocytic/HCC, contradiction exists also regarding gender-outcome correlation [7, 31]. In a study by Chindris et al. (2015), they identified 173 patients with oncocytic/HCC between 2001 and 2012 and reported that male gender and stages III–IV according to the American Joint Committee on Cancer TNM (AJCC-TNM) were independent risk factors for recurrence or death among patients with widely invasive HCC (wiHCC). The cumulative risk of recurrence or death within 5 years of diagnosis was 91% in men with Stages III–IV disease compared to 74% in women with the same stages of disease; the 5-year cumulative probability of recurrence or death in patients with AJCC-TNM Stages I–II was 0% among women compared to 17% among men [30].

Bhattacharyya [16] reported in 2003 that the 5- and 10-year survival for the HCC cohort was 85.1% and 71.1%, respectively. Compared with a matched group of patients with follicular thyroid carcinoma (FTC), the slightly poorer survival for oncocytic/HCC versus FTC was *not* statistically significant ($p = 0.47$). Increasing age (>55 years) at diagnosis, male gender, and increasing tumor size (3.5 cm or more) were each statistically significantly associated with substantially poorer survival on multivariate analysis. Local extent was not a statistically significant predictor of survival on multivariate analysis.

15.6 Microscopic Morphology

The microscopic morphology appears also to correlate with outcome of patients with HCC. Prognosis differs between minimally invasive Hürthle cell carcinoma (miHCC) and widely invasive Hürthle cell carcinoma (wiHCC). In a histopathological appraisal by Stojadinovic et al. (2001) [6], all patients with miHCC exhibited a benign clinical course with no cause-specific mortality while considerable proportions of wiHCC patients developed metastasis, recurrence, or died [6]. These findings are in accordance with those reported by Sanders (1998) [3], and more recently, by Chindris et al. in 2015 [30]. As long as the tumor is minimally invasive and non-angioinvasive, prognosis is excellent with no recurrence observed [30]. If wiHCC is observed in males, older age (>45) with more than four foci of angioinvasion, larger than 4 cm, and/or TNM stage III–IV, prognosis is poor [30, 41]. WiHCCs are significantly associated with the male gender and clinical recurrence or mortality.

On the other hand, Barnabei et al. (1998) [4] stated that vascular invasion (VI), the hallmark of wiHCC, was not associated with worse survival, and Goldstein et al. (2000) [18] reported no statistically significant difference in the number of capsular invasion (CI) or VI foci between metastatic and nonmetastatic oncocytic/HCCs. Tumor encapsulation was associated with improved survival in the study by Lopez-Penabad (2003) [1]. In some series, nuclear aneuploidy is present in as many as 90% of patients with oncocytic/HCC; in some studies, this condition is shown to be associated with an adverse prognosis.

In 2003, Bhattacharyya [16] stated that although oncocytic/HCC is a distinct thyroid histological tumor, it clinically behaves similarly to FTC. Based on risk factor analysis, oncocytic/HCC should be treated aggressively with total thyroidectomy, especially in older patients, men, and those with large tumor size. Extra-thyroidal extension of the primary tumor should *not* preclude aggressive management and does not substantially reduce survival.

In some studies, the oncocytic phenotype has been found by some authors to be prognostic [5, 7, 42, 43]. Hundahl et al. (1998) [42] found that the 5-year overall survival of oncocytic/HCC was similar to that of FTC; however, the 10-year overall survival was worse in oncocytic/HCC (76% versus 85%, respectively). Similar findings were reported by Shaha and colleagues in 1995 [5] and 1996 [14]. Other researchers in studies accounting for other clinicopathological factors such as tumor size and stage, multivariate analysis did not find Hürthle cell morphology to be prognostic [11, 44].

15.7 Impact of Management

Lopez-Penabad et al. (2003) [1] reported that out of 89 patients with oncocytic/HCC, 36 patients (40.4%) died of their cancer as compared to none in 38 patients with oncocytic adenoma (Hürthle cell adenoma—HCA). Univariate analysis identified older age, higher disease stage, tumor size, extra-thyroid extension (ETE), multifocality, lymph node (LN) involvement, distant metastasis, extensive surgery, external beam radiation therapy (EBRT), and chemotherapy as factors that were associated with decreased survival. Although radioactive iodine (RAI) treatment had no overall effect on survival, subgroup analysis showed that patients who received RAI for adjuvant ablation therapy had better outcomes compared either with patients who did not receive RAI or received it for treatment of residual disease. Multivariate analysis indicated that older age and larger tumor size predicted worse survival through an association with worse behaving tumors (multifocal, less encapsulated, and with extra-glandular invasion). The decreased survival in patients with LN metastases may be explained by its association with distant metastases. The association of extensive surgery, EBRT, and chemotherapy with worse survival also disappeared once those factors were analyzed together with other prognostic factors, such as distant metastases.

15.8 Prognostic Nomogram

Several researchers reported that oncocytic/HCC is more aggressive than FTC and is associated with a worse prognosis [6, 45]. Patients with oncocytic/HCC also show a higher metastasis rate and lower overall survival (OS) and disease-specific survival (DSS) [2, 18]. Moreover, oncocytic/HCC is more common than other types of differentiated thyroid cancers (DTC) among men (31.1% versus 23.0%, $P < 0.001$) and older patients (mean age, 57.6 years versus 48.9 years, $P < 0.001$) [12]. Despite the prognostic difference between oncocytic/HCC and FTC, oncocytic/HCC cannot be considered a "highly" aggressive carcinoma. Nishida et al. (1999) [46] used a three-tiered system and classified oncocytic/HCCs as "moderate-grade" to recognize the clinical difference with "low-grade" PTCs and FTCs, and "high-grade" anaplastic thyroid carcinoma (ATC).

At present, the prognostic factors of thyroid oncocytic/HCC remain to be fully elucidated [19, 47]. The early identification of high-risk oncocytic/HCC patients is crucial for improving prognosis. Hence, it is necessary to obtain accurate information on survival-related factors and to develop a prognostic model.

Nomograms are considered a graphical tool that can be used to calculate individual risk by integrating and quantifying prognostic factors [48]. Accordingly, they are widely applied to assess indicators of cancer prognosis, including recurrence, metastasis, and overall survival (OS) [49–51]. A prognostic nomogram has recently (2022) been published to assess both cancer-specific survival (CSS) and overall survival (OS) in oncocytic/HCC, which could assist in making treatment decisions [52]. Data for a total of 3264 patients with oncocytic/HCC (2004–2018) were extracted from the Surveillance, Epidemiology, and End Results (SEER) database. Univariate and multivariate Cox regression analysis was performed to identify significant predictors of prognosis and develop a prognostic nomogram [52].

Females accounted for the majority of the study cohort as compared to males (68.3% versus 31.7%, respectively). The median age of the study cohort was 58 years. The median tumor size was 3.15 cm. Localized metastasis was the most common (2749 patients, 84.2%), followed by regional (11.7%) and distant metastases (4.0%). With respect to tumor stage, 138 patients (4.2%) showed T4 stage disease, 184 (5.6%) showed N1 stage disease, and 90 (2.8%) showed M1 stage disease. Moreover, there were 220 patients (6.7%) with AJCC stage IV disease. Of these patients, 3223 (98.7%) had undergone thyroidectomy, while 41 (1.3%) did not undergo surgery. Multivariate Cox regression analysis showed that age, sex, summary stage, tumor size, N stage, M stage, and treatment with thyroidectomy were independent predictors of OS. Moreover, age, summary stage, tumor size, N stage, M stage, AJCC stage, and treatment with thyroidectomy were significantly correlated with CSS [52].

In a study by Lopez-Penabad [1] (2003), a cohort of 89 HCC patients from the United States, age >45 years was found to be correlated with reduced survival. However, age was not identified as an independent risk factor for poor survival in the multivariate analysis [1]. Many studies show that male gender is predictive of worse outcomes in oncocytic/HCC [16, 47]. In the recent prognostic nomogram developed by Shen et al. (2022) male gender was an independent predictor of OS but *not* CSS [52]. Thyroidectomy is recommended for oncocytic/HCC patients [19, 20, 53, 54] and the multivariate analysis by Shen et al. [52] also indicated that thyroidectomy was the strongest protective factor in oncocytic/HCC. It is widely accepted that tumor size can increase the risk of poor outcomes. Using multivariate analysis, a study by Goffredo et al. (2013) [12] demonstrated that a tumor size ≥4 cm was associated with a higher disease-specific mortality. Another study by Lopez-Penabad (2003) [1] that used 4 cm as the cutoff indicated that a larger tumor size was associated with a worse outcome. The results of the prognostic nomogram [52] confirmed that tumor size was an independent predictor of both OS and CSS.

References

1. Lopez-Penabad L, Chiu AC, Hoff AO, Schultz P, Gaztambide S, Ordoñez NG, et al. Prognostic factors in patients with Hurthle cell neoplasms of the thyroid. Cancer. 2003;97(5):1186–94.
2. Zhang YW, Greenblatt DY, Repplinger D, Bargren A, Adler JT, Sippel RS, Chen H. Older age and larger tumor size predict malignancy in hürthle cell neoplasms of the thyroid. Ann Surg Oncol. 2008;15(10):2842–6.
3. Sanders LE, Silverman M. Follicular and Hürthle cell carcinoma: predicting outcome and directing therapy. Surgery. 1998;124(6):967–74.
4. Barnabei A, Ferretti E, Baldelli R, Procaccini A, Spriano G, Appetecchia M. Hurthle cell tumours of the thyroid. Personal experience and review of the literature. Acta Otorhinolaryngol Ital. 2009;29(6):305–11.
5. Shaha AR, Loree TR, Shah JP. Prognostic factors and risk group analysis in follicular carcinoma of the thyroid. Surgery. 1995;118(6):1131–8.

6. Stojadinovic A, Ghossein RA, Hoos A, Urist MJ, Spiro RH, Shah JP, et al. Hurthle cell carcinoma: a critical histopathologic appraisal. J Clin Oncol. 2001;19(10):2616–25.
7. Kushchayeva Y, Duh Q-Y, Kebebew E, D'Avanzo A, Clark OH. Comparison of clinical characteristics at diagnosis and during follow-up in 118 patients with Hurthle cell or follicular thyroid cancer. Am J Surg. 2008;195(4):457–62.
8. Stojadinovic A, Hoos A, Ghossein R, Urist MJ, Leung DH, Spiro RH, et al. Hürthle cell carcinoma: a 60-year experience. Ann Surg Oncol. 2002;9(2):197–203.
9. Zavitsanos P, Amdur RJ, Drew PA, Cusi K, Werning JW, Morris CG. Favorable outcome of Hurthle cell carcinoma of the thyroid treated with Total thyroidectomy, radioiodine, and selective use of external-beam radiotherapy. Am J Clin Oncol. 2017;40(4):433–7.
10. Nagar S, Aschebrook-Kilfoy B, Kaplan EL, Angelos P, Grogan RH. Hurthle cell carcinoma: an update on survival over the last 35 years. Surgery. 2013;154(6):1263–71.
11. Sugino K, Kameyama K, Ito K, Nagahama M, Kitagawa W, et al. Does Hürthle cell carcinoma of the thyroid have a poorer prognosis than ordinary follicular thyroid carcinoma? Ann Surg Oncol. 2013;20(9):2944–50.
12. Goffredo P, Roman SA, Sosa JA. Hurthle cell carcinoma: a population-level analysis of 3311 patients. Cancer. 2013;119(3):504–11.
13. Kuo EJ, Roman SA, Sosa JA. Patients with follicular and Hurthle cell microcarcinomas have compromised survival: a population level study of 22,738 patients. Surgery. 2013;154(6):1246–53.
14. Shaha AR, Shah JP, Loree TR. Patterns of nodal and distant metastasis based on histologic varieties in differentiated carcinoma of the thyroid. Am J Surg. 1996;172(6):692–4.
15. Ruegemer JJ, Hay ID, Bergstralh EJ, Ryan JJ, Offord KP, Gorman CA. Distant metastases in differentiated thyroid carcinoma: a multivariate analysis of prognostic variables. J Clin Endocrinol Metab. 1988;67(3):501–8.
16. Bhattacharyya N. Survival and prognosis in Hürthle cell carcinoma of the thyroid gland. Arch Otolaryngol Head Neck Surg. 2003;129(2):207–10.
17. Kushchayeva Y, Duh QY, Kebebew E, Clark OH. Prognostic indications for Hürthle cell cancer. World J Surg. 2004;28(12):1266–70.
18. Goldstein NS, Czako P, Neill JS. Metastatic minimally invasive (encapsulated) follicular and Hurthle cell thyroid carcinoma: a study of 34 patients. Mod Pathol. 2000;13(2):123–30.
19. Oluic B, Paunovic I, Loncar Z, Djukic V, Diklic A, Jovanovic M, Garabinovic Z, et al. Survival and prognostic factors for survival, cancer specific survival and disease free interval in 239 patients with Hurthle cell carcinoma: a single center experience. BMC Cancer. 2017;17:371.
20. Mills SC, Haq M, Smellie WJ, Harmer C. Hurthle cell carcinoma of the thyroid: retrospective review of 62 patients treated at the Royal Marsden Hospital between 1946 and 2003. Eur J Surg Oncol. 2009;35:230–4.
21. Kim WG, Kim TY, Kim TH, Jang HW, Jo YS, Park YJ, et al. Follicular and Hurthle cell carcinoma of the thyroid in iodine-sufficient area: retrospective analysis of Korean multicenter data. Korean J Intern Med. 2014;29(3):325–33.
22. Cipriani NA, Nagar S, Kaplan SP, White MG, Antic T, Sadow PM, et al. Follicular thyroid carcinoma: how have histologic diagnoses changed in the last half-century and what are the prognostic implications? Thyroid. 2015;25(11):1209–16.
23. Jillard CL, Youngwirth L, Scheri RP, Roman S, Sosa JA. Radioactive iodine treatment is associated with improved survival for patients with Hürthle cell carcinoma. Thyroid. 2016;26(7):959–64.
24. Ahmadi S, Stang M, Jiang XS, Sosa JA. Hürthle cell carcinoma: current perspectives. Onco Targets Ther. 2016;9:6873–84.
25. Chiapponi C, Hartmann MJM, Schmidt M, Faust M, Burns CJ, Schulteis AM, et al. Hürthle cell carcinoma: single center analysis and considerations for surgical management based on the recent literature. Front Endocrinol (Lausanne). 2022;13:904986.
26. Chiapponi C, Hartmann MJM, Schmidt M, Faust M, Schultheis AM, Bruns CJ, et al. Radioiodine refractory follicular thyroid cancer and surgery for cervical relapse. Cancers (Basel). 2021;13(24):6230.

27. Jin M, Kim ES, Kim BH, Kim HK, Kang YE, Jeon MJ, et al. Clinicopathological characteristics and disease-free survival in patients with Hürthle cell carcinoma: a multicenter cohort study in South Korea. Endocrinol Metab. 2021;36(5):1078–85.
28. Matsuura D, Yuan A, Wang L, Ranganath R, Adilbay D, Harries V, et al. Follicular and Hurthle cell carcinoma: comparison of clinicopathological features and clinical outcomes. Thyroid. 2022;32(3):245–54.
29. McDonald MP, Sanders LE, Silverman ML, Chan HS, Buyske J. Hürthle cell carcinoma of the thyroid gland: prognostic factors and results of surgical treatment. Surgery. 1996;120(6):1000–5.
30. Chindris AM, Casler JD, Bernet VJ, Rivera M, Thomas C, Kachergus JM, et al. Clinical and molecular features of Hurthle cell carcinoma of the thyroid. J Clin Endocrinol Metab. 2015;100(1):55–62.
31. Khafif A, Khafif RA, Attie JN. Hürthle cell carcinoma: a malignancy of low-grade potential. Head Neck. 1999;21(6):506–11.
32. Cooper DS, Schneyer CR. Follicular and Hürthle cell carcinoma of the thyroid. Endocrinol Metab Clin N Am. 1990;19(3):577–91.
33. Besic N, Schwarzbartl-Pevec A, Vidergar-Kralj B, Crnic T, Gazic B, Marolt Music M. Treatment and outcome of 32 patients with distant metastases of Hurthle cell thyroid carcinoma: a single-institution experience. BMC Cancer. 2016;16:162–9.
34. Ghossein RA, Hiltzik DH, Carlson DL, Patel S, Shaha A, Shah JP, et al. Prognostic factors of recurrence in encapsulated Hurthle cell carcinoma of the thyroid gland: a clinicopathologic study of 50 cases. Cancer. 2006;106(8):1669–76.
35. Ito Y, Hirokawa M, Masuoka H, Yabuta T, Kihara M, Higashiyama T, et al. Prognostic factors of minimally invasive follicular thyroid carcinoma: extensive vascular invasion significantly affects patient prognosis. Endocr J. 2013;60:637–42.
36. O'Neill CJ, Vaughan L, Learoyd DL, Sidhu SB, Delbridge LW, Sywak MS. Management of follicular thyroid carcinoma should be individualised based on degree of capsular and vascular invasion. Eur J Surg Oncol. 2011;37:181–5.
37. Petric R, Gazic B, Besic N. Prognostic factors for disease-specific survival in 108 patients with Hürthle cell thyroid carcinoma: a single-institution experience. BMC Cancer. 2014;14:1–9.
38. Xu B, Wang L, Tuttle RM, Ganly I, Ghossein R. Prognostic impact of extent of vascular invasion in low-grade encapsulated follicular cell-derived thyroid carcinomas: a clinicopathologic study of 276 cases. Hum Pathol. 2015;46:1789–98.
39. Mete O, Seethala R, Asa S, Bullock MJ, Carty SE, Hodaket SP, et al. Protocol for the examination of specimens from patients with carcinomas of the thyroid gland, version 4.2.0.0. Northfield: College of American Pathologists (CAP); 2019.
40. Haugen BR, Alexander EK, Bible KC, Doherty GM, Mandel SJ, Nikiforov YE, et al. 2015 American Thyroid Association management guidelines for adult patients with thyroid nodules and differentiated thyroid cancer. Thyroid. 2016;26:1–133.
41. Chen H, Nicol TL, Zeiger MA, Dooley WC, Ladenson PW, Cooper DS, et al. Hürthle cell neoplasms of the thyroid: are there factors predictive of malignancy? Ann Surg. 1998;227(4):542–6.
42. Hundahl SA, Fleming ID, Fremgen AM, Menck HR. A National Cancer Data Base report on 53,856 cases of thyroid carcinoma treated in the US, 1985–1995. Cancer. 1998;83:2638–48.
43. Samaan NA, Maheshwari YK, Nader S, Hill CS Jr, Schultz PN, Haynie TP, et al. Impact of therapy for differentiated carcinoma of the thyroid: an analysis of 706 cases. J Clin Endocrinol Metab. 1983;56:1131–8.
44. Haigh PI, Urbach DR, Singh B, Kebebew E, Chabot JA, Saxe A. The treatment and prognosis of Hürthle cell follicular thyroid carcinoma compared with its non-Hürthle cell counterpart. Surgery. 2005;138:1152–8.
45. Grani G, Lamartina L, Durante C, Filetti S, Cooper DS. Follicular thyroid cancer and Hürthle cell carcinoma: challenges in diagnosis, treatment, and clinical management. Lancet Diabetes Endocrinol. 2018;6:500–14.
46. Nishida T, Katayama S, Tsujimoto M, Nakamura J, Matsuda H. Clinicopathological significance of poorly differentiated thyroid carcinoma. Am J Surg Pathol. 1999;23(2):205–11.

47. Zhou X, Zheng Z, Chen C, Zhao B, Cao H, Li T, et al. Clinical characteristics and prognostic factors of Hurthle cell carcinoma: a population based study. BMC Cancer. 2020;20:407.
48. Iasonos A, Schrag D, Raj GV, Panageas KS. How to build and interpret a nomogram for cancer prognosis. J Clin Oncol. 2008;26:1364–70.
49. Rocco B, Sighinolfi MC, Sandri M, Puliatti S, Bianchi G. A novel nomogram for predicting ECE of prostate cancer. BJU Int. 2018;122:916–8.
50. Jeong SH, Kim RB, Park SY, Park J, Jung EJ, Ju YT, et al. Nomogram for predicting gastric cancer recurrence using biomarker gene expression. Eur J Surg Oncol. 2020;46:195–201.
51. Dong D, Fang MJ, Tang L, Shan XH, Gao JB, Giganti F, et al. Deep learning radiomic nomogram can predict the number of lymph node metastasis in locally advanced gastric cancer: an international multicenter study. Ann Oncol. 2020;31:912–20.
52. Shen C, Zhao Y, Qiu X, Li P, Ding Y, Wang W, et al. Development and validation of a prognostic nomogram for Hürthle cell thyroid carcinoma: a SEER-based study. Gland Surg. 2022;11(3):535–44.
53. McHenry CR, Sandoval BA. Management of follicular and Hürthle cell neoplasms of the thyroid gland. Surg Oncol Clin N Am. 1998;7:893–910.
54. Sulaiman S, Chirukandath R, Krishnan SK, Rajesh N, Antony M, Mohan KSS. Unraveling the enigma: a five-year comprehensive analysis of Hurthle cell tumors in South India's tertiary care center. Cureus. 2024;16(3):e57166.

Oncocytic (Hürthle Cell) Lesions: Conclusions

16

16.1 Nomenclature

The Hürthle cell (HC) is named after the German physiologist and histologist *Karl Hürthle* (March 16, 1860–March 23, 1945), who investigated thyroid secretory function, in canines. However, this is a "misnomer" since what he really described were the "para-follicular" C-cells in the thyroid gland of dogs in 1894 [1]. The oncocytic cells derived from thyroid follicular epithelium (true Hürthle cells) were, in fact, first described in 1898 by the Swiss-German pathologist *Max Ashkanazy* (born on February 24, 1865) in patients with Graves' disease [2]. Despite this historical fact, and despite this being corrected frequently in the literature over the last century, as having been described by Ashkanazy, including a move toward designating these lesions as "oncocytic," more descriptive than ascribed for discovery, the misnomer has taken hold and the term "Hürthle cell" has continued to be used in the literature to refer to thyroid follicular cells with oncocytic features, except in Germany, where the term "Ashkanazy cells" is in use.

Recently, in the "2022 WHO classification of Endocrine and Neuro-endocrine Tumors," the term "oncocytic cell" has replaced "Hürthle cell." Accordingly, oncocytic adenoma and oncocytic carcinoma of the thyroid gland are the new names for Hürthle cell adenoma (HCA) and Hürthle cell carcinoma (HCC), respectively [3].

16.2 Cell of Origin

Despite the recent developments in science, the exact origin of oncocytic (Hürthle) cells in the thyroid gland is unclear, in terms of their physiological function and from which progenitor they arise. Given that the hallmark of oncocytic change is mitochondrial proliferation as an adaptive process to a primary nuclear abnormality [4, 5], it can occur in follicular as well as in parafollicular cells. Thus, oncocytic (Hürthle cell) neoplasms of the thyroid are generally considered to fall into one of

M. Sakr, *Oncocytic (Hürthle Cell) Thyroid Lesions*, https://doi.org/10.1007/978-3-032-03115-0_16

two tumor types, follicular-derived thyroid tumors (FDTT, tumors of thyrocytes) or parafollicular tumors of C-cell/neural crest origin [6]. In conclusion, Hürthle cell/oncocytic change in the thyroid gland occurs mainly in follicular epithelial cells [7, 8], but also can occur in C-cells and their lesions, and in solid cell nests, the embryological remnants of the ultimobranchial bodies [9].

16.3 Pathogenesis and Biological Behavior

The mechanism behind mitochondrial abundance in oncocytic (Hürthle cell) lesions is not completely understood; however, it is likely a reflection of excessive mitochondrial proliferation and/or decreased mitochondrial degradation (mitophagy). Such changes are reported to be a result of mutations in the mitochondrial DNA (mtDNA) encoding for mitochondrial enzymes, leading to proliferation through stimulation of transcription factors encoded by the nucleus [10–12]. Biologically, oncocytic (Hürthle) cells appear to be less active than typical follicular cells, demonstrating lower levels of thyroglobulin production, and oncocytic carcinoma of the thyroid (Hürthle cell carcinoma) have been shown to have markedly lower iodine uptake than their follicular counterparts. Oncocytic thyroid tumors have historically been perceived as carrying a higher risk of malignancy, and in case of malignancy, to carry a worse prognosis than their conventional counterparts [13]. More recent evidence suggests that oncocytic thyroid neoplasms are not more aggressive than usual variants [10, 14].

16.4 Cytology

Oncocytic (Hürthle) cells tend to be polygonal cells with distinct cell borders, larger in size than follicular cells reaching 10-15 μ. The principal features of these oncocytic cells include an eosinophilic granular cytoplasm and a large hyper-chromatic round-to-oval nucleus with a prominent nucleolus [11, 15].

Evaluation of oncocytic/Hürthle cell–predominant fine-needle aspiration (FNA) is often challenging. There is a wide spectrum of conditions that demonstrate oncocytic (Hürthle) cell morphology, from inflammatory or reactive to malignant. Although cytomorphological criteria help distinguish reactive conditions from neoplasia/malignancy to some extent, there remains significant variability in diagnosis and risk of malignancy associated with the oncocytic (Hürthle) cell. The new classification in the fifth edition of the "WHO Classification of Endocrine and Neuroendocrine Tumors" that relates to the thyroid gland has replaced the term "Hürthle cells" with "oncocytic cells" and has categorized Hürthle cell carcinoma (now called "oncocytic carcinoma of the thyroid") as a separate entity under differentiated thyroid carcinoma (DTC) and not as a subtype of follicular thyroid carcinoma (FTC) [3].

The third edition (2023) of "The Thyroid Bethesda System for Reporting Thyroid Cytopathology (TBSRTC)" assigned a single name for each of the six diagnostic categories based on fine-needle aspiration cytology (FNAC): (I) nondiagnostic, (II) benign, (III) atypia of undetermined significance (AUS), (IV) follicular neoplasm, (V) suspicious for malignancy, and (VI) malignant. This resolves the confusion resulting from the prior editions, which assigned alternative names for three of the diagnostic categories. Thus, TBRSTC 2023 discontinued the previously used terms of "unsatisfactory," "follicular lesion of undetermined significance (FLUS)," and "suspicious for a follicular neoplasm." [16].

16.5 Histopathology

Morphologically, oncocytic/HCC demonstrates a distinct feature, which is caused by mitochondrial accumulation. Oncocytic carcinoma of the thyroid (Hürthle cell carcinoma—HCC) has been established as a separate pathological entity and not a subtype of follicular thyroid carcinoma (FTC) in the current WHO classification of Thyroid Tumors (fifth edition—2022) [3].

Traditionally, oncocytic/Hürthle cell neoplasms (HCNs) have been classified into benign (Hürthle cell adenoma—HCA) and malignant (Hürthle cell carcinoma—HCC). In 2000, a third category was added; HCN of uncertain malignant behavior. Based on the degree of capsular invasion and vascular invasion, oncocytic/HCC has been subclassified into two groups: minimally invasive Hürthle cell carcinoma (miHCC) and widely invasive (wiHCC) Hürthle cell carcinoma [17]. In the 2022 WHO classification, "oncocytic cell" has replaced "Hürthle cell." Accordingly, oncocytic adenoma and oncocytic carcinoma of the thyroid are the new names for Hürthle cell adenoma (HCA) and Hürthle cell carcinoma (HCC), respectively [3].

16.6 Diagnosis

One of the most difficult aspects of examining oncocytic/Hürthle cell neoplasms is to determine whether the lesion is benign or malignant. Investigators have thus tried to employ demographic (age, gender, race, ethnicity), clinicopathological criteria (tumor size, radiation history, family history, multifocality, and coexisting thyroid pathology) to better predict the risk of malignancy in oncocytic neoplasms (Hürthle cell neoplasms—HCN). However, examination of factors related specifically to the likelihood of oncocytic (Hürthle cell) carcinoma is limited.

The current definition of a malignant oncocytic/HCN depends on capsular and/or vascular invasion (easy to note in wiHCC and a somewhat subjective diagnosis for miHCC or borderline invasive disease), and the presence of metastasis. This cannot be determined by cytological evaluation and relies on histological examination of a surgically resected specimen. Frozen-section evaluation has been shown to be of little use in the intraoperative evaluation of these lesions. Among its limitations, frozen-section evaluation is compromised by sampling error, variable thickness, irregularity of the capsule, and freezing artifacts [18, 19].

Diagnostic specificity, which has incorporated a sharp increase in molecular genetic studies of thyroid tumor subtypes and the integration of molecular testing into preoperative management protocols, continues to be challenged by oncocytic/Hürthle cell neoplasia. The increasing use of molecular testing during thyroid nodule diagnosis is an important avenue toward understanding the genetic underpinnings of the transition from adenoma to carcinoma as well as the development of specific therapies that target the underlying genetic drivers of these fascinating yet recalcitrant cancers [20].

16.7 Management

There remains significant controversy with regard to optimal management of patients with oncocytic carcinoma of the thyroid (Hürthle cell carcinoma—HCC); it is more pronounced than the management of other forms of differentiated thyroid cancer (DTC), likely due to the relative rarity of the disease and scant high-quality evidence. Preoperative diagnosis is challenging, but indicators of malignancy are male gender, older age, tumor size >4 cm, a solid nodule with an irregular border, or the presence of psammoma calcifications according to ultrasound. Molecular changes involve cellular signaling pathways and mitochondria-related DNA [21].

At presentation, treatment decision should be made by a multidisciplinary team (MDT). It is important for clinicians and pathologists to correlate the entire information collected from clinical history, physical examination, laboratory tests (thyroid function, calcium, thyroglobulin, etc.), fine needle aspiration biopsy (FNAB), immunohistochemistry (IHC), imaging (ultrasonography, computed tomography scan, radioiodine scans, etc.), and histopathology. Thyroid lobectomy alone is sufficient treatment for small, unifocal, intrathyroidal carcinomas, or clinically detectable cervical nodal metastases, but total thyroidectomy is recommended for tumors larger than 4 cm. The effectiveness of radioactive iodine is still debated [21].

External beam radiation therapy (EBRT) may provide palliative relief from symptomatic metastases, control recurrent tumors, and prevent recurrence of advanced resected tumors [22–25]. The role of radiation as an adjuvant therapy in patients who have had complete resection of all locally invasive disease is controversial [26–30].

Salvage treatment of recurrent oncocytic/HCC includes surgery, radioactive iodine (RAI) therapy or radio frequency ablation, ethanol ablation, external beam radiotherapy (EBRT), and systemic treatment.

16.8 Prognosis

Oncocytic carcinoma of the thyroid (Hürthle cell carcinoma—HCC) has been reported to be associated with a more aggressive clinical behavior compared to other differentiated thyroid cancers (DTCs), with a tendency to higher frequency of metastasis and higher mortality rates. Older age, larger tumor size at diagnosis, extra-thyroid extension (ETE), and higher stage (AMES prognostic index) at diagnosis are considered by many authors to be poor prognostic features with lower survival rates for oncocytic/HCCs [31, 32]. With the exception of few studies [33–35], nodal metastasis was correlated with an adverse prognosis [17, 36, 37], while distant metastasis always resulted in a poor prognosis with dismal outcome [36, 37]. Extensive surgery, external beam radiation therapy (EBRT), and chemotherapy were also reported as factors that were associated with decreased survival [31].

With the exception of few studies [33–35], nodal metastasis was correlated with an adverse prognosis while distant metastasis always resulted in a poor prognosis with dismal outcome. Extensive surgery, external beam radiation therapy (EBRT), and chemotherapy were also reported by Lopez-Penabad et al. (2003) as factors that were associated with decreased survival.

In the Surveillance, epidemiology, and End Results (SEER)-9 database (1975–2009), 10-year survival rates of oncocytic/HCC improved dramatically over time; 75% in1975–1979, 81% 1995–1999, and 91% in 2000–2004 [38].

16.9 Future Perspectives

Although very few thyroid nodules are malignant, the possibility of cancer represents the overriding concern when thyroid gland lesions are brought to attention. Neck ultrasound (US) is the central hub in the diagnostic algorithm aimed at stratifying the risk of malignancy (ROM), allowing US-guided FNA, and promoting the individualized management currently advocated. For the vast majority of patients, both tools provide a reliable foundation for defining the initial management strategy, whether follow-up, surgery or nonsurgical treatment with minimally invasive techniques (MITs). However, in a number of cases, the estimates of the ROM will remain uncertain and the subsequent choices unsettled. In such cases, the clinicians' experience and individualized choices based on patient-related factors and preferences represent the way forward.

New tools are emerging in clinical practice, such as molecular/genetic testing. While the analytical and clinical validity have been extensively studied, the ability of the molecular analysis to improve patient outcomes sufficiently to justify its incorporation into real-world clinical practice has yet to be proven. Such studies are warranted for years to come.

Large multi-institutional studies are needed; until that time, utilization of national and nationwide data to assemble an adequate number of cases to inform valid conclusions will need to serve as a surrogate. Important questions that are outstanding include identification of the effect of minimal vascular invasion (1–4 foci) on the risk of recurrence and survival among patients with oncocytic/HCC, as well as measurement of the efficacy of adjuvant radioactive iodine (RAI) in these patients. There also continues to be a need for consensus regarding the criteria needed to establish a diagnosis of minimally invasive Hürthle cell carcinoma (miHCC) in order to avoid potential overtreatment.

References

1. Hurthle K. BeitrÃgezurKenntniss des Secretionsvorgangs in der. SchilddrÃse Pflugers Arch Physiol. 1894;56:10–44.
2. Ashkanazy M. Pathologisch-anatomischeBeitr ÃgezurKenntniss des. MorbusBasedowii, insbesondere Ãmber die dabeiauftretende Muskelerkrankung. Dtsch Arch Klin Med. 1898;61:118–86.
3. Baloch ZW, Asa SL, Barletta JA, Ghossein RA, Juhlin CC, Jung CK, et al. Overview of the 2022 WHO classification of thyroid neoplasms. Endocr Pathol. 2022;33(1):27–63.
4. Katz SM, Vickery AL Jr. The fibrous variant of Hashimoto's thyroiditis. Hum Pathol. 1974;5:161–70.
5. Yang Q, Zhao Z, Zhong G, Jin A, Yu K. Effect of adjuvant radioactive iodine therapy on survival in rare oxyphilic subtype of thyroid cancer (Hurthle cell carcinoma). Peer J. 2019;7:e7458.
6. Jillard CL, Youngwirth L, Scheri RP, Roman S, Sosa JA. Radioactive iodine treatment is associated with improved survival for patients with Hurthle cell carcinoma. Thyroid. 2016;26(7):959–64.
7. Wenter V, Jellinek A, Unterrainer M, Ahmaddy F, Lehner S, Albert NL, et al. Long-term outcome of rare oncocytic papillary (Hurthle cell) thyroid carcinoma following (adjuvant) initial radioiodine therapy. Eur J Nucl Med Mol Imaging. 2019;46(12):2526–35.
8. Goffredo P, Roman SA, Sosa JA. Hurthle cell carcinoma: a population-level analysis of 3311 patients. Cancer. 2013;119(3):504–11.
9. Zhou X, Zheng Z, Chen C, Zhao B, Cao H, Li T, et al. Clinical characteristics and prognostic factors of Hurthle cell carcinoma: a population based study. BMC Cancer. 2020;20(1):407.
10. Schwab M. Encyclopedia of cancer. Berlin/Heidelberg/New York: Springer; 2011.
11. Asa SL. My approach to oncocytic tumours of the thyroid. J Clin Pathol. 2004;57:225–32.
12. Tsybrovskyy O, Rößmann-Tsybrovskyy M. Oncocytic versus mitochondrion-rich follicular thyroid tumors: should we make a difference? Histopathology. 2009;55:665–82.
13. Rosai J, Kuhn E, Carcangiu ML. Pitfalls in thyroid tumour pathology. Histopathology. 2006;49(2):107–20.
14. Carcangiu ML, Bianchi S, Savino D, Voynick IM, Rosai J. Follicular Hürthle cell tumors of the thyroid gland. Cancer. 1991;68:1994–53.
15. Cannon J. The significance of Hurthle cells in thyroid disease. Oncologist. 2011;16(10):1380–7.
16. Ali SZ, Baloch ZW, Cochand-Priollet B, Schmitt FC, Vielh P, VanderLann PA. The 2023 Bethesda system for reporting thyroid cytopathology. Thyroid. 2023;23(9):1039–44.
17. Stojadinovic A, Ghossein RA, Hoos A, Urist MJ, Spiro RH, Shah JP, et al. Hurthle cell carcinoma: a critical histopathologic appraisal. J Clin Oncol. 2001;19(10):2616–25.
18. LiVolsi VA, Baloch ZW. Use and abuse of frozen section in the diagnosis of follicular thyroid lesions. Endocr Pathol. 2005;16:285–93.
19. McHenry CR, Sandoval BA. Management of follicular and Hürthle cell neoplasms of the thyroid gland. Surg Oncol Clin N Am. 1998;7:893–910.
20. McFadden DG, Sadow PM. Genetics, diagnosis, and management of Hürthle cell thyroid neoplasms. Front Endocrinol (Lausanne). 2021;12:696386.
21. Kure S, Ohashi R. Thyroid Hürthle cell carcinoma: clinical, pathological, and molecular features. Cancer. 2021;13(1):26.
22. Foote RL, Brown PD, Garces YI, McIver B, Kasperbauer JL. Is there a role for radiation therapy in the management of Hürthle cell carcinoma? Int J Radiat Oncol Biol Phys. 2003;56(4):1067–72.
23. Tuttle RM, Rondeau G, Lee NY. A risk-adapted approach to the use of radioactive iodine and external beam radiation in the treatment of well-differentiated thyroid cancer. Cancer Control. 2011;18(2):89–95.
24. Romesser PB, Sherman EJ, Shaha AR, Lian M, Wong RJ, Sabra M, et al. External beam radiotherapy with or without concurrent chemotherapy in advanced or recurrent non-anaplastic non-medullary thyroid cancer. J Surg Oncol. 2014;110(4):375–82.

25. Servagi Vernat S, Khalifa J, Sun XS, Kammerer E, Blais E, Faivre JC, et al. 10-year locoregional control with postoperative external beam radiotherapy in patients with locally advanced high-risk non-anaplastic thyroid carcinoma de novo or at relapse, a propensity score analysis. Cancers (Basel). 2019;11(6):849.
26. Farahati J, Reiners C, Stuschke M, Müller SP, Stüben G, Sauerwein W, et al. Differentiated thyroid cancer Impact of adjuvant external radiotherapy in patients with perithyroidal tumor infiltration (stage pT4). Cancer. 1996;77(1):172–80.
27. O'Connell ME, A'Hern RP, Harmer CL. Results of external beam radiotherapy in differentiated thyroid carcinoma: a retrospective study from the Royal Marsden Hospital. Eur J Cancer. 1994;30A(6):733–9.
28. Philips P, Hanzen C, Andry G, Van Houtte P, Früuling J. Postoperative irradiation for thyroid cancer. Eur J Surg Oncol. 1993;19(5):399–404.
29. Kim TH, Yang DS, Jung KY, Kim CY, Choi MS. Value of external irradiation for locally advanced papillary thyroid cancer. Int J Radiat Oncol Biol Phys. 2003;55(4):1006–12.
30. Keum KC, Suh YG, Koom WS, Cho JH, Shim SJ, Lee CG, et al. The role of postoperative external-beam radiotherapy in the management of patients with papillary thyroid cancer invading the trachea. Int J Radiat Oncol Biol Phys. 2006;65(2):474–80.
31. Lopez-Penabad L, Chiu AC, Hoff AO, Schultz P, Gaztambide S, Ordoñez NG, et al. Prognostic factors in patients with Hurthle cell neoplasms of the thyroid. Cancer. 2003;97(5):1186–94.
32. Zhang YW, Greenblatt DY, Repplinger D, Bargren A, Adler JT, Sippel RS, Chen H. Older age and larger tumor size predict malignancy in Hürthle cell neoplasms of the thyroid. Ann Surg Oncol. 2008;15(10):2842–6.
33. Sanders LE, Silverman M. Follicular and Hürthle cell carcinoma: predicting outcome and directing therapy. Surgery. 1998;124(6):967–74.
34. Barnabei A, Ferretti E, Baldelli R, Procaccini A, Spriano G, Appetecchia M. Hurthle cell tumours of the thyroid. Personal experience and review of the literature. Acta Otorhinolaryngol Ital. 2009;29(6):305–11.
35. Shaha AR, Loree TR, Shah JP. Prognostic factors and risk group analysis in follicular carcinoma of the thyroid. Surgery. 1995;118(6):1131–8.
36. Kushchayeva Y, Duh Q-Y, Kebebew E, D'Avanzo A, Clark OH. Comparison of clinical characteristics at diagnosis and during follow-up in 118 patients with Hurthle cell or follicular thyroid cancer. Am J Surg. 2008;195(4):457–62.
37. Stojadinovic A, Hoos A, Ghossein R, Urist MJ, Leung DH, Spiro RH, et al. Hürthle cell carcinoma: a 60-year experience. Ann Surg Oncol. 2002;9(2):197–203.
38. Nagar S, Aschebrook-Kilfoy B, Kaplan EL, Angelos P, Grogan RH. Hurthle cell carcinoma: an update on survivalover the last 35 years. Surgery. 2013;154(6):1263–71.

The manufacturer's authorised representative in the EU is Springer Nature Customer Service Centre GmbH, Europaplatz 3, 69115 Heidelberg, Germany. If you have any concerns regarding our products, please contact ProductSafety@springernature.com

Printed and bound by CPI Group (UK) Ltd, Croydon, CR0 4YY
01/10/2026
02225866-0004